Clinical Measurement in Drug Evaluation

Clinical Measurement in Drug Evaluation

Edited by

Walter S. Nimmo
Inveresk Clinical Research, Edinburgh, UK

and

Geoffrey T. Tucker
University of Sheffield, Department of Medicine and
Pharmacology, The Royal Hallamshire Hospital,
Sheffield, UK

JOHN WILEY & SONS

Chichester · New York · Brisbane · Toronto · Singapore

Other Wiley Editorial Offices

John Wiley & Sons, Inc., 605 Third Avenue,
New York, NY 10158-0012, USA

John Wiley Ltd, 33 Park Road, Milton,
Queensland 4064, Australia

John Wiley & Sons (Canada) Ltd, 22 Worcester Road,
Rexdale, Ontario M9W 1L1, Canada

John Wiley & Sons (SEA) Pte Ltd, 37 Jalan Pemimpin #05-04,
Block B, Union Industrial Building, Singapore 2057

Library of Congress Cataloging-in-Publication Data

Clinical measurement in drug evaluation / edited by Walter S. Nimmo
    and Geoffrey T. Tucker.
        p. cm.
    Proceedings of a symposium held in Edinburgh in Oct. 1993
sponsored by Inveresk Clinical Research.
    Includes bibliographical references and index.
    ISBN 0 471 94391 6
    1. Drugs—Testing—Congresses.   2. Drugs—Physiological effect—
Measurement—Congresses.   I. Nimmo, W. S.   II. Tucker, Geoffrey, T.
III. Inveresk Clinical Research (Firm)
    [DNLM: 1. Drug Evaluation—congresses.   2. Clinical Trials—
congresses.   QV 771 C6407 1995]
RM301.27.C572   1995
615′.1901—dc20
DNLM/DLC
for Library of Congress   94-40650
                                                                   CIP

British Library Cataloguing in Publication Data

A catalogue record for this book is available from the British Library

ISBN 0 471 94391 6

Typeset in 10/12pt Palatino by Acorn Bookwork, Salisbury, Wilts
Printed and bound in Great Britain by Biddles Ltd, Guildford, Surrey

CONTENTS

CONTRIBUTORS

Dr P. Demol
Bayer AG, Pharmaceutical Research Centre, Aprather Weg, Postfach 10 17 09, D-42096 Wuppertal I, Germany

Professor Alvan R. Feinstein
Yale University School of Medicine, 333 Cedar Street, PO Box 3333, New Haven, CT 06510-8025, USA

Dr A. J. Frew
University Medicine, Centre Block, D Floor, Southampton General Hospital, Southampton SO9 4XY, UK

Professor Charles F. George
University of Southampton, Clinical Pharmacology Group, Biomedical Sciences Building, Bassett Crescent East, Southampton SO9 3TU, UK

Dr S. J. Gerhand
University of Aberdeen, Department of Mental Health, University Medical Buildings, Foresterhill, Aberdeen AB9 2ZD, UK

Dr Malcolm F. Hand
University of Edinburgh, Clinical Research Centre, Western General Hospital, Department of Medicine, Edinburgh EH4 2XU, UK

Dr Joerg Hasford
Biometric Centre for Therapeutic Studies, Pettenkoferstrasse 35, 800 Munchen 2, Germany

Dr S. T. Holgate
University Medicine, Centre Block, D Floor, Southampton General Hospital, Southampton SO9 4XY, UK

Dr Eigill F. Hvidberg
University Hospital, Department of Clinical Pharmacy 4042, 9 Blegdamsvej, DK-2100 Copenhagen, Denmark

Dr Peter R. Jackson
Department of Medicine and Pharmacology, University of Sheffield, Royal Hallamshire Hospital, Sheffield S10 2JF, UK

Professor David R. Jones
University of Leicester, School of Medicine, Clinical Sciences Building, Leicester Royal Infirmary, PO Box 65, Leicester LE1 5WW, UK

Professor M. J. S. Langman
Queen Elizabeth Hospital, Medical School, Edgbaston, Birmingham B15 2TH, UK

Professor D. H. Lawson
Glasgow Royal Infirmary, 82–84 Castle Street, Glasgow G4 0SS, UK

Dr Wolfgang Meister
Med. Klinik Innenstadt, University of Munich, Munich, Germany

Dr Colin G. Miller
Bona Fide Ltd, 313 West Beltline Highway, Madison, WI 53713, USA

Dr Gerard B. Nash
University of Birmingham, Medical School, Department of Haematology, Edgbaston, Birmingham B15 2TT, UK

Professor Pertti J. Neuvonen
Department of Clinical Pharmacology, University of Helsinki, Paasikivenkatu 4, Helsinki FIN-00250, Finland

Professor Walter S. Nimmo
Inveresk Clinical Research Limited, Research Park, Roccarton, Edinburgh EH14 4AP, UK

Professor Lawrence L. E. Ramsay
Department of Medicine and Pharmacology, University of Sheffield, Royal Hallamshire Hospital, Sheffield S10 2JF, UK

Dr Tomas Salmonson
SmithKline Beecham Pharmaceuticals, New Frontiers Science Park, Third Avenue, Harlow CM19 5AW, UK

Dr Robert J. Temple
Office of Drug Research and Review, Center for Drug Evaluation and Research, FDA, 5600 Fishers Lane, Rockville, MD 20857, USA

Professor Geoffrey T. Tucker
Department of Medicine and Pharmacology, University of Sheffield, Royal Hallamshire Hospital, Sheffield S10 2JF, UK

Dr John Urquhart
APREX Corporation, 47221 Fremont Boulevard, Fremont, CA 94538-6502, USA

Dr Erica J. Wallis
Department of Medicine and Pharmacology, University of Sheffield, Royal Hallamshire Hospital, Sheffield S10 2JF, UK

Dr David J. Webb
Department of Medicine, University of Edinburgh, Clinical Research Centre, Western General Hospital, Edinburgh EH4 2XU, UK

Professor T. R. Weihrauch
Bayer AG, Pharmaceutical Research Centre, Aprather Weg, Postfach 10 17 09, D-42096 Wuppertal 1, Germany

Dr L. J. Whalley
University of Aberdeen, Department of Mental Health, University Medical Buildings, Foresterhill, Aberdeen AB9 2ZD, UK

Dr Peter Wyld
Inveresk Clinical Research, Research Park, Riccarton, Edinburgh EH14 4AP, UK

Dr Wilfred W. Yeo
Department of Medicine and Pharmacology, University of Sheffield, Royal Hallamshire Hospital, Sheffield S10 2JF, UK

PREFACE

The measurement of the therapeutic and adverse effects of drugs remains an important study. The undoubted success of the first symposium on clinical measurement in the development of new drugs (organised and supported by Inveresk Clinical Research) and the popularity of the published proceedings encouraged us to organise a second conference held in Edinburgh in October 1993.

This volume records the proceedings of the second symposium on clinical measurement in the evaluation of the measurement of drug effects in humans and its role in the development and evaluation of new chemical entities. Emphasis has been given to surrogate endpoints, peripheral vascular disease, the reliability of collection and interpretation of data as well as the identification, predictability and interpretation of drug interactions and adverse effects.

The symposium was organised and supported once again by Inveresk Clinical Research. However, we are grateful to Lothian and Edinburgh Enterprise Ltd and to the Edinburgh Drug Absorption Foundation for some financial support as well as to T. R. Weihrauch and Pierre Demol of Bayer for their advice in the design of the scientific programme. We record our thanks to Gillian Reid and Norma Watson of Inveresk Clinical Research for help with the local organisation of the meeting.

Most of all, we are indebted to the panel of distinguished speakers from academia and the pharmaceutical industry who participated and provided such excellent contributions. Their approach to difficult areas and problematical clinical situations should make this volume helpful to everyone involved in the measurement of drug effects in clinical pharmacology and the appraisal of reports or publications resulting from clinical measurement of drug effects.

We hope that this volume will remind our friends of two happy days spent in Scotland and will encourage clinicians and scientists to give attention to the precision and reproducibility of the measurement of drug effects.

Walter S Nimmo and Geoffrey T Tucker
Edinburgh and Sheffield
September 1994

PART I

SURROGATE ENDPOINTS AS A MEASURE OF DRUG EFFECTS

1 A REGULATORY AUTHORITY'S OPINION ABOUT SURROGATE ENDPOINTS

Robert J. Temple
Food and Drug Administration, Rockville, Maryland, USA

Introduction

We are living and developing drugs in a time of interesting tension. We have, on the one hand, growing impatience with our inability to find treatments for serious illnesses—multiple sclerosis, amyotrophic lateral sclerosis, Alzheimer's disease, most solid tumours, AIDS and AIDS-opportunistic infections. There is a strong sense of 'hurry-up'. All of this drives us towards utilising the earliest, most readily determined evidence of effectiveness, generally evidence of an effect on surrogate or 'intermediate' endpoints.

On the other hand, there are forces urging us towards measuring the ultimate clinical endpoints: survival, disability, capacity for functioning in daily life. These forces are:

- Disappointment in the results of using either surrogate or intermediate endpoints, including some major surprises.
- Recent success in measuring small but very valuable real effects, using larger trials and meta-analyses. These successes are most conspicuous in the cardiovascular area but have also occurred in other settings, such as adjuvant chemotherapy for breast and colon cancer.
- Growing concern with the financial cost of therapy in relation to benefits and increasing interest in the true clinical value of intervention.

In the middle of all this are regulatory agencies, trying hard to get the balance right. The following is an attempt to describe where we are in this

Clinical Measurement in Drug Evaluation. Edited by W. S. Nimmo and G. T. Tucker
© 1995 John Wiley & Sons Ltd

effort, what we have been worried about, what we have done officially, and what we are still considering.

Background, definitions, theoretical reasons for concern about surrogate endpoints

DEFINITIONS

One definition of a 'surrogate endpoint' that we have considered is as follows:

> A surrogate endpoint of a clinical trial is a laboratory measurement or a physical sign used as a substitute for a clinically meaningful endpoint that measures directly how a patient feels, functions or survives. Changes induced by a therapy on a surrogate endpoint are expected to reflect changes in a clinically meaningful endpoint.

It is implicit in this definition that a surrogate endpoint is by itself of no value to the patient. It does *not* make him live longer, function better or feel better—the ultimate reasons for treating patients. It is of value, i.e. a *valid* surrogate, only if an effect on the surrogate does, in fact, lead to a real clinical benefit.

Note that a surrogate endpoint could be valid for one clinical effect but not another. For example, in patients with heart failure, increased cardiac output resulting from treatment with a drug might lead to increased exercise tolerance, a real clinical benefit, but might not lead to improved survival, generally considered the ultimate clinical benefit in a fatal illness.

In addition to surrogate endpoints, which have no immediate clinical value, there are clinical endpoints that are not the 'ultimate' endpoint (e.g. survival or the rate of serious and irreversible morbidity) but that are nonetheless real clinical benefits. These are called, variously, non-ultimate endpoints, intermediate endpoints, lesser endpoints or secondary endpoints. There are many examples of these, such as improved exercise ability and symptom relief in heart failure, reduced symptoms of hyperglycaemia in diabetes, decreased angina in coronary artery disease, improved pulmonary function in chronic lung disease, and weight gain or improved appetite in cancer or HIV-infected patients.

Reliance on these kinds of endpoints is not controversial but raises many of the same problems as reliance on surrogates, with one major exception. Unlike an effect on a surrogate, an effect on one of these endpoints clearly represents a tangible clinical benefit for the patient. This can be weighed against the known and potential risks of therapy, even if the relationship of the intermediate endpoint to ultimate outcome is not clear.

HISTORY OF THE USE OF SURROGATES: WHY THEY ARE ATTRACTIVE

There is nothing new about the use of surrogate endpoints as a basis for approval of drugs. The US Food and Drug Administration (FDA) has:

- Approved drugs that lower cholesterol and triglycerides without evidence that they alter survival or decrease the rate of coronary artery disease.
- Approved drugs that lower arterial pressure, without evidence that those drugs decrease the rate of stroke, heart attacks, heart failure or death.
- Approved drugs for osteoporosis on the basis of change in bone density, without evidence of decreased fractures.
- Approved drugs for acute treatment of heart failure (dobutamine, for example) on the basis of increased cardiac output without evidence of an improvement in symptoms or survival.
- Approved drugs that decrease rates of ventricular premature beats for use in symptomatic patients without evidence of effects on symptoms and without evidence of improved survival.
- Approved drugs that heal gastric or duodenal ulcer without evidence that they reduce ulcer complications and with only small (or in one case, no) effects on symptoms.
- Approved drugs that lower blood sugar and glycosylated haemoglobin concentrations (surrogate endpoints) and decrease symptoms of hyperglycaemia, but without evidence of effects on diabetic complications or on survival.

In all of these cases, there were good bases for approval, i.e., good reason to expect that a real clinical benefit would be associated with the effect on the surrogate, but no direct evidence of clinical benefit for particular drugs (e.g., for antihypertensives other than reserpine, diuretics or beta blockers), or, in some cases (e.g., cholesterol-lowering drugs), no evidence that any drug of the same or different pharmacological class had such a clinical benefit.

It is legal to rely on demonstrated effects on a surrogate endpoint as a basis for approval. The statute does not specifically define effectiveness; rather it describes how effectiveness must be demonstrated. It calls for substantial evidence that the drug will have the effect it is claimed to have in labelling; and it defines substantial evidence as evidence derived from adequate and well-controlled studies. The law does not specifically say that the claimed effect must be clinically meaningful, but it does say that a drug must be safe for its intended use—a phrase the FDA has interpreted to mean that the benefits of a drug must outweigh its risks. Because a meaningless effect would not outweigh *any* risk (and all drugs have some risks), it could be argued that only a clinically meaningful effect could allow a conclusion that a drug was safe. In addition, a critical judicial opinion, in Warner-Lambert v. Heckler, makes it very clear that the FDA can insist that the claimed effect be meaningful. Thus the FDA can rely on surrogate endpoints it considers meaningful.

There are several straightforward, related reasons for the desire to rely on a surrogate endpoint:

- It is often faster and easier to measure an effect of a therapy on a surrogate endpoint than on the definitive endpoint. An effect on arterial pressure or cholesterol can be established in weeks, while the consequences of that effect on survival, stroke rate or heart attack rate would take years to demonstrate. Moreover, the studies needed to show the effect on the surrogate can be small, as every patient will have the surrogate measure (high arterial pressure or cholesterol) and be a candidate for improvement. In contrast, only a small fraction of all patients will have, in any period of several years, a heart attack, death or stroke; to show improvement in these low rates, very large or very prolonged studies are needed.

- Benefits to patients (if the surrogate effect proves in fact to be a benefit) can begin to flow far more rapidly if drugs are made available based on the surrogate. This is of greatest importance where the disease affected by the drug has no recognised effective treatment and is fatal or causes irreversible morbidity, even if only to a small fraction of patients.

- The financial and resource (patient, investigator) costs of drug development may be reduced by reliance on a surrogate endpoint. Apart from the obvious benefits to sponsors, greater efficiency also serves the larger community.

- Finally, the study of the definitive endpoint may be, or seem to be, infeasible. Event rates may be so low that studies of the needed size and duration may be beyond the logistic and financial resources of sponsors and other institutions. In other cases, beliefs about the validity of the surrogate may be so strong that conduct of a definitive study including an untreated group appears ethically infeasible. Views change on such matters, of course. The advent of large simple trials, such as the Physicians Health Study and the ISIS and GISSI studies [1–3], have given a new impression about what is feasible; studies of tens of thousands of patients can now be contemplated. Then too, if an effect is so small as to need a multi-year, multi-thousand patient study, it is becoming of growing interest to ask about its real cost-effectiveness. Also, a number of very surprising results, some described below, have revealed that the untreated group in a clinical trial is not always the disadvantaged group.

THEORETICAL REASONS FOR CONCERN ABOUT SURROGATE ENDPOINTS

There are both theoretical and practical (troubling examples of surrogates gone wrong) reasons for concern about the use of surrogate endpoints.

The fundamental risk of reliance on a surrogate is that, for several reasons, the benefit/risk calculation will be wrong. First, because the effect on the surrogate is of no value to the patient by itself, the risk–benefit judgement for the drug can be made only by attributing some real benefit to the effect on the surrogate and weighing it against known risks. But the actual benefit is not known and, the attribution of benefit may be incorrect. Moreover, because it is usually inherent in the use of a surrogate endpoint that the trials are far shorter and smaller than would be needed to assess low-rate (but serious) or long-term risks, the actual risks are not as well-defined as they could be.

This fundamental risk is manifested in three principal ways:

- The relationship between the surrogate and the true clinical event may not be causal, as supposed, but coincidental or co-related to some third factor.

  Fever or an elevated white count, for example, might be considered potential surrogate endpoints for patients with lobar pneumonia (if we did not understand the nature of infection and the body's response to it) but in fact they do not cause the adverse clinical outcomes of the infection and the infection would not be improved by their treatment. It was not so long ago (the 1960s) that arterial pressure was a highly debatable surrogate; one school of thought held strongly that elevated pressure was an adaptive response to vascular disease and that treating it would lead to greater morbidity. We are sure that that viewpoint is wrong only because studies proved it so. Post-infarction patients with increased ventricular premature beat (VPB) rates have increased mortality. The VPBs *could* be the cause of the mortality or they could reflect underlying cardiac disease that *also* leads to increased risk of ventricular tachycardia. If so, reducing VPB rates might not improve survival.

- They may be other effects of the drug that are unfavourable. These may not be recognized because of the focus on the 'desired effect' (one that influences the plausible surrogate)—the effect thought to be of value. But drugs often have other effects, not as immediate, as prominent, as frequent or as obviously important, that can influence outcome unfavourably, especially in long-term use. These have emerged so frequently that they should be expected. For example:
  - Diuretics lower arterial pressure, but also lower serum and body potassium and raise serum uric acid, glucose and cholesterol.
  - Quinidine lowers VPB rates and can maintain sinus rhythm after cardioversion but prolongs the Q–T interval, causes *torsades de*

> *pointes-type* arrhythmias, and obliterates the activity of cyto-
> chrome P450 2D6 (at doses much lower than the antiarrhythmic
> dose).
> — Many type 1 antiarrythmic drugs lower VPB rates but increase
>   mortality in patients without life-threatening arrhythmias.
> — Several inotropic agents increase cardiac output (a surrogate end-
>   point) and exercise tolerance (a non-ultimate clinical endpoint),
>   but decrease survival.
> — Aspirin prevents thrombosis but provokes bleeding.
> — Thrombolytic agents lyse obstructing clots in coronary vessels but
>   can also provoke intracranial and other haemorrhage by lysing
>   clots that were protecting against internal bleeding.
> — Tricyclic antidepressants are also type 1 antiarrhythmic drugs.
>   Many are anticholinergics, sedatives, hypotensives, inhibitors or
>   inducers of hepatic metabolism, or prolong the Q–T interval.
> — Late, serious, unexpected adverse effects can occur—not very
>   often, but often enough to keep in mind (the practolol syndrome,
>   benoxaprofen renal/hepatic toxicity, amiodarone pulmonary and
>   other toxicity, phenformin lactic acidosis, perhexilene hepatotoxi-
>   city, zimelidine syndrome, etc.).

Most drugs are not as specific as we hope and tend to assume they
will be.

- Whether a drug provides a net gain or loss in a given situation is not
  easy to predict, even if both its desirable and undesirable effects are
  recognised. Both kinds of effects may be dose related (often in a way
  not well defined by surrogates) and may be different, or of different
  importance, in different subsets of the population (e.g., aspirin-
  induced bleeding may be more important than aspirin-prevented
  thrombosis in low-risk people but of lesser importance in high-risk
  patients; susceptibility to proarrhythmic effects of drugs could
  depend on the type and extent of underlying heart disease) and may
  change over time. Moreover, an effect on a surrogate endpoint may
  correlate with one clinical endpoint of a disease but not others.

Examples of 'surrogate surprises': effects on surrogates that did not predict ultimate outcome

ANTIARRHYTHMICS

The Cardiac Arrhythmia Suppression Trial (CAST) [4, 5]

It is not easy to think of a greater medical error, since the practice of therapeutic bleeding, than the use of antiarrhythmic drugs in patients after

myocardial infarction to treat asymptomatic or minimally symptomatic VPBs.

The CAST was a randomised trial of placebo and three type 1C anti-arrhythmics (encainide, flecainide and moricizine) in patients with a recent infarction and more than 10 VPBs per hour but with minimal or no symptoms. It was intended to determine whether antiarrhythmic therapy would reduce the increased mortality known to occur in such patients.

Before randomisation, patients were given open antiarrhythmics; they were excluded from the study if one of the drugs did not achieve at least a 70% reduction of VPBs compared with baseline or appeared to be proar-rhythmic. If patients did respond favourably, they were randomised to the 'successful therapy' or to placebo.

The trial was thus carried out in surrogate responders who seemed free of the risks of therapy. The rationale for the trial seemed sound; indeed, some questioned the ethics of leaving patients at risk of death by failing to use 'recognised effective therapy'.

The results, however, were unexpectedly and markedly adverse, and the trial was stopped before its scheduled end. Instead of reducing mor-tality, encainide and flecainide sharply increased it, with mortality or cardiac arrest rates of 8.4% (63/755) in the treated patients, versus 3.5% (26/743) in the placebo group—roughly a 2.4-fold difference [4]. A third drug, started later in the study, moricizine, also affected survival adversely [5].

Whether this outcome reflects an erroneous theory about the VPB sudden-death relationship or unexpected adverse effects of the drugs used is not known, but studies and meta-analyses of other type 1 antiar-rhythmics in this setting have also tended to be unfavourable.

Quinidine in maintaining sinus rhythm [6]

A meta-analysis pooled six studies comparing the ability of quinidine and placebo to maintain normal sinus rhythm (NSR) after cardioversion of patients with atrial fibrillation. Quinidine was 'effective', giving NSR rates of 58% and 50% at six and 12 months versus placebo rates of 33% and 25%—both significant differences. Unfortunately, mortality was also increased in the quinidine group (2.9% v. 0.8%, odds ratio 2.98, $p <$ 0.05).

Although lack of fibrillation probably represents a significant sympto-matic improvement, this benefit would not seem to outweigh the adverse effect on survival. It seems likely that the proarrhythmic effects of quini-dine and widespread use of anticoagulants in patients with atrial fibrilla-tion (preventing embolic mortality in those patients) led to this net adverse outcome.

Lignocaine (lidocaine) prophylaxis post infarction

Lignocaine prophylaxis post infarction was reviewed in a meta-analysis several years ago [7]. Although prophylaxis was successful in preventing ventricular tachycardia, it did not improve survival and may have reduced it in some circumstances.

CONGESTIVE HEART FAILURE

People with congestive heart failure (CHF) have a low cardiac output and a high left ventricular filling pressure leading to poor exercise tolerance and pulmonary symptoms (dyspnoea, orthopnoea), as well as to increased mortality because of progressive CHF and sudden death. It seems reasonable to expect that improved cardiac output and left ventricular filling pressure, especially if accompanied by improved symptoms, would increase survival and reduce the need for hospitalisation. Moreover, certain angiotension-converting enzyme inhibitors (ACEIs), which produce such effects on CHF by reducing the vascular resistance against which the heart must pump blood, have favourable effects on survival [8–10].

Does that mean that some combination of increased cardiac output and improved CHF symptoms predicts a favourable mortality effect? Unfortunately, it does not.

PROMISE: the Prospective Randomized Milrinone Survival Evaluation [11]

The PROMISE study compared milrinone, a phosphodiesterase-inhibitor inotropic agent, with placebo in patients poorly responsive to diuretics and digoxin. Milrinone improved cardiac output, exercise tolerance and symptoms of CHF but it increased cardiovascular mortality: 29% on milrinone versus 23% on placebo ($p = 0.037$, adjusted). Other drugs related to milrinone have given similar results. Milrinone may have proarrythmic effects but the reason for the adverse outcome is not certain.

PROFILE, the Prospective Randomized Flosequinan Longevity Evaluation

Flosequinan is an arteriovenous vasodilator (not thought to be primarily an inotropic agent) recently approved for treating CHF patients unresponsive to diuretics, digoxin and an ACEI, i.e., a 'last-resort' agent. It showed a clear ability to improve exercise tolerance and symptoms in studies of up to four months duration, although a pooled mortality analysis of controlled trials revealed an adverse trend (but with a wide confidence interval) on survival. The FDA's cardiovascular and renal drugs advisory committee recommended approval despite this, believing that properly informed patients might choose symptomatic improvements even with the possibility of decreased survival. A placebo-controlled mortality trial of flosequinan had been initiated and was ongoing at the time of approval. Labelling for the drug described the mortality analysis of the previous studies. The trial studied a single dose of flosequinan, except that patients with excessive tachycardia on 100 mg per day were randomised separately to 75 mg per day or placebo.

Just as flosequinan reached the market, early results of PROFILE showed a clear adverse effect on survival (Table 1). The effect appeared predominantly in the 100 mg group (but this group was far larger) and was more prominent in NYHA class IV patients. In general, mortality was more prominent in people likely to have higher plasma concentrations (lower renal function) but it was not clear that any of these subsets represented a group that could be treated safely and effectively. A preliminary analysis suggested also that, after three months, the number of hospitalisations increased in the flosequinan group. In the absence of a durable symptomatic benefit the drug was withdrawn by the sponsor.

The explanation for this outcome—a sharp dichotomy between the effects of the drug on function and on survival—is at present obscure. Even if there proves to be a relationship between flosequinan plasma concentrations and mortality—certainly a matter of interest—we will be no nearer to a mechanistic explanation. The pre- and post-marketing treatment populations were somewhat different. Clinical trials before approval had relatively few NYHA class IV patients because, in general, such patients cannot participate in exercise testing. The possibly different

Table 1. Results of PROFILE Study

	Dose of flosequinan		
	75 mg/day	100 mg/day	Total
Mortality of patients randomized to flosequinan	40/206 (19.4%)	201/964 (20.9%)	214/1170 (20.6%)
Mortality of patients randomized to placebo[a]	43/238 (18.1%)	138/937 (14.7%)	181/1175 (15.4%)
Relative risk	1.05	1.48	1.39
95% confidence limits	0.68–1.62	1.19–1.84	1.14–1.68
p value	0.83	0.0004	0.0009

[a]Intent-to-treat analysis.

outcome here could suggest a need in developing a drug for heart failure, to do studies in NYHA class IV patients, relying on symptom assessment or less stressful exercise tests, such as level walking distance.

Vesnarinone [12]

A recent published report (data not reviewed by the FDA at the time of writing) of results with another inotrope/vasodilator (it is often difficult to determine which effect is primary because of reflex responses) adds to the confusion. Vesnarinone at two doses, 60 mg per day and 120 mg per day, was compared with placebo in patients not adequately responsive to digoxin and ACEIs in a study whose primary outcome measure was all-cause mortality plus major cardiovascular morbidity, defined as hospitalisation for CHF requiring intravenous inotropic agents. It is noteworthy that the 60 mg dose has no regularly detectable effects on exercise tolerance or symptoms, while a 120 mg dose does have such effects.

The results were surprising. The 120 mg group had to be stopped prematurely because of sharply increased mortality (Table 2), including several early deaths not seen in the other groups. The 60 mg group continued, however, having no such adverse trend. Final results are shown in Table 3—dramatically improved survival in the treated group, reflecting decreased sudden death and death due to progressive CHF. There was

Table 2. Vesnarinone 60, 120 mg versus placebo

	Deaths		
Total n = 253	Placebo	60 mg	120 mg
	6	3	16 ($p < 0.01$ v. placebo)

Table 3. Vesnarinone 60 mg versus placebo

	Placebo n = 238	Vesnarinone 60 mg n = 239
Mortality, total	33	13*
Sudden death	15	5
Worse CHF	18	7
Non-cardiac	0	1
Mortality from any cause or major CV morbidity	50	26**

*p = 0.002 v. placebo; **p = 0.003 v. placebo.

also a favourable effect on the Sickness Impact Profile, but it seems difficult to separate that from the decreased progression of CHF seen in the
survival data.

The reasons for the favourable effect on survival with little or no effect
on what are thought to be the underlying bases for mortality are obscure,
as are the reasons for so markedly different and adverse an effect of only a
slightly larger dose.

HYPERTENSION

Arterial pressure is a surrogate endpoint in which we generally believe.
Apart from the very well-documented epidemiological relationship of
arterial pressure to adverse outcomes, we have believed in it because Freis
and co-workers showed, at least for a diastolic pressure of >105, that lowering arterial pressure with diuretics and reserpine gave a clear benefit by
reducing stroke, CHF and death. The benefit was greater for higher baseline arterial pressures, and greater lowering of pressure had greater benefit.

We have used diastolic pressure ever since then as the effectiveness endpoint for antihypertensive agents. But it is not a perfect surrogate and
there are doubts that arterial pressure alone tells the whole story.

There is some disparity between the beneficial effects of arterial pressure
lowering on two of the major adverse effects of hypertension: fatal and
non-fatal stroke, and coronary heart disease. There are reasonably parallel
increases in risk for the two outcomes, although somewhat steeper for
stroke, suggesting that a 5–6 mmHg treatment decrement in diastolic pressure for 105 mmHg should give a roughly 25% reduction in coronary heart
disease and a 40–50% reduction in stroke (13). In fact, however, a meta-
analysis of hypertension trials (14) shows that while the overall reduction
in stroke was about 42% (not far from expected) it was just 14% for coronary heart disease.

The arterial pressure surrogate thus seems not to predict equally for
both endpoints. There are many possible explanations. It may be more difficult to reverse the coronary disease process than the pathological process
leading to stroke. Indeed, reduction in haemorrhagic risk might begin at
the same time as treatment, without any delay. It is also possible that the
drugs used in trials are not maximally effective in reversing cardiac hypertrophy, which may have adverse effects on coronary artery disease. It is
also possible that the high doses of diuretics used in many trials lowered
potassium enough to lead to arrhythmias (sudden death would appear as
coronary artery disease deaths in the meta-analysis) or impaired glucose
tolerance and cholesterol sufficient enough to affect coronary artery disease
adversely.

A possible suggestion that this could be so comes from results of the
SHEP (Systolic Hypertension in the Elderly Program) [15]. This placebo-

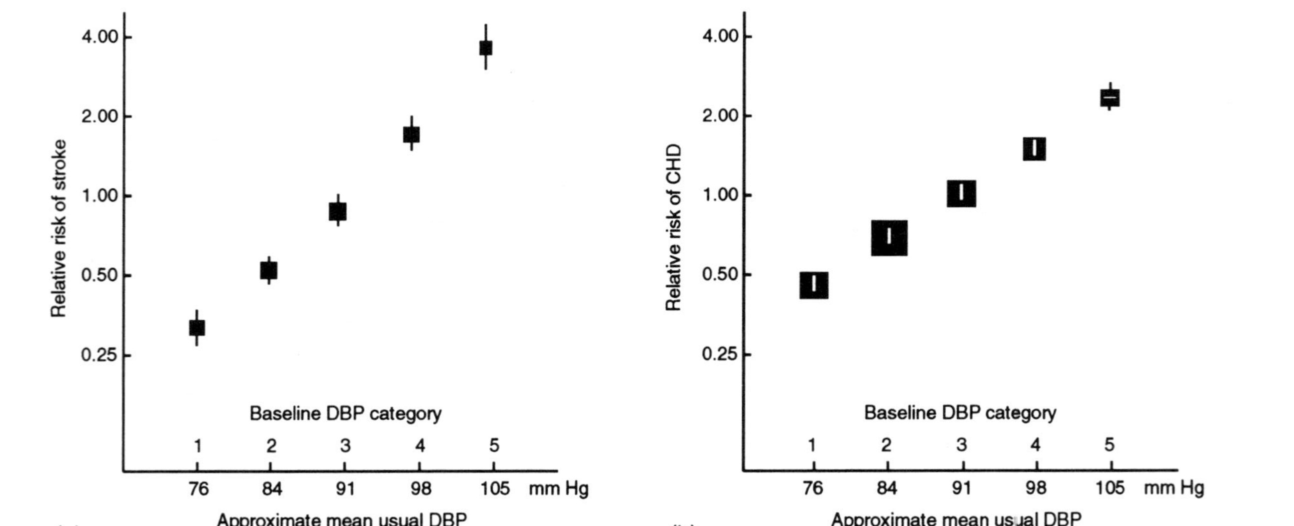

Figure 1. Relative risks of (a) stroke and of (b) coronary heart disease, estimated from combined results. Estimates of the usual diastolic pressure (DBP) in each baseline DBP category are taken from mean DBP values four years post-baseline in the Framingham study. Solid squares represent disease risks in each category relative to risk in the whole study population; sizes of squares are proportional to number of events in each DBP category; 95% confidence intervals for estimates of relative risk are denoted by vertical lines. (a) Stroke and usual DBP (in fire categories defined by baseline DBP); seven prospective observational studies: 843 events. (b) Coronary heart disease (CHD) and usual DBP (in five categories defined by baseline DBP); nine prospective observational studies: 4856 events. Reproduced from MacMahon et al. [13] © by The Lancet Ltd, 1990

controlled trial in patients over 70 with systolic pressure greater than 160 mmHg and normal diastolic ($\leqslant 90$ mmHg) pressure showed a 37% reduction in total stroke and a 33% fall in total myocardial infarctions. This study used very low doses of diuretic (12.5 mg chlorthalidone at first, going to 25 mg if needed)—much lower than past doses. Of course, there are other possibilities; the greater age of patients and the isolated systolic pressure elevation represent a population not previously studied to any great extent.

OTHER SURROGATES

Coronary vessel patency after thrombolysis

Coronary patency has been discussed widely as a surrogate for improved survival of post-infarction patients. The controversy about which thrombolytic agent was best may have obscured matters. High rates of vessel patency are achieved with all three marketed thrombolytics and there is no reason *not* to believe this is the reason for improved survival and less CHF. That is, there is no reason not to believe early vessel patency is a valid surrogate, up to a point. Even a good surrogate, however, poses problems.

We do not really know *which* surrogate measure is best: 90 min patency, some earlier measure of patency, the rate of early patency minus late reocclusion, etc. The result is that the surrogate is imperfect. Thus, in ISIS III [2] and GISSI II [3], two thrombolytics with significantly different effects on patency had the *same* effect on survival; and in ISIS II [16], aspirin, which probably alters early patency little, had as great an effect on mortality as streptokinase, presumably by preventing reocclusion. In addition, of course, early regimens of tissue plasminogen activator that yielded high early vessel patency led also to a higher, unacceptable risk of haemorrhagic stroke—over 1.5%.

Thus, even though patency is a reasonably good surrogate, unintended effects and interactions with aspirin, heparin and other possible anti-thrombin drugs leave one still needing to study the clinical endpoints.

Cholesterol-lowering therapies

The benefits of cholesterol-lowering therapies are complex and still at least somewhat controversial. Although overviews show clear effects on coronary artery disease, survival has not been improved. We await results of studies of drugs that have large effects and that people will take reliably.

All in all, it is difficult to feel wholly comfortable with any surrogate, even where there has been 'confirmation' (i.e., a drug has been shown to affect both the surrogate and the clinical endpoint), because unintended effects of new agents cannot be predicted and can be large and important, and because applicability of results to different populations, stages of disease and clinical situations (other drugs) is difficult to anticipate.

New FDA regulation

Because of the urgent need to make drugs available for conditions without adequate treatment, but reflecting the concerns about the use of surrogates described above, the FDA developed its 'accelerated approval' regulation (21 CFR 314.500), which appeared in the *Federal Register* on 1 December 1992, (FR Vol. 57, No. 239, pp. 58942–58960). The preamble to the final rule contains a detailed discussion of issues related to use of surrogates and US law.

The new rule allows the FDA to approve new drugs or biologicals intended for treatment of serious illnesses and that offer meaningful therapeutic benefits compared with existing treatment on the basis of a documented effect on a surrogate or non-ultimate endpoint. Specifically, approval can be based on evidence from adequate and well-controlled studies of a surrogate endpoint that is 'reasonably likely', based on epidemiological, therapeutic, pathophysiological or other evidence, to predict clinical benefit or on evidence of an effect of the drug other than an effect on survival or irreversible morbidity, on condition that controlled studies to verify and describe the clinical benefits to patients are carried out 'with due diligence'. If the studies fail to show a benefit, or benefits appear not to outweigh risks, there is provision for an accelerated withdrawal procedure.

It is not intended that this procedure should be used for drugs approved on the basis of established surrogates, such as arterial pressure reduction. The preamble to the final rule makes clear that it is intended for use of a surrogate endpoint 'that, while reasonably likely to predict clinical benefit, is not so well established as the surrogates ordinarily used as bases of approval in the past'. It is also clear that the rule is not to be used to base approval casually on any demonstrated pharmacological effect. The rule acknowledges 'that there are well-recognised reasons for caution when surrogate endpoints are relied on'—noting the CAST episode particularly. Reliance on a surrogate and concluding it is 'reasonably likely to predict clinical benefit' is inevitably a matter of judgement that the FDA, with the help of internal and external expertise, will have to make. A sponsor seeking to persuade the FDA that a surrogate should be used is 'likely to be persuasive only when the disease to be treated is particularly severe (so that considerable risk is acceptable) and/or when the surrogate endpoint is well supported'.

Conditions very much like those in the regulation were created ad hoc to support approval of two anti-HIV drugs: didanosine (ddi) and zalcitabine (ddc).

Since it became final, the accelerated approval rule has been used once, in the approval of the use of a biological drug, β-interferon (Betaseron), to reduce the frequency of relapses in multiple sclerosis (MS). In that case, there was a multi-centre study in patients with relapsing–remitting-type MS that showed a statistically significant, clinically meaningful but small effect on annual relapse rate (0.84 v. 1.27 per year, $p = 0.0001$) and time to first relapse (10 v. five months, $p = 0.015$). In view of the relatively small effect, in a single, albeit multi-centre study, and the dependence of the significant result, in part, on a change in definition of relapse during the course of the study (the change was made before any unblinded data were examined), it became important to approval that there was a striking effect on the magnetic resonance image (MRI) of the central nervous system, with a reduction of involved area on β-interferon of 4.2% at the end of the study versus a 19.5% *increase* in the placebo-treated group (a highly significant difference). In the population studied, with little or no disability, this MRI change was not shown to correlate with disability, but the promise of such an effect was considered great and the approval of the drug was based in part on this promise, under the accelerated approval rule. The sponsor agreed to carry out three further studies:

- Randomised, blinded, placebo-controlled trial in patients with chronic progressive MS, of four to six years duration with an endpoint of disability.
- Study in relapsing–remitting MS to assess the value (effect on exacerbation rate) of treatment beyond two years.
- Correlation of MRI parameters and clinical parameters in the first two studies.

Conclusion

Surrogate endpoints will continue to be a basis for drug approval—the ones used historically (arterial pressure, cholesterol) under ordinary procedures; novel ones under accelerated approval procedures. But note that ordinary approval may be with an 'understanding/agreement', if not a requirement, to carry out further studies (as was the case for flosequinan and as is usual for cholesterol-lowering agents) so that there may be less difference than there seems to be between accelerated and ordinary approval. Accelerated approval is limited to those cases where we are *stretching* the use of a surrogate as a basis for approving a drug to treat an untreatable or poorly treated illness.

Suppose, though, that concern arises about a surrogate that has been used widely and where there are already available treatments, e.g. treatment of heart failure or cardiac rhythm abnormalities. Does this mean the FDA would approve a new agent only on the basis of definitive clinical endpoints? That is one possibility but not the only one. Where experience does raise real doubt about the ability of surrogate or intermediate end-points to predict outcome, reliance on the surrogate will, in fact, end. It would be difficult, for example, to imagine approval of a drug for treatment of symptomatic VPB rate elevations without a study of mortality that at least rules out an adverse effect. On the other hand, we continue to accept evidence that a drug can suppress programmed electrical stimulation (PES)-induced ventricular tachycardia as evidence of usefulness in treating life-threatening arrhythmias. Ongoing studies of drugs in patients with ventricular tachycardia or ventricular fibrillation (VT/VF) who have implanted defibrillators may shed new light on that surrogate endpoint.

Recent experience with drugs for heart failure suggests the need for mortality information, possibly except for new ACEIs seeking that claim. On the other hand, we have certainly not decided that mortality data are needed to approve new diuretics for CHF-related fluid retention; and new antihypertensive drugs will, for the present, be approved based on arterial pressure effects. Established surrogates can be used where they remain reasonably credible, even as we ask for more data after approval to show how much clinical benefit really arises from the effect on the surrogate.

Apart from the particular regulatory framework used, certain factors continue to argue for or against their use of surrogates, as reported below.

ARGUMENTS FOR SURROGATES

Biological plausibility

Biological plausibility remains a fundamental argument for reliance on a surrogate. This may take the form of consistent epidemiological evidence, with few or no exceptions, and an appropriate quantitative relation of degree of deviation or amount of exposure to outcome. An animal model of the disease may help support the idea that the aetiology of the disease is known and that the effects of treatment on a surrogate will predict outcome. A particularly unequivocal understanding of disease pathogenesis and an agent that reverses it, e.g. a drug that wholly reverses the consequences of an inborn error of metabolism, would argue for reliance on a surrogate endpoint, especially where study of clinical endpoints would be very delayed.

History of success

Where one member of a well-defined pharmacological class has had a favourable effect on a surrogate endpoint and a clinical outcome, the surrogate gains plausibility, at least for members of that class. Yet caution is needed in defining the class, and class members may differ in important ways; moreover, it may be critical to utilise equivalent doses, not always easy to assess. For example, different results with post-infarction use of different beta blockers could reflect random variation, inadequate study size or different populations, but could also reflect differences in partial agonist activity, beta receptor specificity, degree of penetration of the central nervous system, extent of membrane-stabilising activity, tendency to cause Q–T prolongation, additional pharmacological effects, such as direct vasodilation or alpha-blocking properties, or differences in interaction with other therapy. Beta blockers are a relatively well-defined class of drugs, but even in this case there must be a very substantial discussion before a surrogate (e.g., documented pharmacological effects of beta blockade) would be accepted as a basis for approval. In addition, where one or several members of a pharmacological class are available and known to be effective, there is little sense of urgency with respect to another member of the class.

Where several different drug classes have a favourable effect on a surrogate and on mortality or morbidity, it is tempting to believe something fundamental has been learned. That is the case with hypertension, where diuretics, reserpine and beta blockers can make at least some claim such a relationship and, indeed, we treat arterial pressure as an established surrogate. Even here, however, there can be unexpected effects (e.g., on cholesterol, potassium, Q–T interval) and such matters as dose, time course of effect during the day, tolerability and compliance, and drug–drug interactions could all enhance or undermine clinical effects. Also, the applicability of conclusions to any but well-studied populations is treacherous.

Risk/benefit considerations

The lack of any adequate alternative treatment for a serious disease is an important reason for utilising a surrogate endpoint and is reflected in the accelerated approval regulation. A relatively large safety database at the proposed dose and duration of treatment in reasonably similar patients also limits the risk. Short-term use poses fewer concerns that important adverse effects have been missed; significant long-term exposure data are rarely available from trials relying on surrogate endpoints, even if long-term use is planned.

Finally, the difficulty of studying the ultimate endpoint may argue in favour of relying on a persuasive surrogate; the risk of waiting to find out for certain what the clinical benefit is may seem unacceptable. When cholesterol-lowering drugs and oral hypoglycaemic agents were first introduced, it was not clear, because of practical questions about duration and size of studies, that their ultimate effect could be studied definitively. Indeed, whether they can in all cases remains uncertain, especially with respect to primary prevention. Since that time, on the other hand, we have developed greatly expanded ideas of what is possible.

ARGUMENTS AGAINST SURROGATES

Biological plausibility

Even a single negative therapeutic example greatly undermines the plausibility of a proposed surrogate. Thus the recent adverse outcomes of heart failure drugs and agents to treat elevated VPB rates make reliance on surrogates, or even intermediate endpoints, in those conditions very difficult. While a favourable effect on survival would not be needed if symptomatic improvement was shown, detection of any adverse effect on survival, such as has been seen with several agents, would be important.

Inconsistent epidemiology would also argue against reliance on a surrogate.

Risk/benefit

The existence of a satisfactory alternative known to affect survival argues against acceptance of another agent based on a surrogate (unless, of course, persuasive consistency of effects across several classes exists).

Similarly, surrogates do not seem worth the risk if the endpoint of interest is important and reasonably readily studied, as, for example, thrombolysis and various other post-infarction interventions have proved to be. This is especially true where treatment is long term and is given to people at relatively low risk. Again, views as to what is low risk and what is 'readily' studied change with advancing treatment and new study designs. But when annual event rates fall below, say 5%, a sizeable risk reduction (say 20%) leads to just a 1% salvage. Even a modest rate of a serious adverse unexpected effect could overcome that benefit, and reliance on surrogates in these cases is a very unattractive alternative to defining the true risks and benefits.

The possibility of using a surrogate endpoint arises rarely when a treatment is directed at symptoms because symptoms are easy to study in relatively small, short-term studies. While surrogates will be used, especially where no treatment is available, I believe realisation of the risks involved is critical and growing. The scales have dropped from our eyes, pulled off by CAST, PROFILE, frustration with finding real benefits of cholesterol-lowering drugs, failure to affect survival in most solid tumours, and a growing scepticism about what we get for our health care investment.

Fortunately, we have become more sceptical at the very time when we can do something about it. ISIS, GISSI, GUSTO, SOLVD, SAVE, adjuvant therapy trials in breast and bowel cancer and large simple trials in AIDS have shown us that we can answer therapeutic questions we never dreamed we could because we can carry out trials 10 times the size we thought we could and do so very quickly. Whether such studies are done before or after drug approval, we will, more and more, see clinical trials to explore the real clinical benefits of therapy.

References

1. Steering Committee of the Physicians' Health Study Research Group. Final report on the aspirin component of the ongoing Physicians' Health Study. N Engl J Med 1989; 321: 129–135.
2. The International Study Group. In hospital mortality and clinical course of 20,891 patients with suspected acute myocardial infarction randomized between alteplase and streptokinase with or without heparin. Lancet 1990; 336: 71–75.
3. Gruppo Italiano per lo Studio Della Sopravvivenze Nell'Infarcto Miocardico—GISSI-2: a factorial randomized trial of alteplase versus streptokinase and heparin versus no heparin among 12,490 patients with acute myocardial infarction. Lancet 1990; 336: 65–71.
4. Echt DS, Liebson PR, Mitchell LB et al. Mortality and morbidity in patients receiving encainide, flecanide, or placebo. N Engl J Med 1991; 324: 781–788.
5. The Cardiac Arrhythmia Suppression Trial II Investigators. Effect of the antiarrhythmic agent moricizine on survival after myocardial infarction. N Engl J Med 1992; 327: 227–233.
6. Coplen SE, Antman EM, Berlin JA, Hewitt P, Chalmers TC. Efficacy and safety of quinidine therapy for maintenance of sinus rhythm after cardioversion: a meta-analysis of controlled trials. Circulation 1990; 82: 1106–1116.
7. Hine LK, Laird N, Hewitt P, Chalmers TC. Meta-analytic evidence against prophylactic use of lidocaine in acute myocardial infarction. Arch Intern Med 1989; 149: 2694–2698.
8. The CONSENSUS Trial Study Group. Effects of enalapril on mortality in severe congestive heart failure: result of the Cooperative North Scandinavian Enalapril Survival Study (CONSENSUS). N Engl J Med 1987; 316: 1429–1435.
9. The SOLVD Investigators. Effect of enalapril on survival in patients with reduced left ventricular ejection fractions and congestive heart failure. N Engl J Med 1991; 325: 293–302.
10. Pfeffer MA, Braunwald E, Moye LA et al, on behalf of the SAVE Investigators. Effect of captopril on mortality and morbidity in patients with left ventricular dysfunction after myocardial infarction: results of the Survival and Ventricular Enlargement Trial. N Engl J Med 1992; 327: 669–677.
11. Packer M, Carver JR, Rodehoffer RT et al. Effect of oral milrimone on mortality in severe chronic heart failure. N Engl J Med 1991; 325: 1468–1475.
12. Feldman AM, Bristow MR, Parmley WW et al. Effects of vesnarinone on morbidity and mortality in patients with heart failure. N Engl J Med 1993; 329: 149–155.
13. MacMahon S, Peto R, Cutler J et al. Blood pressure, stroke, and coronary heart disease. Part 1: prolonged differences in blood pressure: prospective observational studies corrected for the regression dilution bias. Lancet 1990; 335: 765–774.
14. Collins R, Peto R, MacMahon S et al. Blood pressure, stroke, and coronary heart disease. Part 2: short-term reductions in blood pressure: overview of randomized drug trials in their epidemiologic context. Lancet 1990; 335: 827–838.
15. SHEP Cooperative Research Group. Prevention of stroke by antihypertensive

drug treatment in older persons with isolated systolic hypertension: final results of the Systolic Hypertension in the Elderly Program (SHEP). JAMA 1991; 265: 3255–3264.

16. ISIS-2 (Second International Study of Infarct Survival) Collaborative Group. Randomized trial of intravenous streptokinase, oral aspirin, both, or neither among 17,187 cases of suspected acute myocardial infarction: ISIS-2. Lancet 1988; ii: 349–360.

2 WHAT TO MEASURE IN DEMENTIA

L. J. Whalley and S. J. Gerhand
The Medical School, Aberdeen, UK

Introduction

The term dementia describes a heterogeneous group of disorders with multiple symptoms and signs. Memory impairment and language disturbance are central features of all types of dementia. Most attempts to measure change in dementia have included items intended to evaluate memory. These are usually adopted from established tests of adult intelligence, for which there are extensive normative data. Tests of language function in dementia are less often used—probably because such tests are not widely understood and there is no consensus on the choice of language test most appropriate to the form of dementia.

It is the aim of many current research programmes in dementia to develop useful measures of change that are valid indicators of altered progress. All retain measures of memory and seek to include other measures that may better elucidate deterioration and its sensitivity to intervention. Examples include measurements of the true extent and location of neuronal loss, impairments of information processing and the frequency of behavioural problems. So far, no single measure or group of measures has achieved this aim. Issues of validity and reliability remain major problems in the development of new scales and in the use of established ones. Because so many scales are primarily subjective, and rely on an observer's impression of what has happened, it is often difficult to obtain objective validation of selected measures of change.

Core symptoms of dementia

CLINICAL–NEUROPATHOLOGICAL CORRELATIVE STUDIES

The core features of dementia are determined by the nature and location of neuronal loss—the pathology—and the resources available to the dement-

Clinical Measurement in Drug Evaluation. Edited by W. S. Nimmo and G. T. Tucker
© 1995 John Wiley & Sons Ltd

ing individual with which to counter this loss. In a landmark series of studies almost 30 years ago, Blessed *et al.* [1] addressed these problems. They showed that clinical measures of the extent of dementia were related to the degree of pathological change, and stated three problems that would confound attempts to measure change in dementia. Although they focused on the relationship between neuropathology and clinical state, their observations remain relevant to the general problem of measurement in dementia:

- What is the relationship between cerebral pathology and psychiatric diagnosis in old age?
- What is the relationship between cerebral pathology and intellectual deterioration in senescence?
- What is the relationship between normal senescence and dementia? Is the latter an acceleration of the former, or is it qualitatively distinct in a pathological sense?

Previously, Roth [2], in his account of the mental disorders of old age, demonstrated by natural history methods the spectrum of psychiatric disorders in senescence to contain several distinct diagnostic entities that differed in mortality and in the coexistence of physical disorder. Corsellis [3] showed that these clinical distinctions were supported by neuropathological examination. Neurofibrillary tangles and senile plaques are the pathognomonic neuropathological features of Alzheimer's disease. There is general agreement among neuropathologists that a post-mortem diagnosis of Alzheimer's disease is supported by identification of significant numbers of senile plaques and, to a lesser extent, neurofibrillary tangles in sections of cerebral cortex in the presence of a clinical history of dementia. Some studies support the Newcastle group's original observations of a direct relationship between the clinical severity of dementia and the density of senile plaques [4–6], while others do not [7–9]. Recently, Arriagadra *et al.* [10] examined prospectively 10 Alzheimer patients and related directly the number of neurofibrillary tangles to the extent of dementia, but not to the density of senile plaques. They suggested that the early features of memory impairment in Alzheimer's disease are associated with pathological disturbance of projections among the entorhinal cortex, hippocampus and amygdala at multiple points in these pathways. They also implicated pathological changes in connections between these areas and cortical and subcortical targets. Other neuropathological–clinical correlative studies have detected strong relationships between parameters of synaptic connectivity (e.g., synaptophysin concentrations) and the degree of dementia [11–13].

Techniques that identify the accumulation in the living brain of neurofibrillary tangles and/or senile plaques would contribute importantly to the measurement of change in dementia. Studies of anatomical change at this microscopic level are, however, not possible during life, but there has been considerable progress in brain imaging and measures of brain function. Positron emission tomographic (PET) studies in Alzheimer's disease reveal deficits in glucose utilisation by neurones in the temporoparietal cortices [14–17]. When retested after two to three years, Alzheimer patients show greater deficits in these brain regions [18]. Compared with macroscopic structural changes detected by CT scan, the degree of increased deficit in glucose utilisation is greater than predicted by the extent of cortical atrophy. It is now important to establish if the progressive decrease in glucose utilisation is a consequence of cell death or secondary to some change in neurotransmitter function. A third possibility is that the glucose deficit precedes neuronal loss in Alzheimer's disease and could be associated with a pathophysiological change that predisposes neurones to early death.

Unfortunately, neuropathological–clinical correlative studies on non-Alzheimer's dementia are sparse and uninformative. There is, as yet, little agreement among neuropathologists on the precise definition of vascular dementia, although in the absence of Alzheimer-type neuropathological change, multiple types of vascular neuropathology, alone or in combination, may account for dementia. ICD-10 suggests four main categories of dementia: Alzheimer's disease, vascular dementia, dementia in diseases classified elsewhere (such as Pick's disease, Creutzfeld–Jakob disease) and 'dementia not otherwise specified'. Alzheimer's disease may be early or late onset, typical or atypical or mixed with vascular dementia. Vascular dementia may be progressive or static, predominantly cortical or non-cortical. When brain cells die because they are diseased and not because of some external event, the term 'primary degenerative dementia' is used. Gustafson [19] summarised recent Swedish agreement on the subtypes of primary degenerative dementia, distinguished by the presence of specific clinical features. When temporoparietal symptoms predominate, the diagnosis of Alzheimer's disease is likely but can be mimicked by head trauma. When frontotemporal symptoms predominate, the diagnosis of Alzheimer's disease is much less likely, and other diagnoses must be considered. These are Pick's disease, frontal lobe dementia [20], motor neurone disease with dementia and certain rare hereditary forms of dementia. Subcortical dementias are associated with pathology of basal ganglia, thalamus and white matter, and are productively investigated by neuro-imaging. There is motor slowing, extrapyramidal and other neurological signs. Features of cortical loss are missing, so dysphasia, dyspraxia and dysgnosia are not seen. Because the frontal lobes are extensively connected to subcortical structures, frontal symptoms are commonplace in Huntington's disease and are not unusual in Parkinson's disease and diffuse Lewy body disease [21].

SENSITIVITY OF SYMPTOMS TO CHANGE

The sensitivity to change of the major signs and symptoms of dementia is unknown. If it is assumed that some features of dementia, e.g. behavioural disturbance, are best understood as consequences of major impairments of memory, language and judgement, then these may be at least partly remediable with available treatments. Such 'secondary' features of dementia are described as behavioural changes that are either loss of acquired behaviours or emergence of new ones ('Sins of commission and sins of omission'). Examples are wandering, shouting, stereotypical behaviours and failure to complete over-learned routines (e.g., dressing, washing). Longitudinal studies of the natural history of Alzheimer's disease show that tests of memory reveal the greatest decrements in function during the progress of the disorder (e.g., the logical memory of the Wechsler Memory Scale [22]). This area of study is of greatest interest to those planning treatment of early or incipient Alzheimer's disease, in the belief that it is at this stage of the disorder that the value of treatment is likely to be the greatest. Obviously, the distinction between early or mild dementia and normal senescence is of considerable relevance to this problem and the questions first posed by Blessed *et al.* [1] and listed above are central to the issues involved.

Berg *et al.* [23] have reported a series of long-term evaluations of a carefully defined sample of late-onset probable Alzheimer patients. Deterioration in this well-described sample contrasted with the stable performances of healthy old people. Premature death was a feature of dementia (much as described by Roth [2]) and those who survive almost invariably become severely demented. Admission to nursing homes was commonplace (63% of 43 subjects within five years). When dysphasia was present early in the disorder, the prognosis was worse, and mortality was higher for men than for women. Of relevance to the problem of choice of measures in dementia was their observation that four of their clinical measures (a global measure of cognitive function over six domains from the Clinical Dementia Rating [24]; the total score and the cognitive subscale of the Dementia Scale [1]; and the Aphasic Battery [25]) were particularly sensitive to longitudinal change. Their observations were extended in a later report [26] by subsequent follow-up of their cohort, and pooling data with a replication sample [27]. Estimates were then made of the entire sample of the measures required to show (a) 100% arrest of the progress of the dementia, (b) 50% slowing, and (c) 25% slowing of the disease. The authors concluded that their clinical global measure (the sum of boxes from the Clinical Dementia Rating Scale) was an appropriate measure in a 12–24-month clinical trial. Among clinical measures, the CDR and the Blessed Dementia Scale performed better than the psychometric tests (subscales of the WAIS (Wechler Adult Intelligence Scale), the Benton and the Boston Naming

Test). Mildly affected Alzheimer patients showed less variability in progression than those who were more severely affected.

NON-COGNITIVE SYMPTOMS OF DEMENTIA

Affective (i.e., mood disorder) and psychotic symptoms occur in dementia. A recent literature review [28] summarised 30 studies on the topic and suggested that 30–40% of Alzheimer patients have depressive or psychotic symptoms. Most commonly, these symptoms are insufficient in duration or severity to merit the diagnosis of a separate psychiatric disorder (e.g., depression). Paranoid features, often of delusional intensity, are the most frequent psychotic symptoms: about 35% of patients had 'at some time' expressed such beliefs. Wragg and Jeste [28] commented that although much of the psychological research effort in Alzheimer's disease focuses on cognitive impairment, the relationship between the extent of cognitive impairment and the occurrence of psychiatric symptoms is little studied and not well understood. They located three studies that agreed delusions are more likely in patients with higher levels of cognitive function, i.e. at an earlier stage of dementia. Plausibly, the emotional reaction to cognitive loss would require higher levels of language function to be retained in order to be expressed. However, Teri *et al.* [29] concluded from a prospective study that cognitive function and frequency of delusions or hallucinations are unrelated. Their data are more compelling than those from retrospective or cross-sectional studies.

Burns *et al.* [30] conducted such a cross-sectional, retrospective survey of delusions, hallucinations and behavioural problems in a large sample ($n = 178$) of Alzheimer patients. Delusions had occurred in 16% and their presence was unrelated to cognitive function. The same authors [31] found a history of perceptual disturbance in 10% (auditory), 13% (visual) and 30% (misidentification syndrome). They concluded that the presence of misidentification syndrome was associated with a lower death rate and hallucinations with a more rapid cognitive decline. The sample was also surveyed for the presence of disorders of moods [32]. Twenty-four per cent were thought to be 'depressed' by a trained observer. Such demented patients tend to be less cognitively impaired, as reported by Reifler *et al.* [33] and Merriam *et al.* [34], and may be related to disturbances of language that invariably accompany severe dementia and the likelihood that retention of judgement in the early stage of illness predisposes to depressive reactions. A history of previous treated depression is more likely in dementia [35].

Clinical trial designs in dementia

When evaluating the effects of drug use, a decision must be made concerning the type of data to be collected and how this should be done. For instance, a study may be cross-sectional or longitudinal. Cross-sectional studies (also referred to as 'independent measures' studies) compare one group of subjects with another group of subjects; for example, a comparison of a group of patients taking a particular drug with a group taking a placebo. Longitudinal or 'repeated measures' studies look at the same group of subjects at different points in time; for example, before and after a period of treatment with a particular drug. However, cross-sectional studies require the two groups of subjects to be carefully matched and, if not done properly, misleading results can be produced because of the influence of confounding variables, such as age, socioeconomic status and education. For instance, the 'Mini-Mental State Examination' (MMSE) [36]—a brief test of cognitive functioning—is widely used as a screening instrument with elderly people. Frequently, a maximum cut-off score is between 22 and 26 points as an entry criterion into a dementia treatment study. However, the MMSE can produce false positive scores, especially with non-demented subjects who are either very elderly or poorly educated [37–39]. Longitudinal studies avoid this problem, as the same subjects are tested on each occasion, but are slow to produce results, and are often more costly. Botwinick *et al.* [40] compared cross-sectional and longitudinal methods for staging in dementia and concluded that comparing patients of different severity provided for the same observations as following up the same subjects over time, although rates of change of individual subjects were lost. Berg *et al.* [27] concluded that cross-sectional research is also likely to underestimate the severity of progression in Alzheimer's disease, as only the less deteriorated subjects are likely to be enrolled in cross-sectional research, whereas longitudinal studies attempt to retain severely demented individuals. A drug trial is often required to use both cross-sectional and longitudinal assessment, as illustrated in a recent study of tacrine in Alzheimer's disease [41]. Subjects were assigned to one of two groups (independent measures), undergoing either a period of treatment with active drug, followed by a period of placebo, or vice versa; cognitive abilities of both groups were assessed each week (repeated measures).

Assessment of individual psychological function requires a comparator against which a patient's performance may be measured. Tests can differ importantly in the origin of their comparator standards. Nomothetic tests compare an individual's performance to the performance of the rest of the population of interest. Ideographic tests use individual comparison standards, such as previous test performance, or current performance on a different test. The choice of comparison standard used depends upon the aspect of functioning to be examined and the rationale underlying that choice. Nomothetic testing is more suited to cross-sectional studies, such as assessment of individual performance and its relationship to the average performance of the population. Lezak [42] points out, however, that this is appropriate only in the measurement of items within the capability of all intact adults and not dependent on education or general intellectual ability. Ideographic testing is required when a change in function is to be evaluated, and is usually more suitable for use in drug trials.

A problem can arise in ideographic measurement, and concerns the availability of individual comparison standards. When comparing functions at the beginning and end of a course of treatment, direct measurement can be employed. However, if a comparison is needed with the patient's ability before the onset of the disease, the necessary measurements have often not been performed, in which case some form of indirect measurement must be made to provide an estimate of pre-morbid ability. Certain tests of word reading ability have been suggested as suitable for this purpose, such as the Schonell Graded Word Reading Test [43] and the National Adult Reading Test [44]. Several studies report that performance on these tests does not deteriorate to the same extent as measurements of other aspects of cognition in Alzheimer's disease [45–47], at least not until the later stages of the disease [48]. It is possible to estimate an individual's likely pre-morbid IQ score from their score on these tests, by use of regression analysis [49].

Choice of measure

Deterioration of cognitive function forms part of every published set of operational criteria for the diagnosis of dementia [50], and consequently the majority of pharmacological treatments focus on improvements of cognitive function [51]. Considering the wide range of cognitive deficits encountered (Table 1), the scope for measurement is very wide indeed. Often the first presenting symptom of Alzheimer's disease is some form of memory deficit, though the impairment is usually non-uniform [52].

MEMORY TESTS

Memory represents a complex phenomenon, and deficits at different stages of processing produce different kinds of memory impairment. The inability to learn new material and retain it for more than 30 s is a registration (or encoding) deficit, and is typically known as 'anterograde amnesia'. This ability is tested either by recall, where the subject produces the 'to-be-remembered' item, or by recognition, where the target item(s) is selected from an array of irrelevant items. A problem of this sort is quite distinct from one of storage, where information can be learned, but is forgotten abnormally quickly; there is some evidence that storage degradation does play a role in the memory problems found in Alzheimer's patients [53]. Even if information is encoded and stored, memory failure can still occur, if it is not possible to retrieve the information [54]. A distinction is possible

Table 1. Range of functions affected in Alzheimer's disease

Function	Element	Reference
Memory	Long-term memory	[52]
	Short-term memory	
	Verbal	[65]
	Visuospatial	[115]
	Attentional	[72]
	Problem solving	[116]
Language	Aphasia	[117]
	Object naming	[76]
	Writing	[77]
	Comprehension	[74]
Perception	Agnosia	[80]
	Hallucinations	[31]
Psychiatric	Behaviour, mood, delusions	[30–32,81]
Psychomotor	Tool use	[95]

between tests of explicit and implicit memory [55], the latter not requiring the subject to be consciously aware of learning the material; and also between procedural and declarative memory, the latter referring to the acquisition of some sort of skill [56]. Within the realms of declarative memory, Tulving [57] proposes a distinction between episodic memory, which is memory for events and experiences, and semantic memory, which covers facts, concepts and language. This is perhaps a particularly relevant distinction, as quite large differences in the degree of impairment of these aspects of memory have been found [46]. Whether these distinctions represent the functioning of separate neural systems or merely different kinds of information within the same system is debated, but the fact that it is possible for subjects to be impaired at some types of these tests and not at others [52,58] requires that these different aspects are assessed separately.

The strongest evidence for separate memory systems is in the distinction between short-term and long-term memory. Short-term memory is regarded as a 'working memory' [59]: a system in which current or ongoing processing takes place. Double dissociations are seen with patients suffering from anterograde amnesia resulting from hippocampal damage, who appear relatively unimpaired on tests of short-term memory [60], and others with apparently intact long-term memory, but deficits on short-term memory tasks [62,63]. A consistent finding is that one thing that distinguishes amnesia from dementia is the impaired short-term memory performance of demented patients [64]. Baddeley [59] views working memory as consisting of a supervisory, attentional system called the central executive, which controls and coordinates the activity of two subsidiary slave systems. One system, called the 'articulatory loop', is specialised for the handling of auditory/verbal material, while the 'visual spatial sketch pad' system deals with visuospatial material. Alzheimer's disease produces deficits in all these areas of functioning, with evidence of impaired digit span [65], problems with visuospatial memory and learning [66,67] and deficits in attentional abilities [68–70]. Certain researchers have suggested that attentional deficits are the underlying factor in many of the other cognitive deficits seen in the disorder [71,72]. Assessment of the relative effects of pharmacological intervention on these various aspects of memory function therefore requires any changes produced to be specified precisely.

LANGUAGE TESTS

Bayles and Tomoeda [73] reported difficulties in object naming in fairly advanced cases of Alzheimer's disease although this appears to result largely from a deterioration of semantic knowledge [74–76]. However, these naming difficulties do not always correlate with the writing difficulties that are also often found [77,78], illustrating the complexity of the language process. An indication of this complexity can be gained from Figure 1, which represents some of the processes involved in recognising and producing words. An inability to perform any one of these processes results in a 'language deficit', each of which can occur independently of any other problems [79]. Therefore, a detailed functional analysis of two patients, apparently with the same problem, might reveal two separate deficits. Alzheimer's appears to affect initially the central processes depicted, but impairment of the more peripheral processes becomes apparent as the disease progresses. Some patients show an ability to read and copy print, without understanding what the words mean [74], but the ability to copy even simple figures eventually becomes impaired (Figure 2). As with memory, the nature of any change occurring in language abilities must be specified precisely to ascertain exactly what is changing.

PERCEPTUAL SYMPTOMS

Before language can be used, the individual must first be able to perceive and make sense of the world. Impairment of this ability is also seen in Alzheimer's disease, and can result in an inability to recognise objects [80]. Hallucinations—the perception of stimuli that are not actually present—

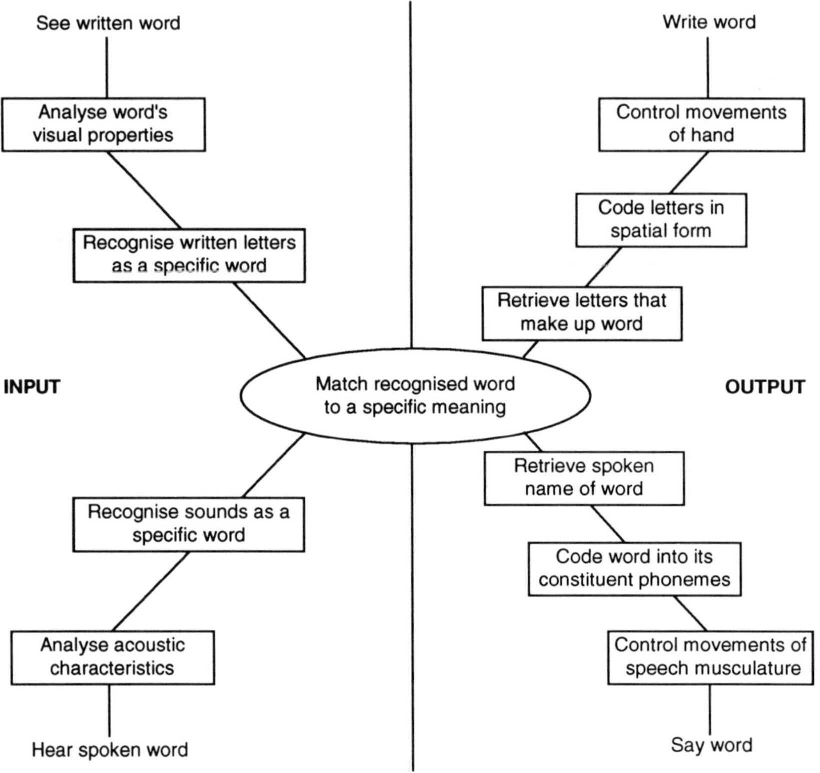

Figure 1. Simplified model of the processes involved in recognition and production of spoken and written words. Alzheimer's disease initially affects the central processes, but the more peripheral processes also become impaired as the disease progresses

also occur in some patients [31], although this may be more properly thought of as a psychiatric problem.

PSYCHIATRIC SYMPTOMS

Alzheimer's disease does not just affect cognition. A number of psychiatric and behavioural problems are also common; for example, depressive and psychotic symptoms occur in 30–40% of Alzheimer patients [28], particularly in the more severely demented patient [32,81]. Delusions occur in 21–31% of cases [82,83], as well as visual and auditory hallucinations [31]. Assessment of these as well as cognitive dimensions must also be addressed, and often use is made of inventories, such as the Beck Depression Inventory [84] and the State-Trait Anxiety Inventory [85]. These contain a

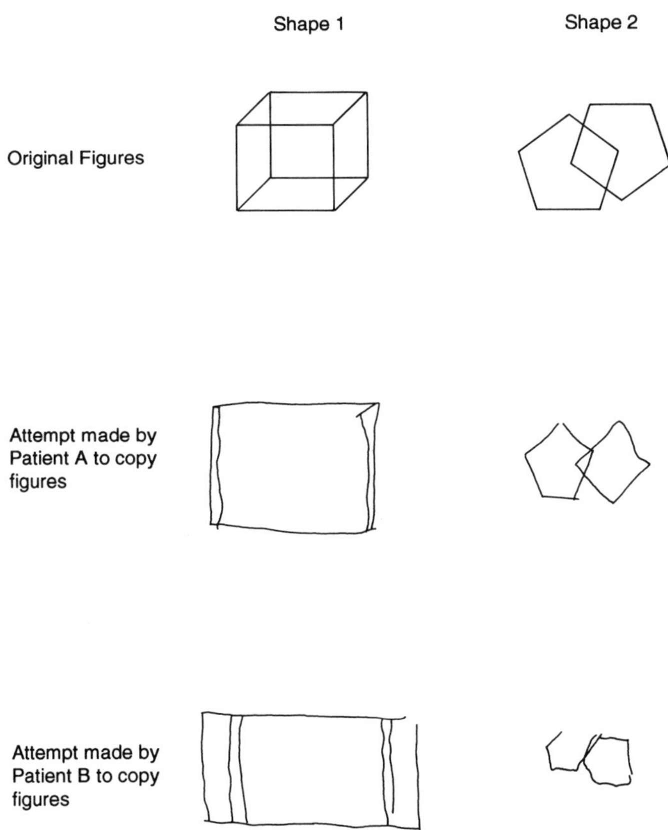

Figure 2. Examples of dysgraphic errors produced by Alzheimer patients. Top figures represent target shapes, and bottom figures are attempts made by Alzheimer patients to draw them

number of sentences relating to a particular problem, for example depression. The subject rates, usually on a five-point scale, how appropriate a particular item is to them, and the ratings for all of the items are then totalled to give an overall score for that particular problem.

Behavioural symptoms can be divided into two categories: positive and negative. Positive symptoms occur in addition to normal behaviour, and include delusions, aggression, wandering and disturbed sleep. Negative symptoms represent a loss or reduction of normal behaviours, and include withdrawal, apathy, loss of initiative and flattened emotional response. The most popular way of assessing behaviour in drug trials is the rating scale [86], which is completed by an observer. For example, the Dementia Behaviour Disturbance Scale [87] requires the frequency of a number of observable behaviours to be rated on a five-point scale. However, there are a number of problems concerning the validity and reliability of rating scales, as accurate ratings require the rater to have a high level of contact with the subject. Patterson *et al.* [88] found an item rating the amount of wakefulness at night was omitted 20% of the time, as night-time observation of the patient had not taken place. Finkel *et al.* [89] compared ratings on three scales by staff working different shifts, and found that, while correlations between scales reached significance for day and evening shifts, they failed to do so during the night shift, which indicates a general problem with night-time behaviour rating. They also found a problem with behaviours such as disrobing and intentional falling, which may be of great importance, but are infrequent and therefore difficult to observe. Another factor to be considered is whether the items in a scale actually cover the behaviours of interest.

A number of other ways of assessing behaviour exist, although they are less commonly used than rating scales. La Porte *et al.* [90] identified methods for measurement of physical activity, which could be grouped into seven categories: mechanical and electronic measures, direct observation, surveys, job classification, dietary assessment, physiological markers, and calorimetry. Unfortunately, there are a number of problems inherent in all these methods that limit their applicability to clinical trials. Dietary assessment, calorimetry and physiological markers are primarily concerned with energy expenditure, and are usually invasive, which makes them difficult to use in a natural setting. Surveys can be useful but usually rely on self-support, which can provide accurate data [91] but are dependent on the willingness and capability of the subject to cooperate.

Direct observation of behaviour originates from ethology, and has been applied successfully to the study of human behaviour, in the fields of developmental psychology and non-verbal communication [92]. However, this type of measurement is mainly of use over short periods of time, and is difficult to apply to long-term monitoring of behaviour, and therefore of limited use. Mechanical and electronic devices are also of use over a limited range of behaviours. For example, devices can be worn on the wrist, which register the overall amount of movement in a given period of time. This can be used to indicate the amount of sleep disruption that a patient suffers [93], which can be validated against EEG readings [94].

PSYCHOMOTOR PROBLEMS

Knowledge of tool use and programmes to control movement can be impaired in Alzheimer patients, with an inability to produce correct gestures when required, which can be separate from any language deficit [95].

The nature of Alzheimer's disease is such that isolated deficits are not found, and there is no one type of deterioration that singles it out from other disorders. What is important is the overall pattern of deterioration, and therefore any attempt at measurement must be multi-dimensional. The effectiveness of pharmacological intervention can only be judged by detailed functional analysis, as non-specific measures do not address the issue of exactly what improves.

Confounding variables

Having decided what aspect of functioning is to be assessed, consideration must be given to other factors which affect performance on a test, so that any incidental change can be distinguished from the effects of pharmacological intervention. Furry and Baltes [96] suggested that age-related differences in test scores are partly caused by fatigue, with more elderly subjects' performance being affected to a greater extent by tiredness than younger subjects. Although later research suggests that this effect is not as strong as initially thought [97], the confounding effect of variables such as fatigue can mean that a discrepancy arises between performance and ability. This problem is well known in assessment of children, where a child may fail to perform at a certain level on a particular test, not because they lack the required ability but because they have not fully understood what they are required to do [98]. As modern testing is becoming increasingly dominated by the use of the computer, problems can arise through elderly subjects not being familiar with computers. Although lower scores may result because of this, the problem can be alleviated by training [99]. This can create further problems, as the apparent effects of pharmacological intervention must be distinguished from practice effects. For instance, Grant *et al.* [100] found that performance on the Digit Symbol test, which was considered to decline with age, is subject to improvement with practice.

Practice effects may be of interest in themselves, as their absence can be used to distinguish the effects of dementia from those of normal ageing. CAMCOG, the cognitive section of CAMDEX [101,102], consists of a computerised battery of cognitive tests, aimed primarily at early detection of dementia. Lineboom *et al.* [103] evaluated the effectiveness of this programme, and concluded that it differentiated well, except when subjects were poorly educated, or were over 75 years of age. However, on a second administration, mildly demented people falling into this category showed less improvement that non-/minimally demented people of similar age and education. The influence of these confounding variables can result in a degree of sampling bias, in particular as cognitive scores are influenced by social class [104] and education [37,39], and poorer, less educated people are often easier to recruit for studies.

Conclusion

To evaluate the effectiveness of a treatment programme, efforts must be made to ensure that the subject is performing optimally, at both the initial and final assessment. The use of devices such as the 'touch screen' makes it easier for the subject to respond, and strategies such as encouragement from the tester can help the subject to feel at ease and reduce the confounding effects of performance anxiety. Elderly subjects are more likely to attempt answers they are unsure about if they feel that risk is low [105]. Therefore, a relaxed testing atmosphere is desirable. However, it is essential that the conditions at the initial test session are as close as possible to those at the follow-up ones.

Any treatment based on a proper understanding of Alzheimer's disease must relate to the primary disease process. At the moment this is not possible, and therefore the main focus of pharmacological intervention is on symptomatic relief. There is strong evidence that the cholinergic neurotransmitter system plays an important role in human memory function [64], and that the extent of reduced cholinergic function in Alzheimer patients is related to the extent of their cognitive impairment [106]. Furthermore, drugs that block the action of acetylcholine cause memory impairments similar to some of those seen in Alzheimer's disease [107]. However, cholinergic therapy, and most other therapies, have not proved to be very effective [51]. Whalley and Starr [108] suggest three reasons for this lack of success:

- Neuronal degeneration may be too advanced for effective use of any treatment requiring a substrate.
- Symptomatic relief only addresses part of the problem, and the remaining symptoms may be just as problematical as those dealt with.
- The accompanying side-effects are particularly distressing, as the Alzheimer patient often cannot fully grasp their circumstances.

These points illustrate the need for precise specification of the effect of any drug used, and also that what is really called for in Alzheimer's disease is to halt the progression of the disorder. Selkoe [109] suggests the most likely pathway to success will involve drugs that inhibit the molecular mechanisms underlying dementia. This will necessarily involve detection of the dementing process before large numbers of neurones have been lost, so that treatment can be implemented while deficits are minimal. Histological markers normally associated with dementia, such as senile plaques and neurofibrillary tangles, are also seen in the brains of non-demented subjects [110], and may represent a pre-clinical stage of the disease [8]. Individuals of high intelligence may perform adequately on cognitive tests, despite having undergone a considerable decline in ability [111], and the distinction between mild dementia and normal ageing may only be apparent in a few selective areas of function [112,113], with considerable overlap between mild dementia and healthy ageing [114]. It is probable that assessment will take place within a range of functioning considered to be normal, and that changes produced by intervention will be quite small. The question of drug use in Alzheimer's disease must therefore address aspects that are sensitive to treatment, and assessment must be made of changes in function that may be very minimal.

Summary

Measurement in dementia has concentrated mainly on memory, and often makes use of items adopted from established tests of adult intelligence. Much current research aims at developing useful measures of change, but it is difficult to overcome the problem of obtaining objective validation. Although there is a relationship between the extent of dementia and the degree of pathological change, a problem remains of how to discern the early effects of dementia from those of normal ageing, as *in vivo* measures of brain pathology currently lack sufficient sensitivity. Whilst neuropathological–clinical studies have identified senile plaques and neurofibrillary tangles in the brains of Alzheimer patients, equivalent markers have not been identified from other types of dementia.

If some of the main behavioural signs and symptoms of dementia result from the underlying cognitive deficits, it is possible that available treatments may provide some remedial effect. Longitudinal studies show memory to be the area of function that declines most in early dementia, and several scales exist, such as the CRR and the Blessed Dementia Scale, which are sensitive to the changes found in mild dementia over a period of 12–24 months. Non-cognitive symptoms, such as depression and paranoia, also occur in dementia, and are related to cognitive symptoms. These are generally more common in the earlier stages of the disease.

Clinical trials can use a number of different designs. Cross-sectional studies compare different subjects at a particular point in time, whereas longitudinal studies consider the same group of subjects at different points in time. Although it is often more costly and slow to produce results, some form of longitudinal assessment is usually required when assessment of change is necessary. Assessment of psychological functioning requires a comparison standard, which can be derived from other people's test performance, or from a measure of the individual's own performance. Individual comparison standards are more suited to longitudinal assessment. However, previous levels of performance may not be known, in which case an estimate must be derived from performance on other tests not sensitive to decline.

It is possible to measure a wide range of psychological function. A function such as memory is not a homogeneous set of abilities and a number of tests exist which measure different aspects of this. Language also represents a complex skill, which can be subdivided, and attempts to measure change in language ability must specify exactly what aspect changes. Perceptual deficits are also found in Alzheimer's disease, and psychiatric and behavioural problems also occur. Assessment of psychiatric and behavioural problems involves the use of inventories, although this is not without complication.

A problem with any measurement in the life sciences is the influence of confounding variables. Factors such as tiredness, practice and education all exert some influence over an individual's test score, and these must therefore be controlled for, in order to be sure that any change produced in a clinical trial is actually caused by the drug. Ultimately, a successful therapy will result from an understanding of the primary disease process. This is not currently possible, and pharmacological intervention currently aims at symptomatic relief. Some symptoms may be more sensitive to change than others, such as attention, and the changes found may be very slight. Measurement should, as far as possible, be multi-dimensional, and sensitive to minimal changes.

References

1. Blessed G, Tomlinson BE, Roth M. The association between quantitative measures of dementia and of senile change in the cerebral grey matter of elderly subjects. Br J Psychiatry 1968; 114: 797–811.
2. Roth M. The natural history of mental disorders in old age. J Ment Sci 1955; 101: 281.
3. Corsellis JAN. Mental Illness and the Aging Brain. London: Oxford University Press, 1962.
4. Wilcock GK, Esiri MM. Plaques, tangles and dementia: a quantitative study. J Neurol Sci 1982; 56: 343–356.
5. Duyckaerts C, Hauw JJ, Bastenaire F et al. Laminar distribution of neocortical senile plaques in senile dementia of the Alzheimer type. Acta Neuropathol (Berl) 1986; 70: 249–256.
6. Delaere P, Duyckaerts C, Brion JP, Poulain V, Hauw JJ. Tau, paired helical filaments and amyloid in the neocortex: a morphometric study of 15 cases with graded intellectual status in aging and senile dementia of the Alzheimer type. Acta Neuropathol (Berl) 1986; 77: 645–653.
7. Neary D, Snowdon JS, Mann DMA et al. Alzheimer's disease: a correlative study. J Neurol Neurosurg Psychiatry 1986; 49: 229–237.
8. Morris JC, McKeel DW, Storandt M et al. Very mild Alzheimer's disease: informant based clinical, psychometric and pathological distinction from normal aging. Neurology 1991; 41: 469–478.
9. Price JL, Davis PB, Morris JC, White DL. The distribution of tangles, plaques and related immunohistochemical markers in healthy aging and Alzheimer's disease. Neurobiol Aging 1991; 12: 295–312.

10. Arriagadra PV, Growdon JH, Hedley-White T, Hyman BT. Neurofibrillary tangles but not senile plaques parallel duration and severity of Alzheimer's disease. Neurology 1992; 42: 631–639.
11. Terry R, Masliah E, Salmon D et al. Structure–function correlations in Alzheimer's disease (abstract). J Neuropathol Exp Neurol 1990; 49: 318.
12. De Kosky ST, Scheff SW. Synapse loss in frontal cortex biopsies in Alzheimer's disease: correlation with cognitive severity. Ann Neurol 1990; 27: 457–464.
13. Masliah E, Terry RD, Alford H, De Teresa R, Hansen LA. Cortical and subcortical patterns of synaptophysin-like immunoreactivity in Alzheimer's disease. Am J Pathol 1991; 138: 235–246.
14. Ferris SH, de Leon MJ, Wolf AP et al. Positron emission tomography in the study of aging and senile dementia. Neurobiol Aging 1980; 1: 127–131.
15. de Leon M, Ferris S, George A et al. Positron emission tomography studies of aging and Alzheimer's disease. Am J Neuroradiol 1983; 4: 568–571.
16. Friedland R, Budinger T, Ganz E et al. Regional cerebral metabolic alterations in dementia of the Alzheimer type: positron emission tomography with fluorodeoxyglucose. J Comput Assist Tomogr 1983; 7: 590–598.
17. McGeer PL, Kamo H, Harrop R et al. Positron emission tomography in patients with clinically diagnosed Alzheimer's disease. Can Med Assoc J 1986; 134: 597–607.
18. Smith GS, De Leon MJ, George AE et al. Topography of cross-sectional and longitudinal glucose metabolic deficits in Alzheimer's disease: pathophysiologic implications. Arch Neurol 1992; 49: 1142–1150.
19. Gustafson L. Clinical classification of dementia conditions. Acta Neurol Scand 1992; Suppl 139: 16–20.
20. Neary D. Dementia of the frontal lobe type. J Am Geriatr Soc 1990; 38: 71–72.
21. Perry RH, Irving D, Blessed G, Fairbairn A, Perry EK. Senile dementia of the Lewy body type. J Neurol Sci 1990; 95: 119–139.
22. Botwinick J, Storandt M, Berg L. A longitudinal, behavioural study of senile dementia of the Alzheimer type. Arch Neurol 1986; 43: 1124–1127.
23. Berg L, Miller JP, Storandt M et al. Mild senile dementia of the Alzheimer type. 2. Longitudinal assessment. Ann Neurol 1988; 23: 477–484.
24. Hughes CP, Berg L, Danziger WL, Coben LA, Martin RL. A new clinical scale for the staging of dementia. Br J Psychiatry 1982; 140: 566–572.
25. Goodglass H, Kaplan E. The Assessment of Aphasia and Related Disorders (2nd edn). Philadelphia: Lea & Febiger, 1983.
26. Berg L, Miller P, Baty J et al. Mild senile dementia of the Alzheimer type. 4. Evaluation of intervention. Ann Neurol 1992; 31: 242–249.
27. Berg L, Smith DS, Morris JC et al. Mild senile dementia of the Alzheimer type: 3. Longitudinal and cross-sectional assessment. Ann Neurol 1990; 28 (5): 648–652.
28. Wragg RE, Jeste DV. Overview of depression and psychosis in Alzheimer's disease: model of the memory deficit in Alzheimer's disease. Psychol Med 1989; 22: 437–445.
29. Teri L, Larson EB, Reifler BV. Behavioural disturbance in dementia of the Alzheimer's type. J Am Geriatr Soc 1988; 36: 1–6.
30. Burns A, Jacoby R, Levy R. Psychiatric phenomena in Alzheimer's disease. 1: Disorders of thought content. Br J Psychiatry 1990; 157: 72–76.
31. Burns A, Jacoby R, Levy R. Psychiatric phenomena in Alzheimer's disease. II: Disorders of perception. Br J Psychiatry 1990; 157: 76–81.
32. Burns A, Jacoby R, Levy R. Psychiatric phenomena in Alzheimer's disease. III: Disorders of mood. Br J Psychiatry 1990; 157: 81–86.

33. Reifler B, Larson E, Harley R. Co-existence of cognitive impairment and depression in geriatric outpatients. Am J Psychiatry 1982; 139: 623–626.
34. Merriam AF, Aronson MK, Gaston P, Wey SL, Kath I. The psychiatric symptoms of Alzheimer's disease. J Am Geriatr Soc 1988; 36: 7–12.
35. Jorm AF, Van Duijn CM, Chandra V et al. Psychiatric history and related exposures as risk factors for Alzheimer's disease: a collaborative reanalysis of case–control studies. Int J Epidemiol 1991; 20 (Suppl 2): S43–S47.
36. Folstein MF, Folstein SE, McHugh PR. Mini Mental State: a practical method for grading the cognitive state of patients for the clinician. J Psychiatr Res 1975; 12: 189–198.
37. Anthony JC, LeResche L, Niaz U, Von Korff MR, Folstein MF. Limits of the Mini-Mental state as a screening test for dementia and delirium among hospital patients. Psychol Med 1982; 12: 397–408.
38. Fillenbaum GG, Hughes DC, Heyman A, George LK, Blazer DG. Relationship of health and demographic characteristics to Mini-Mental State Examination score among community residents. Psychol Med 1988; 18: 719–726.
39. O'Connor DW, Pollitt PA, Treasure FP, Brook CPB, Reiss BB. The influence of education, social class and sex on Mini-Mental State scores. Psychol Med 1989; 19: 771–776.
40. Botwinick J, Storandt M, Berg L, Boland S. Senile dementia of the Alzheimer type: subject attrition and testability in research. Arch Neurol 1988; 45: 493–496.
41. Eagger S, Morant N, Levy R, Sahakian B. Tacarine in Alzheimer's disease: time course of changes in cognitive function and practice effects. Br J Psychiatry 1992; 160: 36–40.
42. Lezak MD. Neuropsychological Assessment (2nd edn). Oxford: Oxford University Press, 1983.
43. Schonell F. Backwardness in the Basic Subjects. London: Oliver & Boyd, 1942.
44. Nelson HE. National Adult Reading Test. Windsor, UK: NFER–Nelson.
45. Cummings JL, Houlihan JP, Hill MA. The pattern of reading deterioration in dementia of the Alzheimer type: observations and implications. Brain Lang 1986; 29: 315–323.
46. Nebes RD, Brady CB. Focussed and divided attention in Alzheimer's disease. Cortex 1989; 25: 305–315.
47. Riddle HV, Bradshaw CM. On the estimation of premorbid intellectual functioning: validation of Nelson & McKenna's formula, and some new normative data. Br J Clin Psychol 1982; 21: 159–165.
48. Fromm D, Holland AL, Nebes RD, Oakley MA. A longitudinal assessment of word reading ability in Alzheimer's disease: evidence from the National Adult Reading Test. Cortex 1991; 27: 367–376.
49. Nelson HE, McKenna P. The use of current reading ability in the assessment of dementia. Br J Social Clin Psychol 1975; 14: 259–267.
50. Huppert FA, Tym E. Clinical and neuropsychological assessment of dementia. Br Med Bull 1986; 42 (1): 11–18.
51. Gottfries CG. Review of treatment strategies. Acta Neurol Scand 1992; Suppl 139: 63–68.
52. Morris RG, Kopelman MD. The memory deficits in Alzheimer-type dementia: a review. Q J Exp Psychol 1986; 38: 575–602.
53. Hodges JR, Salmon DP, Butters N. Semantic memory impairments in Alzheimer's disease: failure of access or degraded knowledge? Neuropsychologia 1992; 30 (4): 301–314.
54. Warrington EK, Weiskrantz L. Amnesic syndrome: consolidation or retrieval? Nature 1970; 228: 628–630.

55. Schacter DL. Implicit memory: history and current status. J Exp Psychol 1987; 13: 501–518.
56. Cohen NJ, Squire LR. Preserved learning and retention of pattern analysing skill in amnesia: dissociation of 'knowing how' and 'knowing that'. Science 1982; 210: 207–209.
57. Tulving E. Episodic and semantic memory. In: Tulving E, Donaldson W (eds), Organization of Memory. New York: Academic Press, 1973; 382–404.
58. Nebes RD. Semantic memory in Alzheimer's disease. Psychol Bull 1989; 106 (3): 377–394.
59. Baddeley A. Working Memory. Oxford: Oxford University Press, 1986.
60. Scoville WB, Miller B. Loss of recent memory after bilateral hippocampal lesions. J Neurol Neurosurg Psychiatry 1957; 20: 11–21.
61. Zola-Morgan et al. Human amnesia and the medial temporal region: enduring memory impairment following a bilateral lesion limited to field CA1 of the hippocampus. J Neurosci 1986; 6(10): 2950–2967.
62. Warrington EK, Shallice T. The selective impairment of auditory verbal short-term memory. Brain 1969; 92: 885–896.
63. Vallar G, Baddeley A. Fractionation of working memory: neuropsychological evidence for a phonological short-term store. J Verbal Learning Verbal Behav 1984; 23: 151–161.
64. Kopelman MD. The cholinergic neurotransmitter system in human memory and dementia: a review. Q J Exp Psychol 1986; 38A: 535–573.
65. Miller E. On the nature of the memory disorder in presenile dementia. Neuropsychologia 1971; 9: 75–81.
66. Sahakian BJ, Morris RG, Evenden JL, Heald A, Levy R, Philpot M, Robbins TW. A comparative study of visuospatial learning in Alzheimer-type dementia and Parkinson's disease. Brain 1988; 111: 695–718.
67. Adelstein TB, Kesner RP, Strassberg DS. Spatial recognition and spatial order memory in patients with dementia of the Alzheimer's type. Neuropsychologia 1992; 30 (1): 59–67.
68. Nebes RD, Brady CB. Focussed and divided attention in Alzheimer's disease. Cortex 1989; 25: 305–315.
69. Freed DM, Corkin S, Growdon JH, Nissen MJ. Selective attention in Alzheimer's disease: characterising cognitive subgroups of patients. Neuropsychologia 1989; 27 (3): 325–399.
70. Parasuraman R, Greenwoon PM, Haxby JV, Grady CL. Visuo-spatial attention in dementia of the Alzheimer type. Brain 1992; 115: 711–733.
71. Jorm AF. Controlled and automatic information processing in senile dementia: a review. Psychol Med 1986; 65 (3): 77–78.
72. Baddeley A, Logie R, Bressi S, Della Sala S, Spinnler H. Dementia and working memory. Q J Exp Psychol 1986; 38A: 603–618.
73. Bayles KA, Tomoeda CK. Confrontation naming impairment in dementia. Brain Lang 1983; 19: 98–114.
74. Schwartz MF, Marin OS, Saffran EM. Dissociations of language function in dementia: a case study. Brain Lang 1979; 7: 277–306.
75. Martin A, Fedio P. Word production and comprehension in Alzheimer's disease: the breakdown of semantic knowledge. Brain Lang 1983; 19: 124–141.
76. Huff FJ, Corkin S, Growdon JH. Semantic impairment and anomia in Alzheimer's disease. Brain Lang 1986; 28: 235–249.
77. Henderson VW, Buckwalter JG, Sobel E, Freed DM, Diz MM. The agraphia of Alzheimer's disease. Neurology 1992; 42: 776–784.

78. LaBarge E, Smith DS, Dick L, Storandt M. Agraphia in dementia of the Alzheimer type. Arch Neurol 1992; 49: 1151–1156.
79. Ellis AW, Young AW. Human Cognitive Neuropsychology. Hove: Erlbaum, 1988.
80. Rapcsak SZ, Kentos M, Rubens AB. Impaired recognition of meaningful sounds in Alzheimer's disease. Arch Neurol 1989; 46 (12): 1298–1300.
81. Burns A, Jacoby R, Levy R. Psychiatric phenomena in Alzheimer's disease. IV: Disorders of behaviour. Br J Psychiatry 1990; 157: 86–94.
82. Reisberg B, Bornstein J, Salob S, Ferris SH, Franssen E, Georgotas A. Behavioural symptoms in Alzheimer's disease: phenomenology and treatment. J Clin Psychiatry 1987; 48 (Suppl 5): 9–15.
83. Rubin E, Drevits W, Burke A. The nature of psychotic symptoms in senile dementia of the Alzheimer type. J Geriatr Psychiatry Neurol 1988; 1: 16–20.
84. Beck AT, Ward CH, Mendelson M, Mock J, Erbaugh J. An inventory for measuring depression. Arch Gen Psychiatry 1961; 4: 561–571.
85. Spielberger CD, Gorsuch RL, Lushene RE. STAI Manual for the State-Trait Anxiety Inventory. Palo Alto, CA: Consulting Psychologists Press, 1970.
86. Sunderland T, Silver MA. Neuroleptics in the treatment of dementia. Int J Geriatr Res 1988; 3: 79–88.
87. Baumgarten M, Becker R, Gautier S. Validity and reliability of the Dementia Behaviour Disturbance Scale. J Am Geriatr Soc 1990; 38 (3): 79–88.
88. Patterson MB, Schnell AH, Martin RJ, Mendez MF, Smyth KA, Whitehouse PJ. Assessment of behavioural and affective symptoms in Alzheimer's disease. J Geriatr Psychiatry Neurol 1990; 3: 21–30.
89. Finkel SI, Lyons TS, Anderson RL. Reliability and validity of the Cohen–Mansfield Agitation Inventory in institutionalised elderly. Int J Geriatr Psychiatry 1992; 7: 487–490.
90. La Porte RE, Montoye HJ, Cappersen CJ. Assessment of physical activity in epidemiological research: problems and prospects. Public Health Rep 1985; 100: 131–146.
91. Klegges RC, Eck LH, Mellon MW, Fulliton W, Somes GW, Hanson CL. The accuracy of self-reports of physical activity. Med Sci Sports Exerc 1990; 22 (5): 690–697.
92. Argyle M. Bodily Communication. London: Methuen, 1988.
93. Aubert-Tulkens G, Culee C, Harmant-van Rijckevorsel K, Rodstein DO. Ambulatory evaluation of sleep disturbance and therapeutic effects in sleep apnea syndrome by wrist activity monitoring. Am Rev Respir Disord 1987; 136 (4): 851–856.
94. Mullaney DJ, Kripke DF, Messin S. Wrist-actigraphic estimation of sleep time. Sleep 1980; 3: 83–92.
95. Ochipa C, Gonzalez Rothi LJ, Heilman KM. Conceptual apraxia in Alzheimer's disease. Brain 1992; 115: 1061–1071.
96. Furry CA, Baltes PB. The effect of age differences in ability-extraneous performance variables on the assessment of intelligence in children, adults, and the elderly. J Gerontol 1973; 28: 73–80.
97. Cunningham WR, Sepkoski CM, Opel MR. Fatigue effects on intelligence test performance in the elderly. J Gerontol 1978; 33 (4): 541–545.
98. Donaldson M. Children's Minds. London: Fontana Press, 1977.
99. Johnson DF, White CB. Effects of training on computerized test performance in the elderly. J Appl Psychol 1980; 65 (3): 357–358.
100. Grant EA, Storandt M, Botwinick J. Incentive and practice in the psychomotor performance of the elderly. J Gerontol 1978; 33 (3): 413–415.

101. Roth M, Tym E, Mountjoy CQ, Huppert FA, Hendrie H, Verma S, Goddard R. CAMDEX: a standardized instrument for the diagnosis of mental disorder in the elderly with special reference to the early detection of dementia. Br J Psychiatry 1986; 149: 698–709.
102. Roth M, Huppert FA, Tym E, Mountjoy CQ. CAMDEX: the Cambridge Examination for Mental Disorders of the Elderly. Cambridge: Cambridge University Press, 1988.
103. Lindeboom J, Ter Horst R, Hooyer C, Dinkgreve M, Jonker C. Some psychometric properties of the CAMCOG. Psychol Med 1993; 23: 213–219.
104. Kittner et al. Methodological issues in screening for dementia: the problem of education adjustment. J Chron Dis 1986; 39 (3): 163–170.
105. Birkhill WR, Schaie KW. The effect of differential reinforcement of cautiousness in intellectual performance among the elderly. J Gerontol 1975; 30 (5): 578–583.
106. Perry EK, Tomlinson BE, Blessed G, Bergman K, Gibson PH, Perry RH. Correlation of cholinergic abnormalities with senile plaques and mental test scores in dementia. Br Med J 1978; ii: 1457–1459.
107. Kopelman MD, Corn TH. Cholinergic 'blockade' as a model for cholinergic depletion: a comparison of the memory deficits with those of Alzheimer-type dementia and the alcoholic Korsakoff syndrome. Brain 1988; 111: 1079–1110.
108. Whalley LJ, Starr JM. Cholinergic therapy. In: Copeland JRM, Abou-Saleh, Blazer DG (eds), The Psychiatry of Old Age. Chichester: Wiley, 1993; 421–426.
109. Selkoe DJ. Aging brain, aging mind. Sci Am 1992; 267 (3): 134–142.
110. Katzman R, Terry R, DeTeresa R et al. Clinical, pathological, and neurochemical changes in dementia: a subgroup with preserved mental status and numerous neocortical plaques. Ann Neurol 1988; 23: 138–144.
111. Jorm AF, Korten AE. Assessment of cognitive decline in the elderly by informant interview. Br J Psychiatry 1988; 152: 209–213.
112. Rubin EH, Morris JC, Grant EA, Vendegna T. Very mild senile dementia of the Alzheimer type I. Clinical assessment. Arch Neurol 1989; 46: 379–382.
113. Flicker C, Ferris SH, Reisberg B. Mild cognitive impairment in the elderly: predictors of dementia. Neurology 1991; 41: 1006–1009.
114. Storandt and Hill. Very mild senile dementia of the Alzheimer type. II. Psychometric test performance. Arch Neurol 1989; 46 (4): 383–386.
115. Grossi D, Becker JT, Smith C, Trojano L. Memory for visuospatial patterns in Alzheimer's disease. Psychol Med 1993; 23: 65–70.

3 TWENTY-FOUR-HOUR AMBULATORY ARTERIAL (BLOOD) PRESSURE MEASUREMENT AND THE ASSESSMENT OF ANTIHYPERTENSIVE DRUG EFFICACY

Joerg Hasford and Wolfgang Meister
University of Munich, Munich, Germany

Introduction

Elevated arterial pressure is an epidemic. Prevalence studies have shown that in Germany about 22.7% of the male and 18.5% of the female population between 30 and 69 years experience elevated arterial pressure, defined as being higher than 160/95 mmHg [1]. Elevated arterial pressure is an important risk factor for stroke and cardiovascular morbidity and mortality. Reduction in pressure decreases the attributable risks. The effectiveness of antihypertensive drug treatment with regard to the reduction of morbidity and mortality had been shown in 1967 for the first time [2]. Since then there have been many types of new antihypertensive drugs. Although arterial pressure has been measured since 1733 when Stephen Hales published his 'statistical essays: containing haemastaticks', and despite its importance, the non-invasive measurement of arterial pressure still presents a challenge for research. This chapter presents a critical review of the three non-invasive techniques to measure arterial pressure for the assessment of antihypertensive drug efficacy in clinical trials: the casual arterial pressure taken by the physician; the home, self-recorded arterial pressure; and the non-invasive 24 h ambulatory arterial pressure monitoring (ABPM).

Clinical Measurement in Drug Evaluation. Edited by W. S. Nimmo and G. T. Tucker
© 1995 John Wiley & Sons Ltd

Time points of measuring arterial pressure in a clinical trial

In an antihypertensive trial the assessment of arterial pressure is crucial at three to four different time points. First, an appropriate target population, i.e. hypertensive patients, have to be identified. Then a baseline measurement just before randomisation is needed. During the treatment and observation phase arterial pressure is recorded repeatedly to assess efficacy of the treatments. At the date specified in the trial protocol when the treatment and the observation phase ends the primary efficacy variable—arterial pressure—is measured again. In the statistical analysis the change of pressure over time is compared between and within the treatment groups. The results of these comparisons are only valid if the measurements of arterial pressure have been reliable and valid and if equality of observation has been secured over time and patients. As arterial pressure is a highly variable biological phenomenon, special attention is necessary to achieve the required quality of its measurement.

Determinants of arterial pressure

Leaving pathophysiology aside, the factors influencing arterial pressure and its measurement can be classified to be related to the investigator, patient or environment.

By far the most important patient-related factor is the so-called 'white-coat hypertension'. This is office-measured elevated pressure, which cannot be reproduced when self-measuring pressure at home or with an abpm device [3]. Thus these patients' arterial pressure is elevated by being measured in a physician's office. The reasons for white-coat hypertension are not well understood but, interestingly, arterial pressure is elevated also when self-measured by the patient in the physician's presence [4]. The proportion of patients with white-coat hypertension varies between 20% and 30% of all patients with office-diagnosed hypertension [5–7]. White-coat hypertension is not a stable phenomenon and tends to decrease with repeated measurements over time [8,9]. Patients with white-coat hypertension must not be admitted to clinical trials. In efficacy trials their inclusion would contribute to the reduction of arterial pressure in the placebo group, thus minimising the difference in endpoint arterial pressure observed between the active and in the control group. In effectiveness or outcome studies the inclusion of 'white-coat hypertensives' would dilute the effects of the antihypertensive treatment as a considerable subsample of the patients only casually experience elevated pressure. Therefore increased sample sizes are necessary to achieve statistically significant results. In addition, the slope of the arterial pressure/risk relationship will be underestimated.

Another important patient-related factor is the patient's activity. It is well established now that arterial pressure does not follow an endogenous circadian rhythm, but rather the physical and emotional activities of a particular person during day and night-time [10]. Food and drinks like coffee or alcohol as well as drugs are not to be forgotten.

There are numerous reports about environmental factors such as temperature, noise, distraction and time of day which can influence arterial pressure in both directions. The literature of investigator and device-related factors again is almost endless [11]. Cuff size, microphone placement, method of inflation, speed of deflation and body posture have been standardised more than once to keep pace with scientific progress, as have been the vessel sounds which count [12]. Random-zero sphygmomanometers have been developed to reduce expectation bias. It still makes a difference, however, whether arterial pressure is measured by a physician, a nurse or the patient himself and whether it is always the same person who does it.

Variability of arterial pressure

Because arterial pressure is a function of mental arousal, emotional and physical activity amongst others, it may not be constant but may be highly variable, reflecting exogenous stimulants. These interactions are shown clearly when arterial pressure data are linked to patient activity data at each measurement point [13] (Figure 1). In this particular patient daytime systolic pressure varied between less than 100 mmHg and about 160 mmHg. Harshfield *et al.* [14] have linked the arterial pressure of normotensive and 644 hypertensive patients with different daily activities to demonstrate the interactions (Table 1). The so-called night-time drop of arterial pressure is related mainly to bed rest, i.e. physical inactivity [10]. It is seen in healthy persons and in patients with essential hypertension, too [15] (Figure 2).

Casual office- or clinic-based arterial pressure measurement

Casual arterial pressure measurement, i.e. the physician measures the patient's arterial pressure in his office or clinic, is the standard method even today. There are many reasons for this: normal and pathological values are defined and almost all we know about the prognostic impact of elevated arterial pressure relies on studies which used casual measurements, e.g. Framingham [16]. The measurement itself and the situation in which it takes place can be standardised, e.g. device, cuff size, vessel sounds, body position, time of day, and thus equality of observation is achievable to a fair degree.

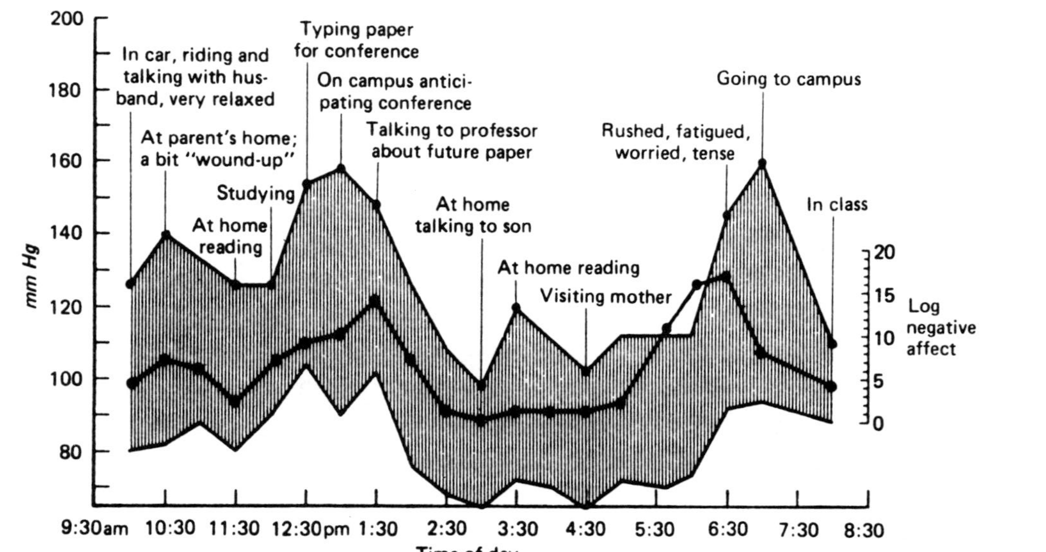

Figure 1. Serial blood pressure obtained with ambulatory blood pressure recordings correlated with patient's activities and emotions. The negative affect scale was derived from the patient's serial entries on an adjective checklist coincident with each blood pressure recording. The peak blood pressure readings, both systolic and diastolic, occurred when the patient was on the university campus, where she returned after a lapse of many years in order to get her PhD. Each time that she was on the campus, the negative affect was greater. She admitted that she really did not want to get her PhD. Reproduced from Sokolow [13]

Table 1. Arterial pressure during activities with either physical or psychological demands [14]

Activity	Normal	Mild	Established
Physical			
Walking	121/78	145/92	164/105
Shopping	119/78	142/93	150/108
Eating	119/78	139/94	166/110
Drinking	122/82	140/92	162/108
Housework	113/78	145/90	162/111
Psychological			
Telephone	118/78	139/94	162/106
Talking	115/78	139/93	158/101
Working (work)	112/78	139/93	159/103
Working (home)	112/76	136/91	155/106
Reading	107/71	131/87	155/104
Television	110/73	130/84	147/98
Relaxation	113/73	130/84	146/96

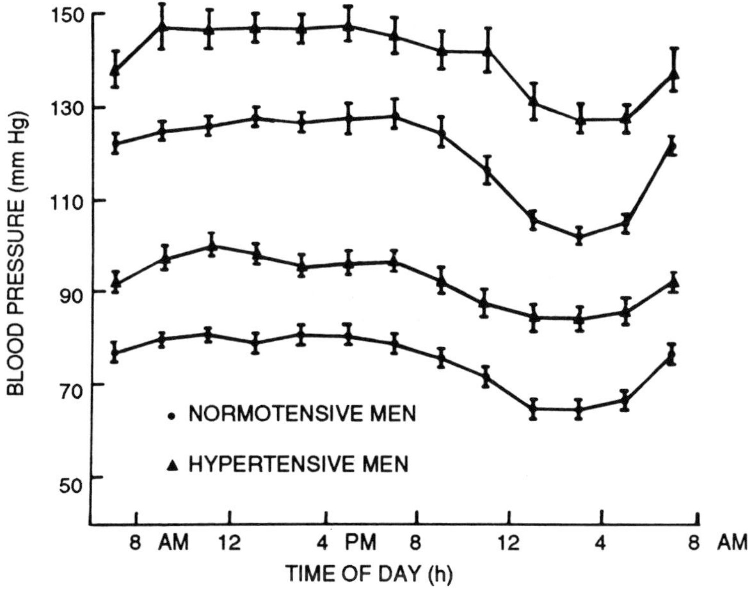

Figure 2. Average systolic and diastolic pressure values of 29 age-matched normotensive–hypertensive pairs of men during whole-day ambulatory blood pressure monitoring. Points shown are the means ($\pm$SD) of the readings obtained during each of 12 2-h periods comprising the day. Reproduced from Weber and Drayer [15]

Casual arterial pressure data can be analysed easily and aggregated to produce summary statistics without problems. The measurement itself is repeatable for many days as it does not impair patients' comfort. Finally, the measurement is simple and inexpensive and thus even large samples can be examined.

The major disadvantage of casual arterial pressure readings is the inherent risk of false positive diagnoses due to the 'white-coat' phenomenon. Thus, the diagnosis of hypertension by means of single casual office-based measurements equals almost a lottery. Armitage and Rose [17] reported as early as in 1966 that if men had been classified as hypertensive on a basis of a single examination, there would have been over one-third of 'false positive' assessments, and 5% of 'false negative'. The only way to minimise this problem is to measure blood pressure repeatably over a period of three to four months [11,18]. For the evaluation of patients' eligibility for a clinical trial this is a rather tedious procedure. Another important disadvantage of casual measurements in the clinical trial setting is its well-described responsiveness to placebo. When arterial pressure drops with placebo treatment, the observed difference compared with the active treatment group decreases and the variance increases. Sample size has to be increased to compensate for this power loss.

In clinical trials, standardisation and equality of observation are a must. In addition, regular and frequent retraining is necessary for the reduction of inter-observer variability [19]. Nevertheless, the need for training of the physicians or the study nurse is often neglected. Reading inaccuracy is a quite common phenomenon: 0 and 5 are the preferred digits. Random-zero sphygmomanometers reduce expectation bias and digit preference for the price of adding computational and machine inaccuracy [20]. It is not only the physician who needs attention, but the measurement device itself has to be cared for and calibrated. Surveys have shown that about half of hospital sphygmomanometers checked were defective [21].

Although casual measurements can be taken repeatedly on different days, it is not possible routinely to do it repeatedly during a single day. Measurements at night-time are limited to inpatients and, even then, are difficult to do.

However, considering these disadvantages, much can be overcome by planning and executing measurements carefully. This reduces the widely assumed advantage that the measurement is simple and inexpensive.

Home or self-measurement of blood pressure

As early as 1940, Ayman and Goldshine [22] reported considerable differences between clinic and home readings in patients with essential hypertension, home readings being considerably lower. The patient measures his arterial pressure himself either with a manual, semi-automatic or fully automatic device. Fully automatic devices are preferred as no effort is required to inflate the cuff—an activity which has been shown to increase arterial pressure [23].

Self-measurement avoids white-coat hypertension to a large degree and thus supports correct diagnosis. Probably as a result of the higher rate of correct diagnoses of hypertension and thus less dilution bias, home-measured arterial pressure correlates better with organ damage than casual readings [24]. There is also less placebo effect [25]—a phenomenon which is not well understood. Also, this procedure allows for multiple measurements during a single day or a longer interval. Thus within-patient variance is decreased, leading to a higher power and reducing the required sample size. Usually the positive effects of self-measurement on patients' compliance are overlooked, although partial compliance is considered to be high in hypertensive patients [26] and can endanger the validity of the trial. Compliance is better in patients who self-monitor their arterial pressure [27].

However, home measurement is difficult to standardise. One has to detail the procedure in the study protocol and to train the patients in the skills necessary to measure and record. It will be impossible to achieve standardisation across a large number of patients with respect to the time of measurement, time of drug administration, body position, food and drinks, physical activity, etc. Between-patient variance will tend to increase. If the data have to be analysed according to the intention-to-treat strategy, missing data are particularly embarrassing. Unreliable patients and missing measurements will always occur. Statistical analysis will become more complicated then.

Home measurement of arterial pressure might not be feasible in placebo-controlled trials as the lack of any relevant pressure reduction will certainly raise the suspicion of the placebo-treated patients. Impaired trust towards the physician and partial compliance are the likely results, neither being a good omen for a successful trial.

Twenty-four-hour ambulatory blood pressure monitoring

The usefulness of invasive monitoring, which is possible over extended periods, is limited for obvious reasons. Thus, we will concentrate on the non-invasive 24 h ambulatory arterial pressure monitoring (ABPM). This uses a portable device with an inflatable cuff, a compressor, an oscillometric or sphygmomanometric gauge and an electronic recorder. The accuracy of the oscillometric technique is regarded to be equivalent to the sphygmomanometric technique, systolic readings being more valid than diastolic readings [6]. At pre-set intervals, e.g. every 15 min in the daytime and every 30–60 min at night-time, the cuff is inflated, and the measurement is taken once and recorded. Typically, 60–80 recordings are made over a 24 h period.

Such arterial pressure data are considerably more representative for the true arterial pressure of a patient. As there is no white-coat hypertension seen with ABPM, correct diagnosis is supported. ABPM is the best procedure available for the proper identification of the target population with regard to hypertension, i.e. checking the eligibility criteria of an anti-hypertension trial. It helps to differentiate essential from secondary hypertension, as the typical night drop tends to disappear in these patients [28]. The use of ABPM in clinical trials is particularly interesting as there seems to be no relevant arterial pressure response to placebo [8,29]. The response to placebo was analysed in 46 hypertensive patients measured with casual clinic measurement and ABPM [29] (Table 2). Clinic-based systolic pressure fell 12.8 mmHg and diastolic pressure 5.6 mmHg on average. With ABPM a relevant response was not to be seen with a decrease in systolic and diastolic pressure of 3.7 mmHg and 1.2 mmHg respectively. The lack of a placebo response means that efficacy can be demonstrated with a smaller sample size. This is especially important in the early phase of drug development and efficacy evaluation.

There is convincing evidence that ABPM data have a higher reproducibility than casual clinic readings. Knowing the variability of arterial pressure, this is what one expects but it has also been demonstrated empirically [8]. One hundred mild to moderate hypertensive patients had their arterial pressure measured twice in a one-month interval with clinic measurement and ABPM. The inter-month correlation of the first with the second month reading for clinic measurement was $r = 0.59$ and for ABPM $r = 0.83$ for diastolic pressure. Averaging the differences of the second month reading minus the first month reading, the standard deviation of the differences was 12.6 mmHg for clinic measurement—twice as high as

Table 2. Arterial pressure before and after placebo (mean $\pm$ SEM) in 46 hypertensive patients [29]

	Baseline	Placebo
Systolic		
Clinic	174.6 $\pm$ 8.1	161.8 $\pm$ 7.6*
Ambulatory	158.3 $\pm$ 6.8	154.6 $\pm$ 7.1
Diastolic		
Clinic	109.8 $\pm$ 3.9	104.2 $\pm$ 4.1
Ambulatory	103.0 $\pm$ 3.6	101.8 $\pm$ 4.1

*$p < 0.001$.

for ABPM, with 6.5 mmHg. The increased reproducibility which accompanies a reduced variance makes statistical tests more powerful. Thus for a given clinically relevant difference smaller sample sizes will suffice.

By its very nature, ABPM is very useful for the assessment of a drug's duration of action. However, it might be necessary to extend the measurement period over the usual 24 h. Precise knowledge of a drug's duration of action is essential for planning the recommended dosage intervals.

Some of ABPM's disadvantages are the same as with home measurement. The situation in which the measurements take place is difficult to standardise, e.g. time since drug administration, starting time point, body position, physical and mental activity may vary. The time of drug administration is highly important for the analysis of the arterial pressure curve and should be recorded as exactly as possible. An electronic medication event monitoring system is very useful for this purpose [30].

The ABPM device usually measures at each time point only once. Armitage and Rose [31] reported that when there are duplicated readings (the interval being shorter than 2 min) the second systolic reading is, on average, 3 mmHg less than the first one. The diastolic second reading is slightly higher, at 0.4 mmHg. That is why some investigators prefer clinic measurements, averaging first, second and occasionally third reading. However, it is doubtful if this is really important in clinical trials as it seems to be a small difference. A more serious disadvantage of measurement performed only once is that data are missing if it fails. Measurement failures are quite common as almost all devices are sensitive to physical activity and position of the arm. Missing values do not present too serious a problem for the inferential analysis, however, even if up to 40% of the readings are missing at random [32]. If there is a systematic bias, fewer missing values can be tolerated (Table 3).

ABPM data may correlate better with cardiovascular risk and target organ damage [24] but there is still a scarcity of epidemiological studies using ABPM. To date only one study has been reported presenting percentiles of arterial pressure over 24 h for 800 healthy persons of both sexes between 17 and 80 years [33]. Correlation and regression procedures using clinic measurements and ABPM data resulted in an upper limit of normal average daytime systolic/diastolic pressure of 135/85 mmHg for ABPM, compared with 140/90 mmHg for clinic measurement [34,35]. This limit is accepted at present but might be changed in the future when epidemiological studies will have yielded more data.

To use an ABPM device properly, careful instruction and training for the physician and patient are needed. The physician has to know how to test, initialise and apply the device; the patient must feel comfortable with it (as far as possible), should stop any physical activity and not move the arm when the cuff is inflating. There is still some inconvenience attached to the ABPM and subsequent drop-outs range from 10% in untreated healthy

Table 3. Changes in overall systolic pressure (mmHg) as measured by 24 h mean, 24 h median and the standardised area under the 24 h profile: mean $\pm$ SD (min., max.) [32]. Reprinted by permission of John Wiley & Sons Ltd

Values missing	24 h mean	24 h median	Standardised area under 24 h profile
10% smallest	2.1 ± 0.6 (0.8, 4.4)	1.3 ± 0.9 (0.0, 4.0)	2.1 ± 1.3 (0.2, 7.9)
10% largest	-2.5 ± 0.7 (−4.4, −1.3)	-1.6 ± 1.2 (−5.0, 0.0)	-1.7 ± 1.0 (−7.7, −0.4)
10% random	0.02 ± 0.6 (−2.3, 2.0)	0.03 ± 0.8 (−2.0, 2.0)	0.09 ± 0.7 (1.2, 4.0)
25% smallest	4.6 ± 1.5 (1.9, 9.2)	3.3 ± 1.6 (0.5, 8.0)	4.9 ± 2.3 (0.9, 11.6)
25% largest	-5.1 ± 1.5 (−9.6, −2.0)	-3.7 ± 2.2 (−9.5, −1.0)	-3.8 ± 1.6 (−11.6, −1.5)
25% random	0.08 ± 0.8 (−1.9, 1.6)	0.05 ± 1.2 (−4.0, 3.0)	0.09 ± 1.2 (2.4, 4.0)
40% smallest	7.2 ± 2.1 (3.2, 13.9)	5.6 ± 2.1 (1.5, 12.0)	7.7 ± 3.3 (2.7, 20.1)
40% largest	-7.5 ± 2.1 (−13.0, −3.5)	-6.0 ± 2.7 (−12.5, −2.0)	-5.7 ± 1.9 (−14.1, −2.5)
40% random	-0.2 ± 1.3 (−3.4, 3.0)	-0.08 ± 1.8 (−7.0, 3.5)	0.05 ± 1.6 (−3.6, 4.2)

volunteers [36] to 33% in treated hypertensive patients [37]. Often patients will not tolerate more than two to three ABPM days. Thus, ABPM cannot easily be repeated several times.

The newer ABPM devices may induce only modest sleep disturbances [38]. However, drop-outs and losses resulting from technical failure of the devices can impair the validity of the trial.

The device itself is very safe; phlebitis or allergic reactions at the site of the cuff have been reported only rarely [24]. The incidence is probably lower than 1:5000. In predisposed patients petechiae can occur. The device is expensive and needs care and calibration.

ABPM AND CLINICAL TRIALS

We are still far from having the ideal device, but the distinct features of ABPM make it almost a necessity in antihypertensive clinical trials. These are as follows.

Reliable identification of the target population

Antihypertensive therapeutic effects can be demonstrated only in hypertensive patients. Thus their correct identification is of utmost importance. Only ABPM allows for the correct diagnosis 'hypertension' as there is no white-coat hypertension. ABPM does so within one measurement day. With home measurement about three days are needed [11] while, with casual clinic measurement, up to three or four months are needed to achieve a similar correct diagnosis. Thus the use of ABPM will shorten considerably the time necessary to identify suitable patients.

There is an ethical reason for the use of ABPM to ensure a correct diagnosis. Patients who are not really hypertensive cannot benefit from antihypertensive treatment but they may be exposed to possible adverse drug reactions, which are not balanced by therapeutic benefit.

Reduction of sample size

ABPM does not respond to placebo and is highly reproducible. Thus the sample size required to show efficacy of an antihypertensive treatment can be reduced markedly. Two studies have shown independently almost identical effects of repeated measurements on the standard deviation of the difference on sample size [8,32] (Table 4). Probably these computations are over-optimistic as one has to allow for losses resulting from drop-outs and technical failures. Nevertheless, a reduction of the required sample size of about 50% seems realistic.

Table 4. Reduction in required sample size with increased measurement frequency for test of antihypertensive effect. The table shows the dependency of standard deviation of the difference (SDD) and the relative sample size for a test of anti-hypertensive effect on the number of measurements made (diastolic pressure before and during the therapy in 15 patients). Measurements were evenly spaced in the time intervals shown and the daytime average was calculated using between 28 and 52 measurements per patient [32]

Number of measurements (time of day)	SDD (mmHg)	Relative sample size (%)
1 (0800–1000)	13.5	100
2 (0800–1000) and (1300–1500)	12.3	83
4 (0800–1200) and (1300–1700)	9.6	51
8 (0800–1200) and (1300–2000)	7.7	33
14 (0800–2200)	6.5	23
daytime average (0800–2200)	6.4	22

Assessment of non-drug therapies

The effect of non-drug therapies on lowering arterial pressure lies in the range of 3–6 mmHg [39]. Such differences have been assumed by many as clinically not relevant. Recent attempts to adjust the data of the Framingham study with regard to regression dilution bias because of casual clinic measurements at baseline indicate strongly that the regression for diastolic pressure and relative risk of stroke is much steeper than had been assumed until then [40]. Thus, a decrease of 5 mmHg in diastolic pressure, for example, can equal a 75% reduction of the relative risk of stroke (Figure 3) [8,40].

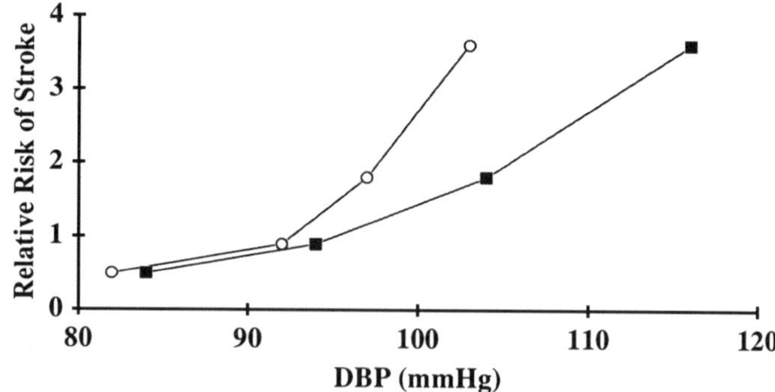

Figure 3. The effect of regression dilution upon the relationship of diastolic blood pressure (DBP) to risk of stroke. ■, Initial clinic DBP; ○, hypothetical line using ambulatory DBP values expected for subjects with initial clinic DBP values as described by the five quintiles in the Framingham study. Data are from the Framingham study. After Coats *et al.* [8]

Recognition of a 3–5 mmHg difference is easier with ABPM [41]—a technique which provides highly reproducible data.

Assessment of dose–response relationship and duration of drug action

The proper assessment of the dose–response curve is easier with ABPM. There is less variability, thus smaller sample sizes and a shorter period of time may suffice. ABPM is a truly elegant way to assess a drug's duration of action and this is not only important for drugs given once daily.

Assessment of night-time blood pressure

Night-time arterial pressure is receiving increasing scientific attention:

- There are reports that night-time arterial pressure correlates more closely with target organ damage than daytime pressure [24]. If these observations can be confirmed in prospective studies, arterial pressure control during night-time will become an important therapeutic objective.
- There are concerns among clinicians that night-time arterial pressure could fall too much with antihypertensive treatment so that regional blood flow, especially in patients with arteriosclerosis, is insufficient. Thus, ABPM at night-time also serves a safety purpose.
- A third indication for measuring night-time pressure is the evaluation of drugs given once daily. Drugs with a once-a-day regimen have to demonstrate that there is adequate arterial pressure control during night-time and especially in the early morning hours before the effect of the next dose is seen.

ABPM is certainly the only reasonable method available to measure arterial pressure during night-time.

ISSUES FOR ABPM IN ANTIHYPERTENSIVE TRIALS

Experience with ABPM in clinical trials is limited. Thus, specific recommendations with regard to the different phases of clinical drug development are difficult. The use of ABPM depends on the aims of a particular study. Some criteria to consider are given in Table 5. We think ABPM is most useful in phase II and phase III studies, both for identification of the target patients and for follow-up and outcome assessment. In phase IV studies ABPM is especially indicated for baseline assessment.

When the decision to use ABPM has been made, some recommendations can be given:

Table 5. Criteria for the use of ABPM in clinical trials phases I–IV

	Objectives	ABPM: useful for	Limited value
Phase I	Assessment of pharmacokinetics and tolerance in healthy volunteers and highly selected patients; dose titration; pharmacokinetic/pharmacodynamic modelling	BP readings at Night-time (safety and efficacy) and for assessment of drug's action duration	Inpatients; often triple measurements; no missing values wanted
Phase II	Assessment of efficacy in selected patients; dose finding; duration of action	Identification of target population; efficacy and safety assessment in small samples; dose and dosage interval finding studies	Within-patient dose titration studies due to inconvenience for patients (tolerated $\leqslant$ 3 times)
Phase III	Assessment of efficacy and safety, placebo-controlled; comparison with therapeutic alternatives	Identification of target population; efficacy and safety—evaluation; assessment of once-a-day drugs; placebo-controlled studies	Expensive with regard to costs and logistics
Phase IV	Assessment of effectiveness and safety, rarely placebo-controlled; comparison with therapeutic alternatives	Identification of target population; assessment of prognostic relevance of 24 h ABPM for clinical endpoints	Expensive with regard to costs and logistics

- Use the same type of ABPM device for the whole trial. Different monitors have different flaws and even the software can change over time in one type of ABPM device [42–44]. Only devices which fulfil the requirements of the Association for the Advancement of Medical Instrumentation should be applied [45].
- Continue to measure arterial pressure in the clinic/office with great care [46]. Clinical measurement will remain the reference.
- Select the investigators and patients carefully and educate them appropriately. To allow for a detailed analysis of the ABPM data, standardise body position, extent of physical activity and time of drug administration. Ask the patient to keep a diary to record these variables and bedtimes. Recording of drug intake should preferentially be done with an electronic medication monitoring system.
- Specify in detail the efficacy variables in the trial protocol. Only then can the results of the analyses be trusted as the multitude of data collected with ABPM and the lack of accepted efficacy variables allow for extensive and successful 'fishing' expeditions for significant p-values.
- Plan the statistical analysis in detail before beginning the trial. Some statistical methods ask for a 26–28 h measurement cycle. Appropriate statistical analysis procedures for antihypertensive clinical trials have been published [32].

Conclusion

The notorious variability of a casual arterial pressure measurement has led to various strategies to capture the 'true' arterial pressure of an individual. Examples are the so-called 'basal' pressure taken immediately after sleep under sedation in a dark, quiet room [47] or the relaxation pressure taken in the supine position after a defined standing period [48]. ABPM is another attempt in the quest for the 'true' arterial pressure. With this wealth of information the question remains which summary value should be used. The golden standard, of course, is the predictive power for hypertensive risks of the value under consideration. These data are still lacking for the ABPM.

The 24 h ABPM provides an improved estimation of the arterial pressure during day and night. White-coat hypertension and pressure response to placebo are effectively reduced. It enables a quick and reliable identification of suitable patients for antihypertensive trials. Smaller samples suffice for proof of efficacy. In the future it might even be possible to omit the placebo group for the evaluation of antihypertensive efficacy as 24 h ABPM data are highly reproducible over time. The US Food and Drug Administration (FDA) has launched a retrospective project to determine if this is feasible [49].

There are also ethical reasons to use ABPM in clinical trials: diagnostic certainty, reduced sample size, less placebo treatment. ABPM yields essential information on the efficacy of antihypertensive drugs which is greater than the information provided by the common office-based measurements. Regulatory authorities have not issued guidelines requesting ABPM data but the inclusion of ABPM data of a subsample of the patients in the registration dossier is likely to be advantageous.

References

1. Härtel U, Keil U, Cairns V. Medical care utilization and self-reported health of hypertensives: results of the Munich Blood Pressure Study. In: Kaplan RM, Criqui MH (eds), Behavioral Epidemiology and Disease Prevention. New York: Plenum, 1985; 201–215.
2. Veterans Administration Cooperative Study Group on Antihypertensive Agents. Effects of treatment on morbidity in hypertension. JAMA 1967; 202: 116–122.
3. World Health Organization/International Society of Hypertension Meeting. 1993 guidelines for the management of mild hypertension. J Hypertens 1993; 22: 392–403.
4. Mengden T, Bättig B, Edmonds D et al. Self-measured blood pressures at home and during consulting hours: are there any differences? J Hypertens 1990; 8 (Suppl 3): S15–S19.
5. Mancia G, Parati G, Pomidossi G, Grassi G, Casadei R, Zanchetti S. Alerting reaction and rise in blood pressure during measurement by physician and nurse. Hypertension 1987; 9: 209–215.
6. Pickering TG, Seymour GB. Blood pressure measurement and ambulatory blood pressure monitoring. In: Laragh JH, Brenner BM (eds), Hypertension: Pathophysiology, Diagnosis and Management. New York: Raven Press, 1990; 1429–1441.
7. Weber MA. White coat hypertension: a new definition. Cardiovasc Drugs Ther 1993; 7 (Suppl 2): 135.
8. Coats AJS, Radaelli A, Clark SJ, Conway J, Sleight P. The influence of ambulatory blood pressure monitoring on the design and interpretation of trials in hypertension. J Hypertens 1992; 10: 385–391.
9. Padfield PL, Lindsay BA, McLaren JA, Pirie A, Rademaker M. Changing relation between home and clinic blood pressure measurements: do home measurements predict clinic hypertension? Lancet 1987; 2: 322–324.
10. Pickering TG. The ninth Sir George Pickering memorial lecture: ambulatory monitoring and the definition of hypertension. J Hypertens 1992; 10: 401–409.
11. Stewart MJ, Padfield PL. Blood pressure measurement: an epitaph for the mercury sphygmomanometer? Clin Sci 1992; 83: 1–12.
12. Joint National Committee on Detection, Evaluation, and Treatment of High Blood Pressure. Fifth report (JNC V). Arch Intern Med 1993; 153: 154–183.
13. Sokolow M. Preliminary studies relating portably recorded blood pressures to daily life events in patients with essential hypertension. Bibl Psychiatr 1970; 144: 164.
14. Harshfield GA, Pickering TG, James GD, Blank SG. Blood pressure variability, and reactivity in the natural environment. In: Meyer-Sabellek W, Anlauf M,

Gotzen R, Steinfeld L (eds), Blood Pressure Measurements. New York: Springer, 1989; 241–251.
15. Weber MA, Drayer JIM. Blood pressure in normal subjects. In: Meyer-Sabellek W, Anlauf M, Gotzen R, Steinfeld L (eds), Blood Pressure Measurements. New York: Springer, 1989; 261–269.
16. Dawber TR. The Framingham Study. Cambridge, MA: Harvard University Press, 1980.
17. Armitage P, Fox W, Rose GA, Tinker CM. The variability of measurements of casual blood pressure. II. Survey experience. Clin Sci 1966; 30: 337–344.
18. British Hypertension Society Working Party. Treating mild hypertension: agreement from the large trials. Br Med J 1989; 298: 694–698.
19. Bruce NG, Shaper AG, Walker M, Wannamethee G. Observer bias in blood pressure studies. J Hypertens 1988; 6: 375–380.
20. O'Brien E, Mee F, Atkins N, O'Malley K. Inaccuracy of the Hawkslay random zero sphygmomanometer. Lancet 1990; 336: 1465–1468.
21. Burke MJ, Towers HM, O'Malley K, Fitzgerald DJ, O'Brien E. Sphygmomanometers in hospital and family practice: problems and recommendations. Br Med J 1982; 285: 469–471.
22. Ayman D, Goldshine AD. Blood pressure determinations by patients with essential hypertension. I. The difference between clinic and home readings before treatment. Am J Med Sci 1940; 200: 465–467.
23. Veerman DP, van Montfraus GA, Wieling W. Effects of cuff inflation on self-recorded blood pressure. Lancet 1990; 335: 451–453.
24. Canzanello VJ, Sheps SG. Emerging clinical roles for ambulatory blood pressure monitoring. Curr Opinion Cardiol 1993; 8: 765–774.
25. Cottier C, Julius S, Gajendragadkar SV, Schork MA. Usefulness of home BP determination in treating borderline hypertension. JAMA 1982; 248: 555–558.
26. Hasford J. Compliance and the benefit/risk relationship of antihypertensive treatment. J Cardiovasc Pharmacol 1992; 20: S30–S34.
27. Edmonds E, Förster E, Greminger P, Groth H, Siegenthaler W, Vetter W. Der Effekt der Blutdruckselbstmessung auf die Compliance des Hypertonikers. Schweiz Rundsch Med Prax 1985; 8: 173–176.
28. Hany S, Baumgart P, Frielingsdorf J, Vetter H, Vetter W. Circadian blood pressure variability in secondary and essential hypertension. J Hypertens 1987; 5 (Suppl 5): 487–489.
29. Waeber B, O'Brien E, Camenzind E, Cox J, Nussberger J, Brunner HR. Efficacy assessment of antihypertensive therapy. In: Brunner H, Waeber B (eds), Ambulatory Blood Pressure Recording. New York: Raven Press, 1992; 145–168.
30. Rudd P, Ahmed S, Zachary V, Barton C, Bonduelle D. Improved compliance measures: applications in an ambulatory hypertensive drug trial. Clin Pharmacol Ther 1990; 13: 471–481.
31. Armitage P, Rose GA. The variability of measurements of casual blood pressure. Clin Sci 1966; 30: 325–335.
32. Dickson D, Hasford J. 24-hour blood pressure measurement in antihypertensive drug trials: data requirements and methods of analysis. Statist Med 1992; 11: 2147–2158.
33. O'Brien E, Murphy J, Tyndall A et al. Twenty-four-hour ambulatory blood pressure in men and women aged 17–80 years: the Allied Irish Bank Study. J Hypertens 1991; 9: 355–360.
34. Consensus document on non-invasive ambulatory blood pressure monitoring. J Hypertens 1990; 8: 135–140.

35. Baumgart P, Walger P, Jürgens U, Rahn KH. Reference data for ambulatory blood pressure monitoring: what results are equivalent to the established limits of office blood pressure? Klin Wochenschr 1990; 68: 723–727.
36. O'Brien E, O'Malley, K. Overdiagnosing hypertension. Br J Med 1988; 297: 1211.
37. Schrader J, Schoel G, Buhr-Schinner H et al. Comparison of the antihypertensive efficacy of nitridipine, metropolol, mepindolol and enalapril using 24-hour blood pressure monitoring. Am J Cardiol 1990; 66: 967–972.
38. Degaute J-P, van de Borne P, Kerkhofs M, Dramaix M, Linkowski P. Does noninvasive ambulatory blood pressure monitoring disturb sleep? J Hypertens 1992; 10: 879–885.
39. National High Blood Pressure Education Program Working Group. National High Blood Pressure Education Program Working Group Report on primary prevention of hypertension. Arch Intern Med 1993; 153: 186–208.
40. MacMahon S, Peto R, Cutler J et al. Blood pressure, stroke, and coronary heart disease. Part I, prolonged differences in blood pressure: prospective observational studies corrected for the regression dilution bias. Lancet 1990; 335: 765–774.
41. Appel LJ, Marwaha S, Whelton PK, Patel M. The impact of automated blood pressure devices on the efficiency of clinical trials. Controlled Clin Trials 1992; 13: 240–247.
42. White WB, Lund-Johansen P, Omvik P. Assessment of four ambulatory blood pressure monitors and measurements by clinicians versus intraarterial blood pressure at rest and during exercise. Am J Cardiol 1990; 65: 60–66.
43. Berardi L, Chau NP, Chanudet X, Vilar J, Larroque P. Ambulatory blood pressure monitoring: a critical review of the current methods to handle outliers. J Hypertens 1992; 10: 1243–1248.
44. Hansen KW, Ørskov H. A plea for consistent reliability in ambulatory blood pressure monitors: a reminder. J Hypertens 1992; 10: 1313–1315.
45. Association for the Advancement of Medical Instrumentation. American National Standard: electronic or automated sphygmomanometers. Washington: AAMI, 1993.
46. Dischinger P, DuChene AG. Quality control aspects of blood pressure measurements in the multiple risk factor intervention trial. Controlled Clin Trials 1986; 7: 137S–157S.
47. Smirk FH. Casual and basal blood pressure. Br Heart J 1944; 6: 176–182.
48. Meesmann W, Stöveken HJ, Billing CP. Die Bestimmung des Basisblutdrucks in der Praxis durch die Ermittlung des sogenannten Entspannungswertes. Dtsch Med Wochenschr 1970; 95: 1–19.
49. Anonymous. FDA–industry project may streamline cardiovascular clinical trials. Appl Clin Trials 2 1993; 9: 8.

4 POTENTIAL MEASUREMENTS IN PATIENTS WITH OSTEOPOROSIS

Colin G. Miller
Bona Fide Ltd, Madison, Wisconsin, USA

Introduction

Osteoporosis is a systemic skeletal disease characterised by low bone mass and microarchitectural deterioration of bone tissue, with consequent increase in bone fragility and susceptibility to fracture [1]. Around 25% of all women by the age of 60 have signs of the disease [2] which are primarily fractures of the vertebrae, distal radius and femoral neck. However, many more women have osteoporosis, as defined by the recent consensus conference on the disease state [1], than have the symptoms. Therefore measurement of this disease state in patients is becoming of increasing importance as this so-called 'silent epidemic' affects more than 200 million individuals in the USA [3] and costs are escalating beyond \$7 billion [4].

Peak bone mass occurs in the fourth decade of life, and then starts declining slowly at a rate of 0.5–0.8% per year [5,6]. In women following the menopause or surgical castration, bone loss may increase to levels of 3% a year [7,8] because of decreased concentrations of circulating oestrogens, for the following 10 years, before returning to a rate of 0.8% per year. Current therapeutic intervention for osteoporosis provides only a cessation in bone loss, and not a true anabolic effect on bone.

Potential measurements

BIOCHEMICAL MEASUREMENTS

The biochemical markers of bone can be subdivided into those that provide information on bone resorption and those that give an indication on bone deposition.

Clinical Measurement in Drug Evaluation. Edited by W. S. Nimmo and G. T. Tucker
© 1995 John Wiley & Sons Ltd

The marker that has been used routinely for a measurement of bone resorption is hydroxyproline. This provides an assessment of by-products from general collagen breakdown. These by-products are formed not only when bone resorption is occurring but also when collagen from other organ systems, e.g. skin, are undergoing biochemical destruction. Therefore a more specific marker has been identified to measure urinary dehydroxypyrodinoline (collagen cross-links). The latter are specific by-products of bone breakdown, and are still under evaluation [9,10,11].

All indications of bone deposition can be obtained by measuring the serum concentrations of alkaline phosphatase, and more recently procollagen peptide (PICP) has been identified to measure turnover or formation.

While biochemical markers provide an immediate 'snapshot' of the relative amount of bone absorption and deposition, they do not provide any indication as to the current quantity of bone or bone mineral content. The values may change because of a host of external influences and therefore a measurement on one day will not be indicative of the serum concentrations of any variable in a few weeks time. They do provide a strong acute indication of the effects of any treatment, unlike bone densitometry which requires 12 months generally. For initial dose-finding purposes, biochemical markers have the potential to provide the relevant information rapidly, but for assessing clinically relevant endpoints bone mineral density measurements remain essential. A more comprehensive critique is provided by Blumsohn and Eastell [9]. The rest of this chapter will therefore concentrate on these other methodologies, for which a comprehensive understanding is required if their use is to be appropriate in the trial setting.

Other clinical laboratory data that may be required are serum calcium and parathyroid hormone (PTH) concentrations to rule out other pathologies such as hypoparathyroidism, vitamin D deficiency and osteomalacia.

PLANAR RADIOGRAPHS

Planar radiographs are the longest-established technique for assessing bone quality and quantity. Reproducibility is the major problem from two sources: firstly the ability of the radiographers to repeat the exact requirements and settings for each film; and secondly the operator evaluation of the radiographs. The three main methodologies for planar radiographic assessments are as follows:

- *Quantification of the trabecular pattern*, principally in the femoral neck region. The most successful of these was the Singh index [12], which was based on a six-point rating scale. The discriminant capabilities of the test are poor and rely on operator interpretation. A similar test was previously developed for the vertebrae [13].

- *Optical densitometry* with planar radiographs by comparison with an aluminium step wedge which is included on the picture [14]. This has recently developed renewed interest using the metacarpals as the anatomical site of interest and computer interpretation of the optical density of the images [15]. This is arguably the least operator dependent of the three techniques.
- *Metacarpal morphometry* involving careful measurement of the cortical bone thickness and medullary cavity has been well evaluated [14,16,17] and is still in vogue with some investigators [18]. This methodology requires measurements of the metacarpals on the radiograph image using callipers.

Currently none of these three techniques has wide acceptance, and although they are potential methods of assessing osteoporosis will not be considered further here.

SINGLE-PHOTON ABSORPTIOMETRY

In 1963, Cameron and Sorenson [19] developed the first direct method for quantifying bone mineral density (BMD) using a technique known as single-photon absorptiometry (SPA). The technique is based on measuring the attenuation of γ-radiation from a monoenergetic radionuclide source (usually iodine-125). Low-energy radiation is required to produce the maximum contrast between the bone and soft tissue. A collimated detector system is scanned in a rectilinear fashion synchronously with the γ-radiation point source across the bone sample being measured. A diagrammatic representation of the technique is given in Figure 1. The variability of the soft tissue thickness is a major problem, which is overcome partly by the

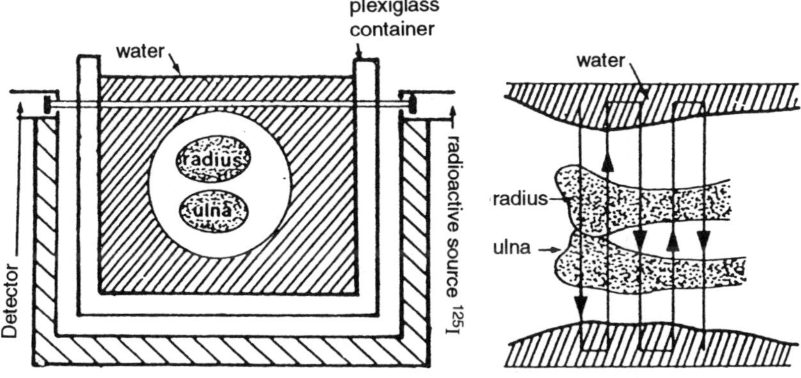

Figure 1. Diagrammatic representation of single-photon absorptiometry

area of the body under assessment being surrounded in a soft tissue
equivalent, such as water. Thus only the distal forearm and infrequently
the calcaneus are measured by SPA.

From the beam attenuation the bone mass can be computed. A series of
point measurements are usually made, the results being summed to
provide the mass per unit length of bone. The figures quoted are usually
bone mineral content (BMC) in grams or BMD in grams per square centi-
metre. The cost of equipment to perform photon absorptiometry was
around £15 000 to £20 000 with running costs in excess of £1000 per annum
for replacement of nuclide sources. Although SPA is still used, it is no
longer available commercially, having been superseded by SXA. Precision
(calculated as the coefficient of variation (CV)) is usually quoted as
between 1% and 3% [20,21].

DUAL-PHOTON ABSORPTIOMETRY

In principle, dual-photon absorptiometry (DPA) is a similar technique to
SPA, the difference being that the photon source has two distinct energies.
The advantage of DPA over its single-photon counterpart is that the thickness of soft tissue and thus the mass of bone mineral in the beam path can
be calculated. Therefore immersion of the measurement site in soft tissue
equivalents is not required, allowing sites of osteoporotic fracture, other
than the distal forearm, to be measured, e.g. the lumbar spine and femoral
neck region. A diagrammatic representation is shown in Figure 2.

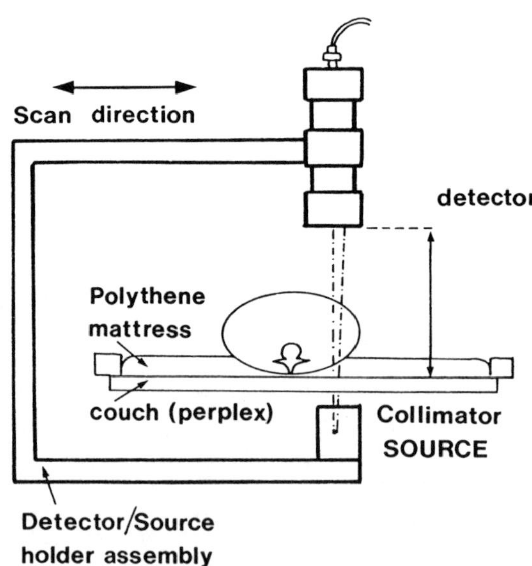

Figure 2. Diagrammatic representation of dual-photon absorptiometry

The calculation of bone mineral content by DPA assumes that there is only a two-component system being measured, i.e. bone and uniform soft tissue. However, this is not the case, particularly where the lumbar spine region is involved. Over the lumbar spine there are varying quantities of muscle, fat and moving volumes of faeces and flatus. These problems are overcome partly by a calculation procedure whereby measurements along the scan line juxtaposition to the bone mass of interest are used to establish a local bone mineral content of zero. Further systematic errors are introduced since the measurement algorithms include the mineral in the spinous processes, osteophytes and any aortic calcification.

The cost of DPA is not considered here since it is no longer available commercially, having been superseded by dual-energy X-ray absorptiometry. The reproducibility of the technique is between 1% and 3% for the vertebrae and 3% and 5% for the femoral neck region [21,22].

DUAL-ENERGY X-RAY ABSORPTIOMETRY

The advent of commercially available dual-energy X-ray absorptiometry (DXA) in 1987 provided a major advance in the assessment of osteoporosis. This measurement technique involves essentially the same algorithms as DPA, but rather than using a decaying ionising radiation source of γ-rays, an X-ray source is employed. The photon flux is higher, which permits scan times to be considerably quicker (of the order of 2–7 min rather than 10–20 min for DPA). Another advantage of DXA over DPA is that the photon source is not decaying and hence does not require regular replacement.

The image quality has improved greatly since the first DXA instruments were introduced, so that the latest generation of equipment will allow the direct visualisation of the vertebrae, enabling accurate determination of deformation. Until recently, a planar radiograph had to be obtained to evaluate fully in the scanning region vertebrae deformity, which would adversely influence the results. It should also be noted that DXA, like SPA and DPA, measures an areal and not a true volumetric density measurement as no assessment is made in the third plane. However, recently attempts have been made with scanners that allow measurement in the lateral projection [23,24].

DXA has become the standard non-invasive measurement of bone quantity in the clinical trial setting. The ease of use and wide acceptance of DXA have assured its use for all phases of clinical trial work. However, a full and complete understanding of the instrument's capabilities and limitations are a prerequisite if it is to be used correctly [25].

DXA, like DPA, involves a two-stage process to obtain the measurement of BMC and BMD. First the raw data from the patient has to be acquired. Care is required both for positioning of the patient on the instrument table and scanning the anatomical area of measurement. Software processing of the scan, or analysis, involving a semi-automated series of calculations by the instrument, requiring operator verification or manipulation can be undertaken either immediately or at a later time.

DXA instruments cost in the region of $60 000 for a basic model to around $160 000 for the latest version, depending on the features required. Running costs are minimal, except for operator time. It should be noted that the algorithms and internal calibration systems differ greatly between the four manufacturers, so that data are not directly transferable between systems. The precision of the measurement is accepted generally as being of the order of 1% for the spine and 3% for the proximal femur [24,26,27]. Precision assessments are undertaken usually on young healthy volunteers and precision will be poorer in those individuals who are elderly and/or suffering with osteoporosis.

SINGLE X-RAY ABSORPTIOMETRY

Single X-ray absorptiometry (SXA) is a recent development which has arisen from the requirement of operator-independent instruments that are sufficiently compact to be of potential use in the primary care physician's office. SXA combines technologies previously used in SPA and DXA. It was therefore only a small step to develop SXA, having had DXA technology around for some years. Although it requires a water bath it is highly automated and simple to use with a precision of around 1% [28].

QUANTITATIVE COMPUTED TOMOGRAPHY

Quantitative computed tomography (QCT) has been studied increasingly over the last 20 years as a method of measuring bone quality. QCT is unique as it has major advantages over the other techniques of allowing very precise three-dimensional anatomical localisation at any site and it can be used to study the trabecular bone of the vertebrae. The *in vivo* precision of QCT is between 0.3% and 5% [29,30].

The capital cost for the computed tomography equipment is around £500 000, with an annual running cost of several thousand pounds per annum [14]. Hence the use of QCT for purely routine detection of osteoporosis is prohibitive due to the cost, and its use is mainly confined to that of a research tool. Alternatively, for a QCT instrument that is being underused for other diagnoses, the extra vertebral software is of the order of £10 000.

Recently a peripheral QCT (pQCT) has been developed which allows the identification of trabecular and cortical bone in just the distal portion of the radius and ulna. It is, like SXA, a potential instrument for use in the primary care physician's office or in the district general hospital setting. It is still being fully evaluated but may prove a useful instrument for assessing osteoporosis in peripheral bone sites.

NEUTRON ACTIVATION ANALYSIS

Neutron activation analysis (NAA) is a method of measuring total body calcium, although it can be used on selected areas of the body, e.g. the appendicular skeleton or the spine. The body, or area under investigation, is bombarded with neutrons, converting a percentage of the naturally occurring calcium-48 in the body to calcium-49. The γ-emission from the calcium-49 decay is only 9 min, and therefore the number of γ-emissions provides information of the quantity of body calcium present.

The disadvantage with NAA is that while the calcium at the site of interest is measured, so is any extra-osseous calcium. The precision of this technique for total body measurement is quoted as being between 1.8% and 8% [14,31,32]. Because of these factors and the radiation dose to the subjects this measurement has never been more than a research technique, and so will not be considered further here.

COMPTON SCATTER TECHNIQUE

The Compton scatter technique is again purely a research tool. The electron density of a tissue sample is estimated by measuring the extent of Compton scattering from an incident beam of radiation. The source is either a monoenergetic radionuclide or filtered X-rays.

The disadvantage with Compton scatter systems is that they measure the density of all the tissues causing the scattering, not just bone. The *in vitro* precision is as high as 1% but for *in vivo* measurements the quoted reproducibility is 2–3% [22]. This technique will not be discussed further because of its rarity of use.

ULTRASOUND

Ultrasound is most commonly known for its applications in obstetrics and other soft tissue imaging. Recently the quantitative ultrasonic assessment of the calcaneum (heel bone) has become a commercially available technique for assessing bone. Two methodologies are used for the assessment of bone; these are the transmitted parameters of broadband ultrasonic attenuation (BUA) and velocity or speed of sound (the acronym SOS will be used here).

BUA, which was first described by Langton *et al.* [33], is the frequency-dependent attenuation measured between 200 and 600 kHz. It has recently been demonstrated to characterise not only the density of the bone but, importantly, the architecture of the trabeculae [34,35]. SOS has been demonstrated to be related to the elasticity of bone and therefore may provide more information than BMD alone of the risk of fracture [34]. One company has combined both BUA and SOS into one all-encompassing algorithm in an attempt to quantify more simply and yet provide diagnostic sensitivity to a complex measure [36]. The calcaneum, being the site of measurement, has high trabecular bone content (about 90%) and is weight bearing, similar to the upper femur. Studies using SPA and DPA suggest that the calcaneum may be the optimum appendicular site of measurement for predicting non-spine fractures [37].

Quantitative ultrasound equipment is the least expensive technique currently available to assess bone. It costs in the region of £14 000 to £25 000. It is also the first instrument that can be described as 'portable', weighing only approximately 20 kg. Although the ultrasonic assessment of bone is still regarded as a research tool, it is rapidly gaining scientific acumen and promises to be one of the first-line instruments for assessment of osteoporosis [35,36,38–41].

Comparison of instruments for clinical trial use

The requirements for efficacy and safety measurements in clinical trials are ultimately defined by the acceptance of the data by regulatory authorities. The currently accepted standard for the measurement of changes in bone quantity is DXA. At present the measurement of DPA, QCT and SPA are also accepted but only as supportive documentation. From a regulatory viewpoint, measures of bone mass are merely a surrogate endpoint for fractures of the spine or hip. Some regulatory authorities, particularly the US Food and Drug Administration (FDA), have questioned the use of DXA, without further supporting evidence that bone quality is not being compromised by some therapeutic interventions [42]. Currently, other European agencies accept bone mass data as surrogate efficacy endpoints alone, but this could change.

With respect to new clinical trials, DPA is now relegated to being an obsolete measurement, so no further discussion on DPA will be entertained here. Because of the costs of QCT and the limited number of sites where it is available, this instrument will not be considered in detail. SPA of the distal forearm has been available for nearly 30 years, but with the advent of software to undertake forearm scans with DXA the future for the use of SPA to obtain clinical trial data can be questioned. However, with the new SXA and pQCT instruments having good precision, the debate on the potential usefulness of a single forearm measurement will be reopened.

Measurements of BUA or SOS are relatively new assessments in this field. Most of the publications using these modalities are cross-sectional and compare results to the recognised standards of SPA, DPA, QCT or

Table 1. A comparison of the precision and discrimination of SPA, DXA and ultrasound measurements (BUA and SOS) with Lunar instruments

	SPA distal radius shaft	DXA spine	DXA hip	BUA calcaneus	VOS calcaneus
Units	g/cm^2	g/cm^2	g/cm^2	dB/MHz	m/s
Range of values (osteoporotic– normal)	0.57–0.71	0.9–1.2	0.7–1.0	90–125	1505–1560
Precision (% CV)	2%	<1%	~2%	1.5%	<0.3%
Discrimination as % SCV	10.1%	4.0%	5.9%	5.4%	8.5%

DXA without therapeutic intervention [39,40,41,43–45], or are studies designed to assess the applicability of ultrasound to predict risk of fracture [33]. These studies suggest that BUA and SOS may have a role in assessing skeletal status, but use in clinical trials is still being evaluated.

With respect to the comparison of precision and discrimination of SPA, DXA and ultrasound (Table 1), SXA and spine DXA measurements have a precision of less than 1% (for information purposes, so does pQCT). For BUA the current value of 1.0–3%, depending upon manufacturer, and has improved from 7% or 8% during the early development [36,46]. The precision of SOS by some ultrasound equipment is now superior to DXA of spine at 0.3% [47]. However, this is now at the operating limits of the equipment and is unlikely to improve much further.

With bone densitometry, there is no absolute measure or definition of bone mineral density, each manufacturer claiming optimum accuracy depending upon its own algorithms. Therefore precision (measured as the percentage coefficient of variation) alone may not provide a correct direct inter-instrument comparison because of scaling differences and thus the concept of standardised coefficient of variation (SCV) has been developed [48].

SCV is defined as:

$$SCV = \frac{SD^*}{Clinical\ range} \times 100 \qquad (1)$$

compared with

$$CV = \frac{SD^*}{Mean} \times 100 \qquad (2)$$

*S.D. of duplicate measurements of normals.

Table 2. A comparison of reliability, relevance, acceptance by regulatory agencies and expense of SPA, SXA, DXA and ultrasound equipment in the clinical trial setting. The question marks denote there is some debate around the statement

	SPA radius	SXA radius	DXA spine	DXA hip	BUA	VOS
Safe	Yes	Yes	Yes	Yes	Yes	Yes
Reliable	?Yes	?Yes	Yes	Yes	?Yes	?Yes
Relevant	?Yes	?Yes	?Yes	?Yes	?Yes	?Yes
Accepted by regulatory agencies	Yes	Yes	Yes	Yes	No	No

This has allowed direct comparisons of the precision of a parameter or instrument using the same population or group of volunteers, regardless of the scaling of the instrument.

As with the percentage coefficient of variation, the lower the value the more precise the instrument. Using SCV, with the same population, DXA of the spine is still the superior assessment compared with SOS.

Table 2 relates the other important characteristics for undertaking clinical trials to each of the instruments already mentioned. The reliability or robustness of an instrument is a mark of its stability in performance over time. This is assessed for DXA by the daily measurement of phantoms: for clinical trials, an instrument quality control (IQC) programme is recommended to allow early identification of problems [25,26]. DXA instruments have a proven track record of reliability and problems can be identified and correct. SXA, because of the similarities with DXA, is likely to prove reliable. The measurement of BUA has currently no recognised calibration standard, although, as with DXA, each manufacturer has developed his own independent phantom.

With respect to the clinical relevance of the measurements, there is now no consensus that any of the measurements alone, is an acceptable surrogate for structural integrity of bone, as previously discussed. However, DXA measurements are the currently accepted standard for the measurement of bone density, the measurement sites being the area of fracture, and the data have proven reliable.

This review has not considered the marketing implications of the development of inexpensive equipment to assess the prevalent risk of skeletal failure or the monitoring of therapeutic intervention. This does play a role in the planning by a pharmaceutical company in the attempt to expand the market size and the company's market share by identifying correctly more patients for treatment. This should then be factored into the phase III planning with the inclusion of the relevant instrumentation in the trials.

Discussion must include the safety and ethical implications of undertaking repetitive measurements of bone density in clinical trials. The increased radiation exposure from DXA, SXA, pQCT and SPA measurements is almost negligible compared to standard radiological techniques and the ethical problems are perceived as being greater than in reality. However, ultrasonic assessments are radiation free and therefore the risk to the patient is absent, making this modality ideal from the ethical standpoint. QCT measurements involve a higher level of radiation exposure than the other modalities and therefore careful assessment as to the quantity of repeated measurements is required, particularly if the patients are having additional planar radiographs.

In all measurements, the key for use in longitudinal clinical trials is to ensure consistency of methodology for each patient. With DXA measurements this means ensuring that for any one patient the same anatomical region is scanned in exactly the same position. The same region of interest is selected each time for each patient and analysed in the same manner. Changes in the values under investigation that are greater or less than those expected should be monitored and a reason for the unexpected deviation identified. Ideally operator training should be given as to the trial requirements and a full data quality control (DQC) programme implemented. This has been demonstrated to improve the precision by up to 50% [23,49].

Conclusion

There is a wide variety of potential measurements that can be undertaken in patients with osteoporosis. Fracture has to be the ultimate endpoint. However, in the clinical trial setting, biochemical assessments must be undertaken to ascertain the acute effects of bone physiology but spine and hip DXA are currently the accepted surrogate standards for the final evaluation of a new chemical entity. SPA of the forearm is of use but to a limited extent, although SXA and QCT may now gain new credence. QCT of the vertebral bodies and spine is used mainly in phase II type trials or perhaps subsets of phase III populations, but its use is limited due to prohibitive costs. The assessment of calcaneal BUA or SOS, while not accepted methodologies for use in clinical trials at present, is being evaluated.

Because of the complexity of the instruments and the operator dependency, more control on clinical trial data is required. Full IQC and DQC programmes need to be implemented by the trial sponsor, which is independent and external to the investigational site's own procedures.

Acknowledgements

The author is grateful to J. Kylstra, N. Pillay and R. Svensen for their helpful input and comments, and to Lorraine Walker for typing the manuscript.

References

1. Consensus Development Conference: Diagnosis, Prophylaxis, and Treatment of Osteoporosis. Am J Med 1993; 94: 646–650.
2. Chesnut CH. Appraisal of the role of oestrogens in the treatment of post-menopausal osteoporosis. J Am Geriatr 1984; 50, 32: 604–608.
3. Dempster DW, Lindsay R. Pathogenesis of osteoporosis. Lancet 1993; 341: 797–801.
4. Lindsay R. The growing problem of osteoporosis. Osteoporosis Int 1992; 2: 267–268.
5. Consensus conference on osteoporosis. JAMA 1984; 252: 799–802.
6. Weavers JK, Chalmers J. Cancellous bone: its strength and changes with ageing and an evaluation of some of the methods for measuring its mineral content. J Bone Joint Surg 1966; 48-A: 389–408.
7. Ruegsegger P, Damsacher MA et al. Bone loss in pre-menopausal and post-menopausal women. J Bone Joint Surg 1984; 66-A: 1015–1023.
8. Parfitt AM. Age related structural changes in trabecular and cortical bone: cellular mechanisms and biomechanical consequences. Calcif Tissue Int 1984; 36: S123.
9. Blumsohn A, Eastell R. Prediction of bone loss in postmenopausal women. Eur J Clin Invest 1992; 22: 764–766.
10. Fledelius C, Riis BJ, Overgaard K, Christiansen C. The diagnostic validity of urinary free pyrodinolines to identify women at risk of osteoporosis. Calcified Tissue Int 1994; 54: 381–384.
11. Blumsohm A, Hannen RA, Al-Dehaimi AW, Eastell R. Short term intra-individual variability of markers of bone turnover in healthy adults. J Bone Miner Res 1994; 9 (Suppl 1): S153.
12. Singh M, Nagrath AR, Maini PS. Changes in trabecular pattern of the upper end of the femur as an index of osteoporosis. J Bone Joint Surg 1970; 52-A: 457–467.
13. Smith RW, Rizek J. Epidemiological studies of osteoporosis in women of Puerto Rico and South Eastern Michigan with special reference to age, race, national origin and to other related or associated findings. Clin Orthop 1966; 45: 31–48.
14. Aitken J. Osteoporosis in Clinical Practice. Bristol, Wright.
15. Cosman F, Herrington B, Himmelstein S, Lindasy R. Radiographic absorptiometry: a simple method for determination of bone mass. Osteoporosis Int 1991; 2: 34–38.
16. Adams P, Davies GT, Sweetnam PM. Observer error and measurements of the metacarpal. Br J Radiol 1969; 42: 192–197.
17. Dequeker J. Precision of the radiogrammatic evaluation of bone mass at the metacarpal bones. In: Dequeker J, Johnston CC (eds), Non-invasive Bone Measurements: Methodological Problems. Oxford: IRL Press, 1982; 27–32.
18. Meema HE, Meindok H. Advantages of peripheral radiogrametry over dual-photon absorptiometry of the spine in the assessment of prevalence of osteoporotic vertebral fractures in women. J Bone Mineral Res 1992; 7 (8): 897–903.

19. Cameron JR, Sorensen J. Measurement of bone mineral in vivo: an improved method. Science 1963; 142: 230–232.
20. Mazess RB. Advances in single and dual photon absorptiometry. In: Christiansen C, Arnaud, CD, Nordin, BEC (eds), Osteoporosis. Glostrup Hospital, 1984; 57–63.
21. Murby B, Fogelman I. Bone mineral measurements in clinical practice. Br J Hosp Med 1987; May: 453–458.
22. Mazess RB. In: Barzel US (ed), Non-invasive Measurement of Bone. New York: Grune & Stratton, 1979; 5–26.
23. Blake GM, Jagathesan T, Herd RJM, Fogelman I. A longitudinal study of supine lateral dual x-ray absorptiometry in peri- and post-menopausal women. In Ring EFJ, Elvins DM and Bhalla AK (eds), Current research in osteoporosis and bone mineral measurement III; 1994: 55–56.
24. Matkovic V, Jelic T, Wardlaw GM et al. Timing of peak bone mass in Caucasian females and its implication for the prevention of osteoporosis. J Clin Invest 1994; 93: 779–808.
25. Miller CG. Bone density measurements in clinical trials: the challenge of ensuring optimal data. Br J Clin Res 1993; 4: 113–120.
26. Orwoll ES, Oviatt SK. Longitudinal precision of dual energy X-ray absorptiometry in a multicenter study. J Bone Mineral Res 1991; 6 (2): 191–197.
27. Ryan PJ, Blake GM, Herd R, Parker J, Fogelman I. Spine and femur BMD by DXA in patients with varying severity spinal osteoporosis. Calcif Tissue Int 1993; 52: 263–268.
28. Kelly TL, Crane G, Baran DT. Single x-ray absorptiometry of the forearm: precision, correlation and reference data. Calcified Tissue Int 1994; 54: 212–218.
29. Genant HK et al. Quantitative computed tomography for spinal assessment. In Christiansen C, Arnaud CD, Nordin BEC (eds), Osteoporosis. Glostrup Hospital, 1984; 65–72.
30. Genant HK. Assessing osteoporosis: CT's quantitative advantage. Diagn Imaging 1985; 8: 52–57.
31. Smith MA et al. The assessment of osteoporosis by total body neutron activation analysis. In: Menczel J et al (eds), Osteoporosis. Chichester: Wiley, 1982; 109–116.
32. Smith MA. Neutron activation analysis: choice of site, precision and accuracy. In: Dequeker J, Johnston CC (eds), Non-invasive Bone Measurement: Methodological Problems. Oxford: IRL Press, 1982; 77–84.
33. Langton CM, Palmer SB, Porter RW. The measurement of broadband ultrasound attenuation in cancellous bone. Eng Med 1984; 13: 89–91.
34. Langton CM, Evans GP, Hodgkinson R, Riggs CM. Ultrasonic, Elastic and Structural Properties of Cancellous Bone. In: Ring EFJ (ed). Current Research in Osteoporosis and Bone Mineral Measurement. London: British Institute of Radiology, 1990; 10–11.
35. Gluer CC, Wu CU, Genant HK. Broadband ultrasound attenuation signals depend on trabecular orientation. An in vitro study. Osteoporosis Int 1993; 3: 185–191.
36. Yamazaki K, Kushida K, Ohmura A et al. Ultrasound bone densitometry of the os calcis in Japanese women. Osteoporosis Int 1994; 4: 220–225.
37. Wasnich RD, Vogel JM, Ross P. Prediction of post-menopausal fracture risk with the use of bone mineral measurements. Am J Obstet Gynecol 1985; 153: 745–751.
38. Porter RW, Miller CG, Grainger D, Palmer SB. Prediction of hip fracture in elderly women: a prospective study. Br Med J 1990; 301: 638–641.

39. McCloskey EV, Murray SA, Miller C et al. Broadband ultrasound attenuation in the os calcis: relationship to bone mineral at other skeletal sites. Clin Sci 1990; 78: 227–233.
40. Baran DT, McCarthy CK, Leahey D, Lew R. Broadband ultrasound attenuation of the calcaneus predicts lumbar and femoral neck density in Caucasian women: a preliminary study. Osteoporosis Int 1991; 1: 110–113.
41. Stewart A, Reid DM, Porter RW. Broadband ultrasound attenuation and dual energy x-ray absorptiometry in patients with hip fractures: which technique discriminates fracture risk. Calcified Tissue Int 1994; 54: 466–469.
42. Food and Drug Administration, Division of Metabolism and Endocrine Drug Products. Guidelines for pre-clinical and clinical evaluation of agents used in the prevention of treatment of post-menopausal osteoporosis (Draft). Rockville: FDA, April 1994.
43. Agren M, Karellas A, Leahey D et al. Ultrasound attenuation of the calcaneus: a sensitive and specific discriminator of osteopenia in postmenopausal women. Calcif Tissue Int 1991; 48: 240–244.
44. Bernecker P, Resch H, Pietschmann et al. Broadband ultrasound attenuation of the calcanous in women with osteoporotic vertebral fractures: comparative measurements with QCT and SPA. Am J Roentgenol 1990; 155: 825–828.
45. Baran DT, Kelly AM, Karellas A et al. Ultrasound attenuation of the os calcis in women with osteoporosis and hip fractures. Calcif Tissue Int 1988; 43: 138–142.
46. Stevenson JC, Lees B, Ramalingam T, Blake GM. Precision and sensitivity of a new ultrasound bone densitometer. Bone Res 1992; 7 (Suppl 1): 5187.
47. Collet P, Vico L, Alexandre C. Ultrasound measurement in the os calus: relationships to bone mineral at other skeletal sites. J Bone Mineral Res 1993; 8 (1): 921.
48. Miller CG, Herd RJM, Ramalingam T, Fogelman I, Blake GM. Ultrasonic velocity measurements through the calcaneus: which velocity should be measured? Osteoporosis Int 1993; 3: 31–35.
49. Gluer CC, Faulkner KG, Estilo MJ, Engelke K, Rosin J, Genant HK. Quality assurance for bone densitometry research studies: concept and impact. Osteoporosis Int 1993; 3: 227–235.

5 ARE BRONCHIAL CHALLENGE STUDIES INDICATORS OF ANTIASTHMATIC ACTIVITY?

A. J. Frew and S. T. Holgate
Southampton General Hospital, Southampton, UK

Introduction

Bronchial asthma is a chronic inflammatory condition of human airways characterised by marked variation in the calibre of the intrapulmonary airways over short periods of time. Some patients may have mild intermittent disease. In addition, asthmatic individuals often experience acute episodes of asthma on exposure to non-specific irritants such as cold air, inorganic dusts, cigarette smoke, perfumes, paint, etc. These are not allergic responses but are exaggerated responses of the airways to the non-specific irritant. This phenomenon is termed non-specific bronchial hyperresponsiveness and can be formally documented by the response to the non-specific bronchoconstrictors methacholine or histamine.

In experimental studies, a wide range of non-specific stimuli have been used to induce bronchospasm in asthmatic patients: some agents act directly on the airways smooth muscle (e.g., histamine, methacholine) while others act indirectly, either by inducing the release of mast cell mediators (e.g., hypertonic saline, adenosine) or through neural reflex mechanisms (e.g., sulphur dioxide, sodium metabisulphite). Some of these agents will also induce bronchoconstriction in non-asthmatic individuals, but the increase in non-specific responsiveness is characteristic of asthma and correlates with disease severity. Other pharmacological agents have no direct bronchoconstrictor effect but increase bronchial responsiveness by increas-

Clinical Measurement in Drug Evaluation. Edited by W. S. Nimmo and G. T. Tucker
© 1995 John Wiley & Sons Ltd

ing epithelial permeability or increasing post-receptor sensitivity of smooth muscle. There is more to bronchial asthma than bronchial hyperresponsiveness but symptoms such as exercise-induced asthma, nocturnal asthma, cough and variability of peak flow measurement are largely manifestations of bronchial hyperresponsiveness.

Specific bronchial responsiveness

As well as increased non-specific responsiveness, many asthmatic patients have hypersensitivity to airborne allergens (pollens, house dust mites, animal danders, etc). This specific responsiveness is due to the presence of immunoglobulin E (IgE) antibody directed against the relevant allergen, and in these individuals acute exposure to allergens will lead to bronchoconstriction. When sensitised asthmatic subjects are exposed to allergen under standardised conditions, they show a characteristic pattern of physiological response as assessed by dynamic spirometry. Bronchoconstriction begins to develop within 5–10 min with measurable reductions in forced expiratory volumes and peak expiratory flow rates. Generally, this early asthmatic response (EAR) peaks between 15 and 20 min after allergen exposure and then resolves over 1–2 h. Subsequently a proportion of subjects will go on to develop a secondary or 'late-phase' asthmatic response (LAR) with recurrence of their bronchoconstriction between 3 and 9 h after exposure. The LAR usually evolves slowly and can last a few hours or continue for several days [1]. Subjects who experience LAR often report destabilisation of their asthma following challenge and will have increased non-specific bronchial responsiveness for up to two weeks after challenge, even though their spirometric values have returned to baseline [2,3]. Patients who experience an isolated EAR do not usually show alterations in non-specific bronchial responsiveness (NSBR) or destabilisation of their asthma.

The propensity to develop LAR is associated with worse clinical status [4,5] and, interestingly, patients with seasonal asthma are more likely to develop LAR during or after the natural pollen season than in the winter [6].

Reproducibility of early- and late-phase asthmatic responses

Comparative studies have indicated that the magnitude of the EAR depends on two main variables. These are the concentration of allergen-specific IgE and the level of non-specific bronchial responsiveness. If all other factors are kept constant, it is possible to predict accurately the magnitude of response or, alternatively, to predict the dose of allergen which will induce an EAR of fixed magnitude [7].

The factors that determine the magnitude of the LAR are less well defined [8]. There are considerable difficulties in comparing studies from different centres, owing to variation in the methods and endpoints used [9]. In most instances, LAR are preceded by EAR, but there is no direct correlation between the magnitude of the EAR and the subsequent LAR [10,11]. Similarly, there is only a very limited association between serum concentrations of allergen-specific IgE, bronchial responsiveness or cutaneous sensitivity to allergen and the magnitude of the LAR [7,12,13]. Nevertheless, within individuals, LAR do appear to be dose-dependent phenomena in terms of the dose of allergen administered [14,15].

When using bronchoprovocation tests for drug evaluation, it is essential to maximise the reproducibility of the response within each individual. To do this requires careful attention to the several parameters that are known to influence response [9]. These include patient factors and methodological factors (Table 1). Baseline lung function, drug usage and intercurrent infections all influence the patient's response to allergen. In addition, bronchial responsiveness varies randomly and in relation to the pollen season. Most importantly, allergen challenge itself can alter bronchial reactivity for up to two weeks [2]. This becomes particularly important when drug studies demand serial challenges.

The dose of allergen administered is another obvious potential source of variation. Standard allergen extracts should be used, preferably from the same batch. Dilutions used for challenge should be made in a standard manner and ideally should be checked for activity by skin testing on the patient prior to inhalation. The total dose delivered can be affected by the delivery system and the breathing pattern (Table 1). Accurate interpretation of drug effects requires that these factors be as standard as possible. When it comes to measuring the physiological response, definitions of LAR vary between centres. Different physiological measures have different inherent variability and, moreover, different spirometers may give different results, so it is vital that the physiological measurements are made in the same way on each occasion using the same spirometric devices. If different devices are used, accurate formal comparison must be made to ensure comparability.

Even if these variables are carefully considered, responses to allergen are always less reproducible than responses to histamine and other non-specific bronchoconstrictors. Group mean responses are generally reproducible [16]. For all these reasons, it is important that study design is carefully considered before assessing the efficacy of drugs against allergen bronchoprovocation. Special consideration must also be given to appropriate randomisation and the use of control or placebo days. Challenge

Table 1. Sources of variability in allergen challenge

Patient factors
Degree of sensitisation (allergen-specific IgE)
Baseline lung function
Baseline NSBR
Recent infection (esp. viral)
Drug treatment (antihistamines, theophyllines, steroids, etc.)

Allergen factors
Seasonal exposure
Source and composition of allergen extract
Dilution
Diluents

Methodological factors
Environmental conditions (temperature, humidity)
Delivery system
   Type of nebuliser, mouthpiece
   Air flow rate
   Stability of output with changing volume
   Droplet size
Breathing pattern
   Tidal breathing v. forced inhalation
   Dosimeter
   Sitting v. standing position
   Noseclip
Physiological measurement
   Inherent reproducibility of spirometric parameter used
   Definition of provoking dose
   Definition of endpoint

---

days need to be separated by sufficient time to allow the effect of previous challenges to wear off, and baseline lung function and non-specific sensitivity should be measured on each occasion.

Cellular and biochemical correlates of early- and late-phase asthmatic responses

The EAR to allergen is accompanied by the release of a range of mediators from bronchial mast cells. Chief among these are histamine, prostaglandin D_2, and the leukotrienes (LTC_4, LTD_4 and LTE_4). These agents induce contraction of smooth muscle, microvascular leakage (oedema) and mucus secretion, and stimulate neural reflexes (Table 2).

Early studies suggested that the late-phase response to allergen was dependent on immune complex-mediated (type III) hypersensitivity [17]

Table 2. Actions of mast cell mediators

	Leukotrienes	Histamine	PAF	Prostanoids
Bronchoconstriction	$LTD_4 > C_4 > E_4$	+++	++	PGD_2, $PGF_{2\alpha}$, $9\alpha11bPGF_2$, TxA_2
Mucosal oedema	LTC_4, D_4	+++	++	PGE_2, PGI_2, TxA_2
Mucus secretion	LTC_4, D_4	±	++	+
Chemotaxis and cellular activation	LTB_4	+	++++	−
Increased NSBR (duration)	LTB_4, LTE_4 transient	−	variable (1/5 studies)	PGD_2 transient only

but subsequent studies have confirmed that LAR are IgE-dependent [18,19] and that IgG is probably not relevant [20,21]. In addition to the late effects of mast cell mediators (especially leukotrienes), LAR are associated with the influx of inflammatory cells including neutrophils, eosinophils, lymphocytes and monocytes, and the consequent development of chronic inflammatory changes in the respiratory epithelium [22,23]. These inflammatory cells augment the inflammatory response by generating and releasing additional pro-inflammatory mediators, especially mediators which activate endothelial cells and promote microvascular leakage.

Pharmacology of the early and late asthmatic response

Careful pharmacological dissection of the EAR indicates that approximately 50% of the bronchoconstriction is attributable to histamine, with the remainder due to the combined actions of the newly generated mediators (prostaglandins, leukotrienes, platelet activating factor) [24].

Over the past 25 years many studies of the pharmacology of the LAR have been carried out to try to delineate the pathophysiological mechanisms of the LAR. Sodium cromoglycate (SCG) consistently inhibits the development of the early and late asthmatic responses when administered prior to allergen inhalation [25–27]. However, SCG does not influence the magnitude of the LAR if given after the evolution of an EAR [28]. Pretreatment with SCG prevents the allergen-induced increase in bronchial responsiveness [29] and the recruitment of eosinophils [30]. The precise mechanism(s) through which SCG exerts its effect on the EAR and LAR is not known. Initial suggestions that SCG acted by inhibiting degranulation of pulmonary mast cells have not been fully supported by comparison with other, more effective inhibitors of mast cell degranulation [31]. However, it is possible that SCG reduces the release of mast cell-associated cytokines (IL-4, IL-5, TNF-α, IL-6) that are involved in the upregulation of endothelial adhesion molecules and leucocyte recruitment into the airway during the LAR [32].

Nedocromil sodium attenuates the allergen-induced EAR and LAR when administered before allergen exposure and, like SCG, nedocromil sodium also prevents the subsequent increase in non-specific bronchial responsiveness [33,34]. As with SCG, the mechanism by which nedocromil sodium inhibits the LAR is not known. *In vitro* both drugs have a variety of actions against inflammatory cells as well as being mast cell stabilisers [35,36]. However, nedocromil sodium is significantly superior to SCG in conferring protection against other non-specific bronchoconstrictor stimuli such as sulphur dioxide, adenosine and neurokinin A [37–39].

CORTICOSTEROIDS

Corticosteroids are the most effective antiasthma drugs available at present, although their use is limited by their potential side-effects. When given as a single dose before allergen exposure, corticosteroids have little effect on the early asthmatic response, although they do attenuate the EAR when given over several weeks prior to challenge [40], probably by depleting mast cell numbers [41]. In contrast, corticosteroids are extremely effective against the LAR [28,29]. As with SCG, successful abolition of the LAR prevents the rise in bronchial responsiveness that usually follows the LAR [29]. Corticosteroids have no direct effect on mast cell mediator release [42] and it is likely that their effect on the LAR is due to a combination of direct effects on vascular endothelium and cellular recruitment [42] and indirect effects on cellular activation by inhibition of phospholipase A_2 [43]. Longer-term steroid treatment (e.g., 14 days treatment with inhaled budesonide) decreases airway response to methacholine, sodium metabisulphite and adenosine, with a greater effect against adenosine than the other two stimuli [44], which is probably due to the effect of long-term steroid therapy in reducing mast cell numbers as well as airways inflammation [45].

β_2-ADRENERGIC AGONISTS

β_2-Adrenergic agonists are widely used to treat asthma and act rapidly to relieve bronchospasm. When administered prior to allergen challenge, salbutamol attenuates the immediate response to allergen and the associated rise in plasma histamine [46] but has no effect on the subsequent development of the late-phase response or the subsequent increase in NSBR [29]. If given after allergen challenge, some reversal of the LAR is observed

[34,47,48]. Another β_2-agonist, fenoterol, also prevented the EAR and partially attenuated the LAR, whereas orciprenaline (the precursor of fenoterol) did not affect the LAR [28]. In addition to its bronchodilator properties, salbutamol is a very potent mast cell stabiliser, being about 1000 times more potent than SCG in inhibiting degranulation of human pulmonary mast cells [31]. This suggests that prevention of the LAR by other drugs cannot simply be attributed to prevention of mast cell degranulation.

Salmeterol and formoterol are long-acting β_2-receptor agonists which produce bronchodilatation in man for 12–24 h after a single administration [49,50]. *In vitro*, salmeterol and formoterol inhibit anti-IgE-mediated degranulation of human basophils and pulmonary mast cells for up to 12 h [51,52]. Both salmeterol and formoterol shift the methacholine dose–response curve to the right for over 24 h, but they do not abolish the usual circadian variation in FEV_1 (forced expiratory volume in 1 s) [50]. Pretreatment with salmeterol or formoterol prevents the development of both the EAR and the LAR after allergen challenge [53–55]. Unlike salbutamol, salmeterol prevented the usual increase in NSBR. With formoterol some parameters of allergen-induced cellular activation were also partially attenuated [55].

THEOPHYLLINES

Theophylline (1–3-dimethylxanthine) and related xanthines have been used for many years to treat asthma. Some controversy remains about their precise mode of action [56] but they have retained an important role in the treatment of nocturnal asthma and acute severe asthma. In provocation tests, theophylline attenuates the responses to sulphur dioxide, histamine and adenosine [57–59]. Xanthines have modest effects on the EAR to allergen but significantly attenuate the LAR even at concentrations below those that cause bronchodilatation [28,60,61]. However, theophylline does not alter the post-challenge increase in bronchial responsiveness [62].

ANTIHISTAMINES

Despite the clear role of histamine in acute responses to allergen, histamine H1-receptor antagonists (antihistamines) have not generally proved effective in treating clinical asthma, nor do they alter bronchial responsiveness over a four-week period [63]. When used in challenge studies, antihistamines given by mouth or by inhalation prevent the response to histamine but not to methacholine [64,65]. Antihistamines also prevent bronchoconstriction induced by exercise, hyperventilation, or inhalation of hypotonic or hypertonic saline [66–68]. This emphasises the importance of histamine as a mediator of these indirect bronchial responses. Antihistamines partially attenuate the immediate response to allergen [28,69,70]. Effects on the LAR are more variable: early studies showed that mepyramine given after the EAR reduced the magnitude of the LAR by up to 50%. Azelastine, a modern non-sedating antihistamine, attenuated the EAR and LAR, with greater efficacy against the LAR [69]. In contrast, loratidine given as a single 10 mg dose had little or no effect on the LAR [70]. In another study, terfenadine was able to abolish the EAR, but if the allergen dose was increased to achieve a 20% early fall in FEV_1 after terfenadine, LARs developed in some patients who had had isolated EARs to the lower dose of allergen that was required to induce a 20% EAR without antihistamine treatment [71].

INHIBITORS OF ARACHIDONIC ACID METABOLISM

Indomethacin and other cyclooxygenase inhibitors have no demonstrable effect on clinical asthma [72]. Investigators have found no direct effect on responses to histamine or methacholine [73] and have reported variable effects on the EAR and LAR. The EAR is partly attenuated by pre-treatment with flurbiprofen [74,75]. Inhibition of the LAR has been reported with indomethacin, benoxaprofen and flurbiprofen [74,76,77] but others have found no effect on the LAR, although indomethacin did nevertheless inhibit the increase in non-specific bronchial reactivity following allergen challenge [78].

Specific antagonists for leukotrienes have been actively investigated since the identification of 'slow-reacting substance of anaphylaxis' (SRSA) as the sulphidopeptide leukotrienes LTC_4, LTD_4 and LTE_4 [79]. A number of drugs have been developed which are all effective against inhalation of LTD_4, but have variable effects on the response to allergen inhalation. Some studies have reported attenuation of the EAR but no effect on the LAR [80], while others have reported blockade of the LAR [81–83]. Interestingly, ICI 204 219 blocked both LAR and the allergen-induced increase in bronchial responsiveness [82], while MK 886 blocked the LAR but not the change in bronchial responsiveness [83]. Some leukotriene antagonists have proved effective in preventing exercise-induced asthma [84,85] and these agents are presently undergoing trials in clinical asthma.

A number of selective thromboxane receptor antagonists have also been developed. These agents are active against prostaglandin D_2 inhalation [86,87] but had no effect on exercise-induced bronchostriction. One agent has been tested against allergen challenge and significantly attenuated the EAR [86]. Further evaluation of these agents is needed.

PLATELET ACTIVATING FACTOR ANTAGONISTS

Platelet activating factor (PAF) is a recently discovered lipid mediator, which is generated as a product of phospholipid breakdown and is highly active upon eosinophils. PAF inhalation causes bronchoconstriction in man and can induce bronchial hyperreactivity for several days after inhalation, although this has not been a consistent finding [88,89]. A number of specific PAF receptor antagonists have been developed: these inhibit the effects of PAF in the skin and attenuate the response to inhaled PAF [90,91]. PAF antagonists have variable effects in animal models of anaphylaxis and asthma [92]. In man, pre-treatment with oral PAF antagonists reduces the duration but not the magnitude of bronchoconstriction after exercise [93]. PAF antagonists have no effect on the EAR or LAR to allergen and do not affect the subsequent increase in bronchial responsiveness [94–98] although they do alter *ex vivo* platelet and granulocyte responses. In clinical trials, PAF antagonists have not demonstrated any steroid-sparing effect when used as an adjuvant treatment in asthmatic patients who require inhaled corticosteroids to control their disease [99].

ANTICHOLINERGIC AGENTS

Ipratropium bromide is an anticholinergic agent which is active by the inhaled route and produces equivalent bronchodilation to salbutamol in mild asthmatics. As expected, ipratropium is highly effective against methacholine challenge, displacing the airways dose–response curve up to 200-fold. Ipratropium is active against exercise-induced asthma but has not been studied extensively in the allergen challenge model. Although a study using atropine has reported some protection against allergen-induced bronchoconstriction [100], a study that combined physiological and biochemical measurements found no effect on either the early response to allergen or the release of mast cell mediators [46].

FRUSEMIDE

The loop diuretic frusemide has never been used to treat asthma but has interesting effects on the bronchoconstrictor responses to different agents. Inhalation of nebulised frusemide almost completely abolishes the airway responses to exercise and to hypotonic 'fog' (nebulised distilled water) [101]. Pre-treatment with frusemide blocked the EAR and LAR to allergen [102,103]. However, frusemide did not affect the development of increased NSBR after allergen challenge, nor did it have any direct bronchodilator effect in patients with reversible airflow obstruction [103]. *In vitro,* frusemide has no effect on contraction of bronchial smooth muscle to a range of spasmogens, suggesting that its effect *in vivo* may be due to an affect on mast cells or on nerve endings. This pattern of response is similar to that observed with SCG but clearly SCG and frusemide do not have comparable efficacy in clinical disease.

Use of bronchial provocation tests to predict drug efficacy in asthma

Since the discovery of the EAR and LAR to allergen, there has been considerable interest in the possible use of inhalation challenge tests to predict drug activity against clinical asthma. Initial studies in the late 1960s and early 1970s were aimed at dissecting the pathophysiological mechanisms of asthma, by using drugs which were already established in clinical practice. More recently, efficacy in bronchoprovocation tests has become one of the essential milestones in development of new anti-asthmatic drugs. Few drugs that are ineffective in bronchoprovocation tests are likely to undergo further development. It is therefore difficult to ascertain whether any drug is ineffective in models of asthma but effective in clinical disease. The only exception to this route of drug development is where drugs that are already established for other indications are tried in asthma, e.g. the recent use of methotrexate and cyclosporin A in chronic severe asthma [104,105]. These drugs are too toxic for use in mildly affected asthmatic subjects and so it is unlikely that we will ever know their efficacy in bronchoprovocation tests in man. In guinea-pigs, treatment with cyclosporin A during sensitisation attenuates the induction of bronchial responsiveness to trimellitic anhydride inhalation [106], but this appears to be an effect on induction of sensitisation rather than on the subsequent response [107].

The central question posed here is whether efficacy in bronchoprovocation tests is a reliable predictor of efficacy in clinical disease. There is also the subsidiary question of whether a particular pattern of response in bronchoprovocation tests may predict efficacy in a selected subset of asthmatic patients.

Three distinct types of challenge tests have been used:

- Specific mediator challenge (histamine, leukotriene, methacholine).
- Indirect challenge (exercise, cold air, SO_2, distilled water, hypertonic saline, adenosine, etc.).
- Allergen challenge.

Specific mediator challenges are generally used to determine the known activity of a drug (e.g., the efficacy of a leukotriene antagonist against inhaled leukotrienes or of an antihistamine against inhaled histamine). Sometimes the question at issue is the efficacy of a new drug preparation (e.g., a powdered aerosol) against a standard challenge. Such challenges are useful parts of drug development in firmly demonstrating that the pharmacological responses shown in pre-clinical studies can be reproduced in normal or asthmatic humans at the doses selected and by the specific route chosen for administration.

Indirect challenges have received considerable attention because they can be standardised more easily than allergen challenges and remove the variability due to differential sensitisation to allergens. Some of these act by neural reflexes and are independent of mast cell numbers, while others act by triggering mast cells and thus offer an integrated measure of mast cell responsiveness to the challenge agent and pre-existing non-specific bronchial responsiveness. Differential activity in these tests can thus be a useful indicator of site and mode of drug action. In general, drugs which are active in these models are likely to work well in exercise-induced asthma but may not predict response in more severe forms of the disease.

Allergen challenge is considered to be the model that is closest to clinical asthma, based on the association of LARs with clinical disease and NSBR, together with the inhibition of the LAR by drugs which are known to be effective in asthma. As might be expected, good activity against allergen challenge is associated with efficacy in patients who have a prominent allergic component to their disease. However, not all drugs which are effective against allergen challenge are equally effective in clinical disease—older patients and patients with non-allergic asthma rarely respond to SCG and a minority respond to nedocromil sodium, while other drugs (e.g., antihistamines) may be active against allergen challenge but are either ineffective in clinical disease or offer little marginal benefit when combined with existing best treatment options. It is important to remember that the LAR is still an acute response to allergen and in real-life asthma there are additional elements of chronic inflammation that may not be directly related to the evolution or pathophysiology of the LAR (Table 3). Thus drugs may be active against the inflammatory component of the LAR but less effective in the chronic inflammatory state observed in long-standing active asthma. Certainly it is clear that some drugs can block the bronchoconstriction response to allergen but not the associated increase in non-specific bronchial responsiveness. Some of these limitations may be overcome by local (segmental) allergen challenge, which evokes a greater degree of inflammation than conventional inhalation challenge [108,109]. Even this model has limitations in terms of time-scale and requires further validation against clinical disease. In conclusion, bronchoprovocation tests are valuable tools for dissecting the pathophysiological mechanisms of asthma and for determining the activity and mode of action of new drugs. Such tests are a useful indicator of activity against some forms of asthma,

Table 3. Pattern of activity of drugs against various types of bronchial challenge

Drug class	Non-specific provocants					Allergen challenge		
	Histamine	Methacholine	Exercise	Adenosine	SO$_2$	EAR	LAR	↑NSBR
DSCG	−	−	++	+	±	+++	+++	+++
Nedocromil	−	−	++	++	++	+++	+++	+++
Corticosteroids	−	−	−	−	−	−	++++	++++
(longer term)				+++	+	+	++++	++++
β$_2$-Agonists	++	++	+++	+++		+++	++/±	−
β$_2$-Agonists (long acting)	++	++	+++	+++		+++	++/±	++
Xanthines	++	−	+	++	++	+	+++	−
Antihistamines	++++	−	+++	++		++	±/+	−
NSAIDs	−	−	?	?		+	Variable	++
LT antagonists	−	−	++	?		+/±	++	Variable
PAF antagonists	−	−	±	?		−	−	−
Ipratropium	−	++++	±?	?		−	?	?
Frusemide	−	−	++++	?++		++	++	−

?, not clear; ±, equivocal responses.

but at the end of the day efficacy in clinical disease has to be confirmed by carefully controlled studies of patients with active asthma.

References

1. Pepys J, Hutchcroft BJ. Bronchial provocation tests in the etiologic diagnosis and analysis of asthma. Am Rev Respir Dis 1975; 112: 829–859.
2. Cockcroft DW, Ruffin RE, Dolovich J, Hargreave FE. Allergen-induced increase in non-allergic bronchial reactivity. Clin Allergy 1977; 7: 503–513..
3. Durham SR, Graneek BJ, Hawkins R, Newman-Taylor AJ. The temporal relationship between increases in airway responsiveness to histamine and late asthmatic responses induced by occupational agents. J Allergy Clin Immunol 1987; 79: 398–406.
4. Herxheimer H. The late bronchial reaction in induced asthma. Int Arch Allergy Appl Immunol 1952; 3: 323–328.
5. Warner JO. Significance of late reactions after bronchial challenge with house dust mite. Arch Dis Child 1976; 51: 905–911.
6. Boulet LP, Cartier A, Thomson NC, Roberts RS, Dolovich J, Hargreave FE. Asthma and increases in non-allergic bronchial responsiveness from seasonal pollen exposure. J Allergy Clin Immunol 1983; 71: 399–406.
7. Cockcroft DW, Ruffin RE, Frith PA et al. Determinants of allergen induced asthma: dose of allergen, circulating IgE antibody concentration and bronchial responsiveness to inhaled histamine. Am Rev Respir Dis 1979; 120: 1053–1058.
8. Durham SR. Late asthmatic responses. Respir Med 1990; 84: 263–268.
9. Aas K. Standardization of bronchial challenge with allergen. In Melillo G, Norman PS, Marone G (eds), Respiratory Allergy. Toronto: Decker, 1990; 171–177.
10. Metzger WJ, Hunninghake G, Richerson H. Late asthmatic responses: inquiry into mechanisms and significance. Clin Rev Allergy 1985; 3: 145–165.
11. Durham SR, Lee TH, Cromwell O et al. Immunologic studies in allergen-induced late-phase asthmatic reactions. J Allergy Clin Immunol 1984; 74: 49–60.
12. Boulet LP, Roberts RS, Dolovich J, Hargreave FE. Prediction of late asthmatic responses to inhaled allergen. Clin Allergy 1984; 14: 379–385.
13. Crimi E, Brusasco V, Losurdo E, Crimi P. Predictive accuracy of late asthmatic reactions to *Dermatophagoides pteronyssinus*. J Allergy Clin Immunol 1986; 78: 908–913.
14. Ihre E, Axelson IGK, Zetterstrom O. Late asthmatic reactions and bronchial variability after challenge with low doses of allergen. Clin Allergy 1988; 18: 557–568.
15. Venables KM, Newman-Taylor AJ. Exposure–response relationships in asthma caused by tetrachlorophthalic anhydride. J Allergy Clin Immunol 1990; 85: 55–58.
16. Twentyman OP, Finnerty JP, Holgate ST. Reproducibility of the late asthmatic reaction: comparisons with the histamine bronchoprovocation test. Thorax 1989; 44: 867 (abstract).
17. Pepys J, Turner-Warwick M, Dawson P, Hinson KFW. Arthus (type III) reactions in man: clinical and immunopathological features. Allergology. Excerpta Med Int Congr Ser 1968; 211–235.
18. Dolovich J, Hargreave FE, Chalmers R, Shier KJ, Gauldie J, Bienenstock J. Late

cutaneous allergic responses in isolated IgE-dependent reactions. J Allergy Clin Immunol 1973; 52: 38–46.

19. Solley G, Gleich GJ, Jordan R, Schroeter AL. The late phase of the immediate weal and flare skin reaction: its dependence upon IgE antibodies. J Clin Invest 1976; 58: 408–420.

20. Zetterstrom O. Dual skin test reactions and serum antibodies to subtilisin and *Aspergillus fumigatus* extracts. Clin Allergy 1978; 8: 77–91.

21. Frew AJ, Kay AB. Failure to detect deposition of complement and immunoglobulins in allergen-induced late-phase skin reaction in atopic subjects. Clin Exp Immunol 1991; 85: 70–74.

22. Frew AJ, Kay AB. Eosinophils and T-lymphocytes in late-phase allergic reactions. J Allergy Clin Immunol 1990; 85: 533–539.

23. Bentley AM, Meng Q, Robinson DS, Hamid Q, Kay AB, Durham SR. Increases in activated T lymphocytes, eosinophils and cytokine mRNA expression for interleukin-5 and GM-CSF in bronchial biopsies after allergen challenge in atopic asthmatics. Am J Respir Cell Mol Biol 1993; 8: 35–42.

24. Holgate ST, Mann JS, Church MK, Cushley MJ. Mechanisms and significance of adenosine-induced bronchoconstriction in allergic asthma. Allergy 1987; 42: 727–730.

25. Booij-Noord H, Orie NGM, DeVries K. Immediate and late bronchial obstructive reactions to inhalation of house dust and protective effects of disodium cromoglycate and prednisolone. J Allergy Clin Immunol 1971; 48: 344–354.

26. Pepys J, Davies RJ, Breslin ABX, Hendrick DJ, Hutchcroft BJ. The effects of inhaled beclomethasone diproprionate and sodium cromoglycate on asthmatic reactions to provocation tests. Clin Allergy 1974; 4: 13–24.

27. Hegardt B, Pauwels R, van der Straeten M. Inhibitory effect of KWD2131, terbutaline and DSCG on the immediate and late allergen-induced bronchoconstriction. Allergy 1981; 36: 115–122.

28. Booij-Noord H, DeVries K, Sluiter HJ, Orie NGM. Late bronchial obstructive reaction to experimental inhalation of house dust extract. Clin Allergy 1972; 2: 43–61.

29. Cockcroft DW, Murdock KY. Comparative effects of inhaled salbutamol, sodium cromoglycate, and beclomethasone diproprionate on allergen-induced early asthmatic responses and increased bronchial responsiveness to histamine. J Allergy Clin Immunol 1987; 79: 734–740.

30. Diaz P, Galleguillos FR, Gonzalez MC, Pantin CFA, Kay AB. Bronchoalveolar lavage in asthma: the effect of disodium cromoglycate on leukocyte counts, immunoglobulins and complement. J Allergy Clin Immunol 1984; 74: 41–48.

31. Church MK, Young KD. The characteristics of inhibition of histamine release from human lung fragments by sodium cromoglycate, salbutamol and chlorpromazine. Br J Pharmacol 1983; 78: 671–679.

32. Bradding P, Roberts JA, Britten KM et al. Interleukins-4, -5, -6 and TNF-α in normal and asthmatic airways: evidence for the human mast cell as an important source of these cytokines. Am J Respir Cell Mol Biol 1994; 10: 471–480.

33. Aalbers R, Kauffman HF, Groen H, Koeter GH, de Monchy JGR. The effect of nedocromil sodium on the early and late reaction and allergen-induced bronchial hyperresponsiveness. J Allergy Clin Immunol 1991; 87: 993–1001.

34. Twentyman OP, Sams VR, Holgate ST. Albuterol and nedocromil sodium affect airway and leukocyte responses to allergen. Am Rev Respir Dis 1993; 147: 1425–1430.

35. Wells E, Jackson CG, Harper ST, Mann J, Eady RP. Characterisation of primate bronchoalveolar mast cells. II. Inhibition of histamine, LTC4 and PGD2 release from primate bronchoalveolar mast cells and a comparison with rat peritoneal mast cells. J Immunol 1986; 137: 3941–3945.

36. Moqbel R, Cromwell O, Walsh GM, Wardlaw AJ, Kurlak L, Kay AB. The effects of nedocromil sodium (Tilade) on activation of human eosinophils, neutrophils and histamine release from mast cells. Allergy 1988; 43: 268–276.

37. Dixon CMS, Fuller RW, Barnes PJ. Effect of nedocromil sodium on sulphur dioxide-induced bronchoconstriction. Thorax 1987; 42: 462–465.

38. Richards R, Phillips GD, Holgate ST. Nedocromil sodium is more potent than sodium cromoglycate against AMP-induced bronchoconstriction in atopic asthmatic subjects. Clin Exp Allergy 1989; 19: 285–291.

39. Joos GF, Pauwels RA, van der Straeten ME. The protective effect of nedocromil sodium on neurokinin A-induced bronchoconstriction. Bull Eur Physiopathol Respir 1987; 23: 312S.

40. Burge PS, Efthimiou J, Turner-Warwick M, Nelmes PTJ. Double blind trials and inhaled beclomethasone diproprionate and fluocortin butyl ester in allergen-induced immediate and late asthmatic reactions. Clin Allergy 1982; 12: 523–531.

41. Djukanovic R, Wilson JW, Britten KM et al. The effect of inhaled corticosteroids on airway inflammation and symptoms of asthma. Am Rev Respir Dis 1992; 145: 669–674.

42. Schleimer RP. Effects of glucocorticosteroids on inflammatory cells relevant to their therapeutic applications in asthma. Am Rev Respir Dis 1990; 141 (2 pt 2): S59–S69.

43. Blackwell GJ, Carnuccio R, di Rosa M, Flower RJ, Parente L, Persico P. Macrocortin: a polypeptide causing the anti-phospholipase effect of glucocorticoids. Nature 1981; 287: 147–149.

44. O'Connor B, Ridge SM, Barnes PJ, Fuller RW. Greater effect of inhaled budesonide on adenosine monophosphate-induced than on sodium metabisulphite-induced bronchoconstriction in asthma. Am Rev Respir Dis 1992; 146: 560–564.

45. Holgate ST, Djukanovic R, Wilson JW, Roche WR, Britten K, Howarth PH. Allergic inflammation and its pharmacologic modulation in asthma. Int Arch Allergy Appl Immunol 1991; 94: 210–217.

46. Howarth PH, Durham SR, Lee TH, Kay AB, Church MK, Holgate ST. Influence of albuterol, cromolyn sodium and ipratropium bromide on the airway and circulating mediator responses to allergen bronchial provocation in asthma. Am Rev Respir Dis 1985; 132; 986–992.

47. Malo JL, Ghezzo H, L'Archeveque RT, Cartier A. Late asthmatic reactions to occupational sensitising agents: frequency of changes in nonspecific bronchial responsiveness and of response to inhaled β2-adrenergic agents. J Allergy Clin Immunol 1990; 85: 834–842.

48. Twentyman OP, Finnerty JP, Holgate ST. The inhibitory effect of nebulised albuterol on the early and late asthmatic responses and increase in airways responsiveness provoked by inhaled allergen in asthma. Am Rev Respir Dis 1991; 144: 782–787.

49. Ullman A, Svedmyr N. Salmeterol, a new long acting inhaled β2-adrenoceptor agonist: comparison with salbutamol in adult asthmatic patients. Thorax 1988; 43: 674–678.

50. Rabe KF, Jörres R, Nowak D, Behr N, Magnussen H. Comparison of the

effects of salmeterol and formoterol on airway tone and responsiveness over 24 hours in bronchial asthma. Am Rev Respir Dir 1993; 147: 1436–1441.

51. Mita H, Shida T. Anti-allergic activity of formoterol, a new β-adrenoceptor stimulant and salbutamol, in human leukocytes and human lung tissue. Allergy 1983; 38: 547–552.

52. Butchers PR, Cousins SA, Vardey CJ, Salmeterol: a potent long acting inhibitor of the release of inflammatory and spasmogenic mediators from human lung. Br J Pharmacol 1987; 92: 745P.

53. Twentyman OP, Finnerty JP, Harris A, Palmer J, Holgate ST. Protection against allergen-induced asthma by salmeterol. Lancet 1990; 336: 1338–1342.

54. Palmqvist M, Balder B, Löwhagen O, Melander B, Svedmyr N, Wåhlander L. Late asthmatic reaction decreased after pretreatment with salbutamol and formoterol, a new long-acting β2-agonist. J Allergy Clin Immunol 1992; 89: 844–849.

55. Wong BJ, Dolovich J, Ramsale EH et al. Formoterol compared with beclomethasone and placebo on allergen-induced asthmatic responses. Am Rev Respir Dis 1992; 146: 1156–1160.

56. Pauwels R. New aspects of treatment potential of theophylline in asthma. J Allergy Clin Immunol 1989; 83: 548–553.

57. Clarke H, Cushley MJ, Persson CG, Holgate ST. The protective effects of intravenous theophylline and enprofylline against histamine and adenosine 5'monophosphate-provoked bronchoconstriction: implications for the mechanisms of action of xanthine derivatives in asthma. Pulm Pharmacol 1989; 2: 147–154.

58. Seppälä OP, Iiasalo E. Measuring the bronchial effects of bronchodilating drugs in healthy subjects with methacholine provocation: theophylline protects against induced bronchoconstriction in a dose-dependent manner. Int J Clin Pharmacol Ther Toxicol 1990; 28: 380–386.

59. Koenig JQ, Dumler K, Rebolledo V, Williams PV, Pierson WE. Theophylline mitigates the bronchoconstrictor effects of sulphur dioxide in subjects with asthma. J Allergy Clin Immunol 1992; 89: 789–794.

60. Pauwels R, van Renterghem D, van der Straeten M, Johannessen N, Persson CGA. The effect of theophylline and enprofylline on allergen-induced bronchoconstriction. J Allergy Clin Immunol 1985; 76: 583–590.

61. Ward AJM, McKenniff M, Evans JM, Page CP, Costello JF. Theophylline: an immunomodulatory role in asthma? Am Rev Respir Dis 1993; 147: 518–523.

62. Cockcroft DW, Murdock KY, Gore BP, O'Byrne PM, Manning P. Theophylline does not inhibit allergen-induced increase in airway responsiveness to methacholine. J Allergy Clin Immunol 1989; 83: 913–920.

63. Ruffin RE, Latimer KM. Lack of effect of four weeks treatment of oral H1 histamine receptor antagonist on bronchial responsiveness. Eur Respir J 1991; 4: 575–579.

64. Brik A, Taskin DP, Gong H, Dauphinee B, Lee E. Effect of cetirizine, a new histamine H1 antagonist, on airway dynamics and responsiveness to histamine in mild asthma. J Allergy Clin Immunol 1987; 80: 51–56.

65. Patel KR. Effect of terfenadine on methacholine-induced bronchoconstriction in asthma. J Allergy Clin Immunol 1987; 79: 355–358.

66. Patel KR. Terfenadine in exercise-induced asthma. Br Med J 1984; 288: 1496–1497.

67. Badier M, Beaumont D, Orehek J. Attenuation of hyperventilation-induced bronchospasm by tefenadine. J Allergy Clin Immunol 1988; 81: 437–440.

68. Rodwell LT, Anderson SD, Seale JP. Inhaled clemastine, an H1 antihistamine, inhibits airway narrowing caused by aerosols of non-isotonic saline. Eur Respir J 1991; 4: 1126–1134.

69. Rafferty P, Ng WH, Phillips G et al. The inhibitory actions of azelastine hydrochloride on the early and late bronchoconstrictor responses to inhaled allergen in atopic asthma. J Allergy Clin Immunol 1989; 84: 649–657.

70. Town GI, Holgate ST. Comparison of the effect of loratidine on the airway and skin responses to histamine, methacholine and allergen in subjects with asthma. J Allergy Clin Immunol 1990; 86: 886–893.

71. Lai CKW, Beasley R, Holgate ST. The effect of an increase in inhaled allergen dose after terfenadine on the occurrence and magnitude of the late asthmatic response. Clin Exp Allergy 1989; 19: 209–216.

72. Smith AP. Effect of indomethacin in asthma: evidence against the role of prostaglandins in its pathogenesis. Br J Clin Pharmacol 1975; 2: 307–309.

73. Fish JE, Ankin MG, Adkinson NF, Peterman VI. Indomethacin modification of immediate-type immunologic airway responses in allergic asthmatic and non-asthmatic subjects. Am Rev Respir Dis 1981; 123: 609–614.

74. Hamid M, Rafferty P, Holgate ST. The inhibitory effect of terfenadine and flurbiprofen on early and late-phase bronchoconstriction following allergen challenge in atopic asthma. Clin Exp Allergy 1990; 20: 259–265.

75. Curzen N, Rafferty P, Holgate ST. Effects of a cyclo-oxygenase inhibitor, flurbiprofen and an H1 histamine receptor antagonist, terfenadine alone and in combination on allergen-induced immediate bronchoconstriction in man. Thorax 1987; 42: 946–952.

76. Fairfax AJ, Hanson JN, Morley J. The late reaction following bronchial provocation with house dust mite allergen. Clin Exp Immunol 1983; 52: 393–398.

77. Shephard EG, Malon L, Macfarlane CM, Monton W, Joubert JR. Lung function and plasma levels of thromboxane B2, 6-ketoprostaglandin F1α and β-thromboglobulin in antigen-induced asthma before and after indomethacin pretreatment. Br J Clin Pharmacol 1985; 19: 459–470.

78. Kirby JG, Hargreave FE, Cockcroft DW, O'Byrne PM. Effect of indomethacin on allergen-induced asthmatic responses. J Appl Physiol 1989; 66: 578–583.

79. Lewis RA, Austen KF. The biologically active leukotrienes: biosynthesis, metabolism, receptors, functions and pharmacology. J Clin Invest 1984; 73: 889–897.

80. Rasmussen JB, Eriksson LO, Tagari P, Margolskee DJ, Girard Y, Andersson KE. Urinary LTE4 excretion in antigen-provoked asthmatic patients treated with the inhaled LTD4 antagonist L-648,051. Allergy 1992; 47: 599–603.

81. Delehunt JC, Perruchoud AP, Yerger L, Marchette B, Stevenson JS, Abraham WM. The role of slow reacting substance of anaphylaxis in the late bronchial response after antigen challenge in allergic sheep. Am Rev Respir Dis 1984; 130: 748–754.

82. Taylor IK, O'Shaughnessy KM, Fuller RW, Dollery CT. Effect of the cysteinyl-leukotriene receptor antagonist ICI 204,219 on allergen-induced bronchoconstriction and airway hyperreactivity in atopic subjects. Lancet 1991; 337: 690–694.

83. Friedman BS, Bel EH, Buntinx A et al. Oral leukotriene inhibitor (MK 886) blocks allergen-induced airway responses. Am Rev Respir Dis 1993; 147: 839–844.

84. Robuschi M, Riva E, Fuccella LM et al. Prevention of exercise-induced bronchoconstriction by a new leukotriene antagonist (SK&F 104353). Am Rev Respir Dis 1992; 145: 1285–1286.

85. Makker HK, Lau LC, Thomson HW, Binks SM, Holgate ST. The protective effect of inhaled leukotriene D4 receptor antagonist ICI 204,219 against exercise-induced asthma. Am Rev Respir Dis 1993; 147: 1413–1418.
86. Beasley CRW, Featherstone RL, Church MK et al. The effect of a thromboxane receptor antagonist GR.32191 on prostaglandin D2 and allergen-induced bronchoconstriction. J Appl Physiol 1989; 66: 1685–1693.
87. Magnussen H, Boerger S, Templin K, Baunack AR. Effects of a thromboxane receptor antagonist (BAYu 3405) on prostaglandin D2 and exercise-induced asthma. J Allergy Clin Immunol 1992; 89: 1119–1126.
88. Barnes PJ, Chung KF, Page CP. Platelet activating factor as a mediator of allergic disease. J Allergy Clin Immunol 1988; 81: 919–934.
89. Kaye MG, Smith LJ. Effects of inhaled leukotriene D4 and platelet activating factor on airway reactivity in normal subjects. Am Rev Respir Dis 1990; 141: 993–997.
90. Roberts NM, McCusker M, Chung KF, Barnes PJ. Effect of a PAF antagonist BN52063 on PAF-induced bronchoconstriction in normal subjects. Br J Clin Pharmacol 1988; 26: 65–72.
91. Adamus WS, Heuer H, Meade CJ, Schilling JC. Inhibitory effects of the new PAF acether antagonists WEB 2086 on pharmacologic changes induced by PAF inhalation in human beings. Clin Pharmacol Ther 1990; 47: 456–462.
92. Lohman IC, Halonen M. Effects of the PAF antagonist WEB 1086 on PAF-induced physiologic alterations and IgE anaphylaxis in the rabbit. Am Rev Respir Dis 1990; 142: 390–397.
93. Wilkens JH, Wilkens H, Uffmann J, Bovers J, Fabel H, Frolich JC. Effects of a PAF antagonist (BN52063) on bronchoconstriction and platelet activation during exercise-induced asthma. Br J Clin Pharmacol 1990; 29: 85–91.
94. Coyle A, Sjoerdsma K, Page CP, Brown L, Metzger WJ. Modification of the late asthmatic response and bronchial hyperreactivity by BN52021, a platelet activating factor antagonist. Clin Res 1987; 35: 254.
95. Bel EH, de Smet H, Rossing TH, Timmers MC, Dijkman JH, Sterk PJ. The effect of a specific oral PAF antagonist, MK-287, on antigen-induced early and late asthmatic reactions in man. Am Rev Respir Dis 1991; 143: A811.
96. Freitag A, Watson RM, Matsos G, Eastwood C, O'Byrne PM. The effect of treatment with an oral platelet activating factor antagonist (WEB 2086) on allergen-induced asthmatic responses in human subjects. Am Rev Respir Dis 1991; 143: A157.
97. Wilkens H, Wilkens JH, Bosse S et al. Effects of an inhaled PAF antagonist (WEB 2086 BS) on allergen-induced early and late asthmatic responses and increased bronchial responsiveness to methacholine. Am Rev Respir Dis 1991; 143: A812.
98. Hopp RJ, Eda R, Bewtra AK, Kinberg KA, Dowling PJ, Townley RG. The in vivo and ex vivo effect of an oral platelet activating factor antagonist (RP 59227) against antigen-induced bronchospasm and chemotaxis. Am Rev Respir Dis 1993; 147: A295.
99. Johnston S, Spence D, Calverley et al. WEB 2086, a platelet activating factor antagonist has no steroid sparing effect in asthmatic patients requiring inhaled corticosteroids. Thorax 1992; 47: 871P.
100. Yu DYC, Galant SP, Gold WM. Inhibition of antigen-induced bronchoconstriction by atropine in asthmatic subjects. J Appl Physiol 1972; 32: 823–828.
101. Bianco S, Vaghi A, Robuschi M, Pasargiklian M. Prevention of exercise-induced bronchoconstriction by inhaled frusemide. Lancet 1988; ii: 252–255.

102. Robuschi M, Pieroni M, Refini M et al. Prevention of antigen-induced early obstructive reaction by inhaled furosemide in atopic subjects with asthma and actively sensitised guinea pigs. J Allergy Clin Immunol 1990; 85: 10–16.
103. Bianco S, Pieroni MG, Refini RM, Rottoli L, Sestini P. Protective effect of inhaled frusemide on allergen-induced early and late asthmatic reactions. N Engl J Med 1989; 321: 1069–1073.
104. Mullarkey MF, Blumenstein BA, Andrade WP et al. Methotrexate in the treatment of corticosteroid-dependent asthma: a double-blind crossover study. N Engl J Med 1988; 318: 603–607.
105. Alexander AG, Barnes NC, Kay AB. Cyclosporin A in corticosteroid-dependent chronic severe asthma: a randomized double-blind placebo-controlled crossover trial. Lancet 1992; 339: 324–328.
106. Lötvall J, Arakawa H, Kawikova I, Andius P, Löfdahl CG, Skoogh BE. Treatment of guinea pigs with glucocorticoids and cyclosporin A during sensitisation: effects on allergen induced airway responses three weeks later. Am Rev Respir Dis 1993; 147: A294.
107. Andersson P, Ottoson P. Effect of cyclosporin A, budesonide, and a protein kinase C inhibitor on allergic reactivity in sensitised guinea pigs. Eur Respir J 1992; 5 (S15): 112s.
108. Gratzion C, Carroll MP, Walls AF, Howarth PH, Holgate ST. Early changes in T-lymphocytes recovered by BAL following local allergen challenge of asthmatic airways. Am Rev Respir Dis 1992; 145: 1259–1264.
109. Calhoun WJ, Jarjour NN, Gleich GJ, Stevens CA, Busse WW. Increased airway inflammation with segmental versus aerosol antigen challenge. Am Rev Respir Dis 1993; 147: 1465–1471.

PART II
DRUGS AFFECTING BLOOD FLOW TO THE PERIPHERAL CIRCULATION

6 MEASUREMENTS OF BLOOD RHEOLOGY FOR THE EVALUATION OF PHARMACOLOGICAL AGENTS

Gerard B. Nash
Medical School, University of Birmingham, Birmingham, UK

Introduction

Blood is a transport organ whose circulation depends on its physical properties, as well as the characteristics of the vessels. To be more formal, blood flow is determined by rheological and vascular components of resistance. This review deals with the rheological properties of the blood (i.e., those properties relating to deformation and flow) which influence circulation and which may be targets for pharmacological modification in circulatory disorders. More specifically, the evaluation of pharmacological compounds (e.g., efficacy, mode of action) via measurements of blood rheology is discussed. It is not aimed to give a detailed methodological primer or description of clinical conditions where rheological intervention might be warranted. Rather, the areas of rheology which might be investigated are described first, along with an overview of relevant variables and measurements. Next, the rationale for rheological and pharmacological studies is considered, along with problems of design and interpretation. At the same time, examples are given to illustrate how the rheological evaluation of drugs might be approached.

Clinical Measurement in Drug Evaluation. Edited by W. S. Nimmo and G. T. Tucker
© 1995 John Wiley & Sons Ltd

Rheological parameters and their assessment

OVERVIEW

The rheological behaviour of the blood can be considered at the level of the whole organ, its constituent cells or at the molecular structural level. Figure 1 illustrates the major factors influencing the circulation at these levels, which are evidently interrelated. It is immediately apparent that, in general, one cannot hope to investigate the effects of a particular pharmacological agent at all levels, although in a disorder such as peripheral vascular disease the whole range of rheological parameters has been studied over the years. It follows that early in any study one needs to define the target(s) relevant to the compound or pathology under consideration. There are some simplifying generalisations that make this task easier.

Blood appears liquid at the macroscopic level, and in large vessels it behaves as a continuous fluid (albeit a complex one). The major overall resistance to circulation occurs in vessels of this type and the rheological component can be thought of as determined at the 'whole organ' level, dominated by blood viscosity. However, at the microscopic level blood is particulate, and in microvessels with diameters of the order of the dimensions of the blood cells circulation depends on the properties of the particles themselves. Thus local obstruction and distribution of flow, and oxygen delivery are dependent on the physical properties of the cells. Finally, the cellular resistance to flow depends on molecular structure, changes in which can also feed back to the organ level, so that ultimately many circulatory problems or attempts at rheological modification must refer to molecular processes.

BLOOD VISCOSITY

The viscosity of a liquid defines its rate of flow for a given driving force and is the dominant rheological property of the blood flowing through vessels with a diameter that is large compared with the size of the blood cells (e.g., greater than or about 0.2 mm compared with 0.01 mm respectively). The factors affecting the viscosity of the blood are shown in Figure 1 [1].

Determinants

The major physiological changes in blood viscosity come about because of variations in the concentration of red cells and in plasma viscosity. Blood viscosity increases by about 4% for each per cent increase in haematocrit (i.e., the percentage of the blood volume occupied by red cells), and the effect is even greater at low shear rates [2]. Viscosity thus varies widely

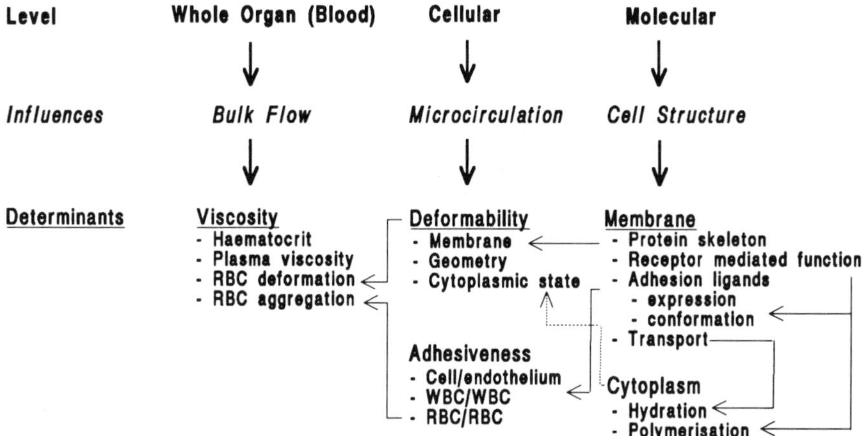

Figure 1. Schematic representation of the different levels at which rheological investigations may be carried out, and of the major factors affecting blood rheology at these levels

even within the normal range for haematocrit. The less numerous white blood cells and platelets have a negligible effect on viscosity, except under exceptional circumstances.

It must be remembered that oxygen delivery depends on the oxygen-carrying capacity of the blood as well as its rate of flow. The oxygen-carrying capacity is proportional to the haematocrit, but for a given driving force (blood pressure) the flow rate will be reduced as haematocrit increases, because of its effect on blood viscosity. The quotient haematocrit/viscosity may be used to quantify the rate of oxygen supply. If this quotient is plotted as a function of haematocrit, a bell-shaped curve results, and an optimal haematocrit can be defined where the supply rate should be optimal [2]. This value is between 30% and 50% in adult humans. Thus, within a certain range, increased blood viscosity resulting from increased haematocrit is not necessarily detrimental.

Plasma viscosity is determined by the concentration of plasma proteins, and has a narrow range of values for healthy individuals (being about 60% greater than the viscosity of water) [3]. However, plasma viscosity can vary more widely in disease, and, in general, blood viscosity increases in proportion with plasma viscosity. In addition, the major proteins associated with increased plasma viscosity (fibrinogen and macroglobulins) can also induce red cell aggregation, so that their effects on blood viscosity are even greater at low shear rates (see below).

Blood is not a simple Newtonian fluid, and as the shear rate decreases so the viscosity increases. The phenomena of red cell aggregation and deformation underlie this shear dependence of blood viscosity. Blood is a crowded milieu, and at low flow rates the cells form interconnected stacks or rouleaux. These aggregates disturb the flow and increase blood viscosity. Conversely, as flow rate increases the rouleaux are broken up, until a dispersed but randomly orientated suspension develops and viscosity decreases. As the flow rate continues to increase, the red cells deform and align with the flow, leading to more efficient packing and further reduction in viscosity.

The links within rouleaux are not generally strong, and for flowing blood they are disrupted if the shear rate rises above about 50 s^{-1} [4]. The average shear rate in most major vessels is above this level (about 100–1000 s^{-1}) [2], but is lower in the centre of a vessel and high near the walls. Thus, aggregation may occur in large vessels [5], especially on the venous side where flow rates are at their lowest, or in regions of intermittent or fluctuating flow, where it may increase flow resistance.

Because alignment and elongation of red cells reduce blood viscosity with increasing flow rate, impaired ability to deform can lead to increased viscosity. However, this effect is not large in any known clinical conditions, and abnormal deformability of red cells is believed to have a more significant effect at the microcirculatory level.

Measurement

The measurement of blood viscosity and its major contributing factors are not problematic. Blood and plasma viscosity can be measured precisely by a range of viscometers [1]. If plasma viscosity and haematocrit are known, the viscosity of the blood, relative to normal values, can be deduced [1].

Red cell aggregation can be quantified directly by measuring the intensity of light transmitted through (or reflected from) sheared blood [6]. When the shearing is stopped, aggregates form and light transmission increases (reflection decreases). The typically exponential variation in intensity with time can be integrated to obtain a measure of total aggregation, or the rate of aggregation can be calculated.

The erythrocyte sedimentation rate (ESR) is measured commonly in hospital diagnostic laboratories, and reflects the degree of red cell aggregation in the blood (the greater the aggregation the more rapid the sedimentation). However, ESR is also influenced by haematocrit and plasma viscosity. It is used generally as an indicator of elevation of plasma proteins as part of the acute-phase response to inflammatory processes [7], rather than for rheological information.

CELLULAR RHEOLOGY

Red blood cells (RBC) and white blood cells (WBC) can influence the microcirculation because of their resistance to entry and flow through capillaries with diameters less than the cell dimensions, and because of their ability to obstruct microvessels (mainly venules) by adhering to the vascular endothelium. Although greatly outnumbered by RBC, WBC are much more resistant to deformation and potentially more adhesive, so that their contribution to microvascular resistance is not necessarily negligible [8].

Deformability and its determinants

Deformability is a rather loose term used to characterise the passive ability of cells to alter and recover their shape under the action of circulatory forces. In the case of WBC, it should be divorced from the ability to change shape actively and relatively slowly during migration. For either cell type, deformability can generally be considered to be determined by the cell geometry (i.e., volume, surface area, shape), membrane resistance to deformation (i.e., viscoelasticity) and cytoplasmic state (i.e., internal viscosity, cytoskeletal structure). It is probably true to say that, whereas all factors appear to influence RBC deformation and may be altered in pathological conditions, for leucocytes the great resistance to deformation arises from the high viscosity of the cytoplasm and its associated structures. Not only this, but the neutrophilic granulocyte responds to activating stimuli by polymerising cytoplasmic actin, which increases greatly internal viscosity and rigidity [9]. Other types of WBC have been studied less, although the large size of the relatively scarce monocytes makes them particularly resistant to flow through pores [10].

Cellular adhesiveness

Red blood cells are not considered generally to be adhesive to the vessel wall, although they may become so after malarial parasitisation, and to a lesser extent in sickle cell disease and diabetes [11–13]. On the other hand, it is an essential part of the function of WBC to adhere to and migrate through the vascular endothelial layer. For either type of cell, the adhesive phenomenon is a rheological one, in that it is highly dependent on the rate of flow of the cells and the forces acting on them, and in that it may obstruct microvascular flow. For WBC, it is mediated by a series of endothelial receptors and matching leucocyte ligands, which appear to play separate but complementary roles in a process of slowing cells down, capturing them and allowing locomotion over the endothelial surface [14]. Although a natural part of inflammatory and immune responses, such adhesion may be provoked inappropriately in chronic and acute inflammatory and vascular disorders, causing vascular obstruction and mediating a series of cellular–biochemical interactions which damage the vessel wall and surrounding tissue. Activated leucocytes also have the potential to form aggregates, and granulocyte aggregation may be an additional cause of vascular obstruction [15].

Measurements

Methods for analysing cellular rheology have been reviewed [6]. In general, clinical and pharmacological studies have focused on measurement of RBC filterability, using resistance to flow of suspensions through multipore filters as a way of modelling microcirculatory flow. Although guidelines regarding methodology for measuring red cell filterability exist [16], methods reported remain far from standardised. Interpretation can be problematic, for example, potentially being influenced by small subpopulations of poorly deformable cells and particularly any white cells left in the red cell suspension. Whole blood filterability is still in use, but interpretation of results is difficult, and the method should not be equated with measurement of red cell deformability. Although possibly useful as a general measure of blood rheology, results are bound to be dominated by RBC and/or WBC count. Filtration tests have also been used to evaluate deformability of isolated WBC, and are sensitive to cellular activation [17]. Newly developed filtration essays comparing purified red cells and diluted blood offer the possibility of assessing flow resistance of both red and white cells relatively simply [18]. Also, recent development of a device (cell transit analyser) to measure pore transit times for large numbers of individual red or white cells holds out the possibility of a precise form of measurement which can evaluate the presence of poorly deformable subpopulations of cells [6].

More specific measurements take the form of testing the individual factors determining cell deformability. Red cell volume and internal haemoglobin concentration can be routinely measured by automated cell counters. The membrane viscoelasticity of red cells and the structural resistance to deformation of WBC can be evaluated by micropipette techniques. Here, the cell, or a portion of it, is aspirated into a pipette with internal diameter in the range 1–5 μm, depending on the exact variable under investigation [19].

RBC and WBC adhesiveness have not been investigated extensively in pharmacological studies. Methods incorporating flow are complex generally, although we have used them to test compounds thought likely to modify adhesion of sickle cells and neutrophils to cultured endothelium [20]. Static assays, where red or white cells are allowed to settle on to adhesive surfaces before non-adherent cells are washed off, are less complex and more widely used [12,13]. Other forms of adhesion may be assayed in pharmacological studies, for example, granulocyte–granulocyte aggregation in whole blood [21] or granulocyte–platelet adhesion using isolated cells [22].

INVESTIGATIONS AT THE MOLECULAR LEVEL

The cellular properties that influence deformation and adhesion are controlled at the molecular level. In terms of red cell deformability, the membrane protein skeleton gives the cell its elastic properties and is a major contributor to resistance to deformation [23]. Membrane transport of cations controls cellular hydration, and, for example, clinically relevant dehydration of sickle cells occurs because of activation of membrane channels [24]. The deformability of leucocytes, as well as sickle cells, depends on polymerisation of cytoplasmic proteins—actin and haemoglobin respectively. These polymerisation processes can be quantified and correlated with changes in cellular mechanics. Actin polymerisation and loss of deformability of neutrophils follow activation by inflammatory mediators such as bacterial toxins and activated complement [9], and is a receptor-mediated function of the cells. Thus, one can identify possible molecular rheological targets in the blocking of receptor binding or of the second-messenger system that transduces the signal.

Cellular adhesion is regulated at the level of adhesion molecules present on the blood cells and endothelium. The actions of these cell adhesion molecules and their levels of expression in response to stimulating factors are targets for modification. In terms of assay, an alternative to cell–cell adhesion studies is to quantify the level of expression of cell adhesion molecules by immunofluorescence [25]. Although such levels of expression reflect neutrophil activation, they do not necessarily correlate exactly with adhesiveness of these cells [26]. This is because the conformation as well as the quantity of ligands can influence adhesion [27]. Again, expression of adhesion molecules is a receptor-mediated function of activated leucocytes and endothelium. In addition to modulating this process, an alternative indirect approach to rheological improvement at the molecular level may be to inhibit the release of the cytokines that mediate these processes [28].

OVERVIEW OF RHEOLOGICAL MEASUREMENTS AND TARGETS

The previous sections allow us to identify rheologically relevant targets for pharmacological modification and methods that might be used for evaluation (Table 1). The complexity of methodology tends to increase as one moves from the whole blood, to the cellular, to the structural molecular level. It is also true generally that standardisation and quality control of

Table 1. Rheological targets and methods for their evaluation

Targets	Methods
Blood viscosity	
Reduction of haematocrit	Cell counter
Reduction of plasma viscosity	Capillary viscometry
Inhibition of red cell aggregation	Light reflection/transmission aggregometer
Cellular rheology	
Improved red cell deformability	Filterability of isolated cells or blood or
Improved white cell deformability	Cell transit analysis
Inhibition of adhesion to endothelium	Adhesion assays, with or without flow
Inhibition of cell–cell adhesion	Aggregation assays in whole blood or with isolated cells
Molecular/structural rheology	
Membrane structure/viscoelasticity	Protein analysis and micropipette aspiration
Membrane transport	Analysis of flux and content of cations
Polymerisation of cytoplasmic proteins	Fluorescence quantitation of actin polymer
Expression of adhesion molecules	Immunofluorescence
Receptor–function coupling	Assessment of intracellular Ca^{2+}

methodology become more difficult. Overall, one is faced with a wide range of possible technical approaches and it follows that the choice of methodology depends on the targets chosen for modification. This may appear self-evident, but it is probably true to say that past studies of putative rheologically active drugs have often suffered from poor definition of targets, as well as poor choice of methodology. The other major factor influencing choice of methodology is the stage of evaluation of the compound (e.g., screening v. clinical trial). These matters are considered further below.

Rheological and pharmacological study design

RATIONALE FOR STUDY OF BLOOD RHEOLOGY

The main reason for carrying out studies of rheological factors is that these factors are believed to influence disease processes and, therefore, that their pharmacological modification will be of therapeutic benefit. Nevertheless, the number of disorders where abnormalities in blood rheology are proven primary factors is not great (Table 2), and evidence of therapeutic benefit from drug treatment in these is scarce. However, this is not the only reason for rheological studies, because rheological changes may occur in disease without being the primary cause. A range of disorders are characterised by an acute-phase response or haematological stress syndrome (Table 2), typically with raised concentrations of plasma proteins such as fibrinogen, and an associated increase in red cell aggregation, blood and plasma viscosity, or leucocytosis and neutrophil activation. In this situation, rheological changes could be secondary factors affecting disease progress (e.g., exacerbating an underlying pathology, such as atherosclerosis or thrombosis), or may act as markers of disease progress and/or inflammation.

Having established that rheological factors are relevant to a pathological process and their modification desirable, a case has still to be made for their measurement, rather than relying entirely on clinical endpoints. To some extent, this depends on the history of development of a particular drug. In the case of a compound with known physiological action, rheological measurements may be required to establish the mode of action. If a compound has been developed specifically with a rheological action in mind, this action must be verified and quantified. Thus rheological measurements can provide objective and quantitative evidence of drug action *in vitro* and *ex vivo*. *Ex vivo*, these actions may not be the primary target of the drug, because rheological endpoints could act as markers of an effect on the disease process via another route. Situations during drug development when rheological endpoints can be useful are considered in the next section.

WHEN TO USE RHEOLOGICAL ENDPOINTS

From the foregoing, there are several basic reasons why rheological endpoints might be used in pharmacological studies. The way in which rheological measurements are applied depends on the stage of the development of the compound under investigation (Table 3).

Tests of blood rheology may be used *in vitro* for screening of novel compounds which have been designed or are hoped (based on actions of structurally similar agents) to modify one of the parameters outlined above, under 'Rheological parameters and their assessment'. At a more detailed level, a selected compound might have a broad rheological profile evaluated *in vitro*, either to investigate its mode of action more precisely or to evaluate its range of actions. The latter information might be useful in targeting of the compound (i.e., choice of clinical application for a potent agent). In addition, dose–response studies at this stage may be needed to predict whether an active agent is likely to be useful *in vivo*.

Table 2. Primary and secondary rheological disorders

	Basis	Rheological treatment
Primary disorders		
Hyperviscosity syndromes		
Polycythaemia	Excess of red cells	Venesection
Paraproteinaemia	Excess of abnormal immunoglobulins	Plasmapheresis
Hyperleukocytic leukaemia	Excess of leucocytes	Leucopheresis
Genetic defects in red cells		
Haemolytic anaemias	Defect in membrane structure	–
Sickle cell disease	Defect in haemoglobin (Hb) structure	Inhibit Hb polymerisation
		Inhibit cell dehydration
		Promote production of HbF
Acquired defects in red cells		
Falciparum malaria	Abnormal deformability and adhesion of parasitised cells	Inhibit adhesion?
Secondary disorders		
Acute-phase response in vascular disorders		
Acute myocardial infarction	Increased fibrinogen, red cell aggregation and blood viscosity	Inhibition of acute-phase response mediated by cytokines?
Stroke	Leucocytosis	Inhibit change in neutrophil deformability and adhesiveness
	Neutrophil activation	
	Endothelial activation	
Haematological stress syndrome in chronic vascular disorders		
Peripheral vascular disease	Increased fibrinogen, red cell aggregation and blood viscosity	Same as acute response
Diabetes	Mild leucocytosis	
Raynaud's syndrome	Neutrophil and endothelial activation	
Chronic heart disease	— chronically or during acute episodes?	

Table 3. Use of rheological endpoints in pharmacological studies

---

Rationale
Relevant to pathological process
Objective and quantitative markers for drug action
Information on mode of action
Dose finding
Monitoring of treatment
Correlation with clinical endpoints

When and why	
Screening of new compounds	Markers for drug action
In vitro rheological profile	Mode and range of action
	Dose prediction
Ex vivo testing	Markers for drug action
(in animals or humans)	Mode of action
	Dose finding
Adjunct to clinical trials	Surrogate endpoints
	– Markers for drug action
	– Dose finding
	Mode of action
	Monitoring of treatment
	Correlation with clinical endpoints

Proven rheologically active compounds need also to be tested *ex vivo*, in animal models and/or in humans. Such studies are needed to verify whether an *in vitro* action can be reproduced and may, again, be used to define dose response. At this stage it may become apparent whether metabolism of the compound obviates its *in vitro* action, although it is also possible that a drug metabolite will induce a greater or different response from that expected from *in vitro* studies. Thus, *ex vivo* studies could show the rheological action of a compound that has physiological effects but no influence on blood rheology *in vitro*.

Rheological tests will be useful not only in the earlier stages of development of new pharmacological compounds, but also in clinical studies. Rheological endpoints may supplement, and in some situations even replace, clinical endpoints. At an early stage, verification of drug action may be required in particular patient groups, to support evidence from animals and/or healthy volunteers. Here, rheological measurements can act as surrogate endpoints which give evidence that trials of clinical efficacy are worthwhile. In this situation, dose finding may also be possible, using rheological measurements to predict optimum treatment regimens.

At later stages of clinical evaluation, rheological endpoints may be correlated with clinical endpoints. It might or might not be found that rheological effects in the patient population are linked with improvement of symptoms. This will distinguish a rheological mode of action from fortuitous or irrelevant coincidence between averaged changes in blood rheology and the clinical outcome. From another point of view, rheological measurements might be useful for monitoring of treatment even when the pharmacological action is not primarily rheological. For example, alleviation of disease might abolish an acute-phase response and influence blood rheology. Then, measurements act as an objective sign of improvement, supporting clinical evidence.

CHOICE OF METHODOLOGY AND STUDY DESIGN

Having established the potential usefulness of rheological measures for evaluation of pharmacological agents, one is faced with the question of what to measure, when and how. As noted earlier, there are several levels at which measurements can be carried out, and choice of procedures will depend on both the stage of evaluation of a compound and the rationale of its use. Choice is also conditioned by time available, the level of sample throughput, the expense and complexity of methodology and the availability of laboratory expertise in the more specialised tests.

In testing a new compound, it is important to define the target(s) for drug action. Thus, at the most general level, circulatory improvement may be desired, changes in a known rheological factor required or a specific molecular process may be the target for modification. Design of rheological studies becomes easier as the goals become better defined. At the whole organ or gross circulatory level, a wide range of targets present themselves and screening may be lengthy. Conversely, test procedures for structural or molecular action can be very well defined and tested precisely.

In the clinical context, as there is likely to be evidence of mode of action from *in vitro* tests and animal studies, one is usually in a better position to define the measurements to be carried out. An agent which improves deformability of red cells or inhibits adhesion of neutrophils *in vitro* will presumably be tested for the same actions in patients. Nevertheless, the choice of methods is still likely to depend on the stage of development of a compound and the specific goals of the study. This is because of the constraints of cost, time and sample throughput mentioned earlier. In small studies, e.g. for dose finding or seeking evidence of efficacy, a complex protocol might be developed to screen a series of measures. Even here, choice will be restricted if multiple sampling is required or time courses are to be determined. It is likely to be beyond the capability of any laboratory to carry out complex measures, e.g. of leucocyte adhesion to endothelium, on several samples per day over a prolonged period. In larger clinical trials carried out on a routine basis or over a long period, complex tests are not suitable because of the expertise they require (which is unlikely to be available at reasonable cost) and more simple measures are necessary.

Because of the various possible rheological targets and dependence on stage of development, it is difficult to make specific recommendations on how pharmacological studies should be carried out. However, the next section gives illustrative examples of previous rheological studies of drugs, and some typical problems that arise.

EXAMPLES OF STUDIES OF 'RHEOLOGICALLY ACTIVE' COMPOUNDS

There have been many studies of putative, rheologically active compounds [29]. In this section, examples will be given of investigations at the various levels (whole blood, cell, molecular) and stages of drug development (*in vitro*, *ex vivo*, clinical trial). These are drawn particularly from our own experience, so that problems of design or interpretation can be highlighted.

Pentoxifylline is the best known and most widely investigated drug with rheological action, initially found to improve whole blood and red cell filterability, and reduce plasma fibrinogen and blood viscosity [30]. The improvement in red cell deformability may be in doubt, because in many studies the variables measured were influenced by other factors, such as white cells. Subsequent work showed that filterability of neutrophils could be improved by this agent [31] and pentoxifylline has been shown to inhibit neutrophil functional responses to stimulus [32], reduce adhesiveness and surface expression of adhesion molecules of monocytes [33] and inhibit release of the inflammatory mediator, tumour necrosis factor, by these cells [28]. These studies illustrate that a single agent may have a wide range of rheological actions and also the problems of interpretation that can arise when loosely defined rheological endpoints and methods are initially chosen. Pharmacological studies based on whole blood filterability continue to be carried out, but these can rarely be definitive.

Ex vivo studies of leucocytes from patients receiving pentoxifylline have shown variable efficacy [34,35], so that *in vitro* studies may not necessarily be a good guide to *in vivo* action. We carried out *ex vivo* studies of leucocytes from patients with critical ischaemia receiving pentoxifylline and found that filterability of mononuclear cells (lymphocytes and monocytes) was improved by short infusions, but that there was only evidence of improved granulocyte filterability in those patients who had the worse filterability initially (Figure 2) [36]. This might not be surprising, and raises the possibility that rheological studies could be used to define a target patient population likely to benefit from treatment.

A series of rheological investigations (incorporating whole blood and cellular measurements) was carried out in a subset of centres participating

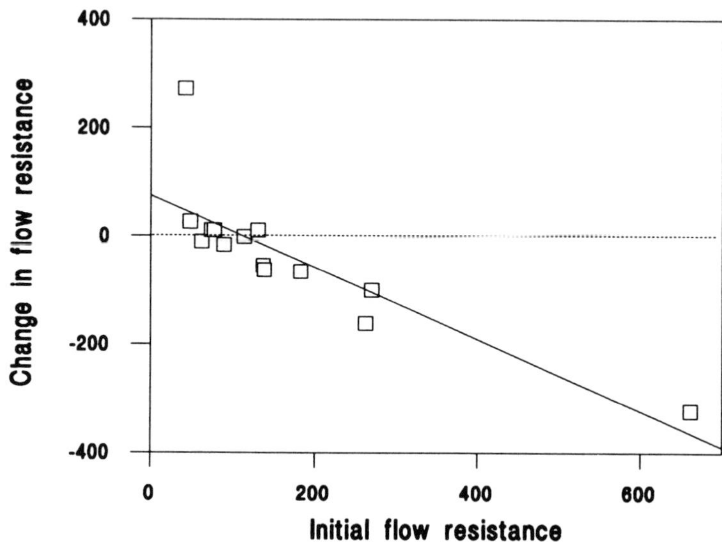

Figure 2. Effect of infusion of pentoxifylline on the filterability of granulocytes derived from 14 patients with critical leg ischaemia (data derived from Nash *et al.* [36]). The graph shows the change in resistance of granulocytes to flow through 8 μm pore filters (arbitrary units; a negative value represents improved flow) on a patient-by-patient basis, as a function of the initial value for the resistance. There was a significant correlation between improved flow and the existence of initially impaired flow, suggesting that only those with abnormal granulocyte filterability benefited from treatment

in the large-scale PACK study of claudicants (prevention of atherosclerotic complications by ketanserin) [37]. Based on a small study that suggested reduction of filter pore blocking by white cells after *in vitro* treatment with ketanserin [38], six international centres carried out parallel studies, but found no improvement in blood or plasma viscosity, or in red or white cell filterability [39]. Again, this may be taken to illustrate the difference between small *in vitro* studies and larger *ex vivo* clinical ones, but the clinical study also illustrated the problems of multi-centre quality control. Although the methods were standardised by exchange of laboratory personnel before the trial, results from the different centres were not in good agreement (Figure 3).

Improvement in red cell deformability has rarely been demonstrated clearly, probably because this variable is not greatly abnormal in most disorders. However, in sickle cell disease, attempts to improve red cell flow have been based *in vitro* on inhibiting polymer formation at low oxygen

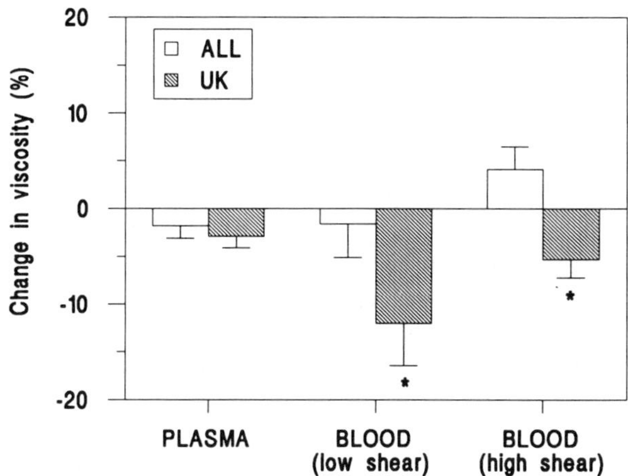

Figure 3. Changes in the viscosity of plasma and blood from patients with intermittent claudication after treatment with ketanserin. Data are from a multi-centre investigation of rheological parameters, carried out as part of the PACK study [37, 39]. The results illustrate that although a single group (UK) found significant reduction of blood viscosity (*), this was not the case when the data from all centres (ALL) were analysed. This illustrates that standardisation and quality control of measurements are essential parts of clinical trials with rheological end-points

tension [40] or the dehydration of cells during sickling [41]. Unexpectedly, a series of calcium channel blockers inhibited dehydration, not by influencing calcium entry but by blocking calcium-induced potassium loss [42]. Unfortunately, the most potent agent (nitrendipine) failed to have any effect in a small-scale patient study, probably because an insufficient level of the free compound (i.e., unbound by plasma proteins) could be achieved [43]. The molecular studies of this class of compound supported the concept that structural analogues of an active agent are worth screening, because relative potency is not otherwise predictable.

In addition to pentoxifylline, non-steroidal inflammatory agents may influence neutrophil activation [44], while we have found that the calcium channel blocker nitrendipine partially inhibits the increase in neutrophil adhesion to endothelial cells induced by bacterial toxin analogue [20]. However, the molecular mechanism remains uncertain. Rheological improvement based on inhibition of adhesion might be obtained by indirect action, if an agent alters the surface properties of endothelium or of other adhesive cells such as platelets. The stable prostacyclin analogue Iloprost almost completely ablates the adhesive interaction between platelets and neutrophils by action on the platelets [22], and this illustrates the possibility of indirect inhibition of vascular immobilisation of leucocytes.

PROBLEMS OF RHEOLOGICALLY BASED STUDIES

The first problems to be considered relate to interpretation of results: do the rheological parameters measured define *in vivo* circulation and, if so, do the *in vitro* measurements accurately reflect the *in vivo* behaviour of the blood? The former questions the basis of the measurements (e.g., is tissue perfusion determined by blood viscosity or is this a minor problem compared with vascular abnormalities?). The latter questions whether the blood is altered by removal and processing (e.g., are leucocytes functionally normal when isolated from plasma or interacting cell types?). These are questions that must be considered at the very start, so that the rheological contribution to a disorder is defined, and the procedures used are justified.

Drugs are unlikely to improve the normal rheological properties of the blood. Abnormal rheological behaviour may occur only when the blood is exposed to some form of stress, which may be relevant to *in vivo* processes but hard to reproduce *in vitro*. Even in patients, changes in blood rheology may be dependent on stress, such as exercise in claudicants [45,46]. Problems may also arise when moving from the *in vitro* to *ex vivo* stage of evaluation. Concentrations of agents shown to be active *in vitro* may not be attainable *in vivo*, effective concentration may be reduced by binding to plasma proteins, and metabolism of drugs may abolish *in vitro* effects.

In clinical trials, choice of patients may be problematic. Although all may have a clinically identifiable condition, the contribution of rheological factors may not be equal in all. As noted earlier, definition of subpopulations of patient may be possible in advance, using rheological criteria. Another problem in clinical trials is standardisation and quality control of methodology, particularly if multi-centre studies are planned. There is no general agreement on the methods and parameters suitable for evaluation of leucocyte behaviour. Although standardisation of viscometric and red cell filtration methods has been attempted [16], many studies apparently ignore published advice. Standardised preparations are not available for quality control of most methods. Our own experience [39] has shown that results from quite simple tests can vary widely between laboratories, and a major goal of haemorheological research must be to define more precisely how clinical and pharmacological studies can be quality controlled.

IMPROVING STUDY DESIGN

Various methods of improving the interpretability, quality and sensitivity of pharmacological studies can be suggested. Wherever possible, measures of blood rheology should be supported by relevant haematological, bio-chemical and structural assays. These might range from automated blood analysis (white cell count, haematocrit, mean cell volume (MCV), mean cell haemoglobin concentration (MCHC)) to plasma protein determinations, or molecular investigations of the basis of cellular behaviour. For red cells, altered deformability might be explained by changes in simple indices such as MCV and MCHC, as well as by factors such as membrane protein structure, which can be assessed independently. Measures of white cell mechanics or adhesiveness could be supported by measures of actin poly-merisation and cell shape, and surface expression of adhesion molecules. Such investigations may reveal how drugs alter rheology, and also supply additional, often well-controlled, independent confirmation of an action.

In terms of methodology, it is preferable usually to make direct mea-surements of rheological variables of interest, rather than to infer informa-tion from indirect measurements. For example, reduced blood viscosity might be attributed to altered aggregation or red cell deformability. However, if the latter are the targets for modification, they should be mea-sured directly. Altered whole blood filterability might be attributed to changes in red cell deformability—again, this must be directly verified. It may be adequate, and in fact necessary, at initial stages of drug studies to use simple measures, but these should be followed up to obtain support-ing evidence and explain any action.

With the caveat that they should be clearly interpretable, use of whole blood measures have a number of advantages, particularly for clinical studies. The cells are manipulated less, cell–cell interactions can occur, and complexity, cost and time of procedures may be reduced. As examples, recent improvements in theory and methods of blood filtration hold out hope that measurements of red and white cell deformability may become possible with minimal sample manipulation [18]. The morphology, surface adhesion molecules and aggregation of white cells can also be tested in whole blood [21,25,47].

Demonstration of rheological abnormalities or pharmacological actions may require application of stress models relevant to the disease process—either *in vitro* or *in vivo*. *In vitro*, this might take the form of exposing sickle cells to cycles of deoxygenation and reoxygenation, or exposure of normal red cells to hypertonic or acidotic conditions, exposure to oxidants, etc. For white cells, and particularly neutrophils, well-defined stimuli such as bacterial toxin analogues, activated complement or phorbol esters may be used to cause rheological change and activation relevant to *in vitro* inflammatory conditions. *In vivo*, ischaemia and rheological changes can be induced in normal volunteers using tourniquet or inflatable cuffs, in animals by vessel ligation and in claudicants by exercise. In such models, it will be the changes induced by the stress that the test compounds must act against. Not only does this improve the possibility of detecting rheological actions, but quality control may be improved because of the well-matched internal control given by the measurements before stress.

Summary

Rheological tests can be carried out at various levels—organ, cellular, molecular. From the pharmacological point of view, different stages of rheological testing can be identified: *screening* of a number of potentially useful compounds (e.g., variants on a known structure), more detailed *in vitro tests* of a promising compound (possibly with relatively well-defined putative action), *ex vivo tests* of a compound with known *in vitro* action (either in humans or animal models), *clinical studies with rheological endpoints* (possibly at an early stage to aid design of therapeutic studies or objectively verify efficacy), or to verify *mode of action in clinical studies* which primarily have therapeutic endpoints. General prescriptions as to use of rheological methodology are impossible, but Figure 4 shows how a particular type of agent acting on sickle cells has been studied in our laboratory and with collaborators, and illustrates systematic testing at various levels.

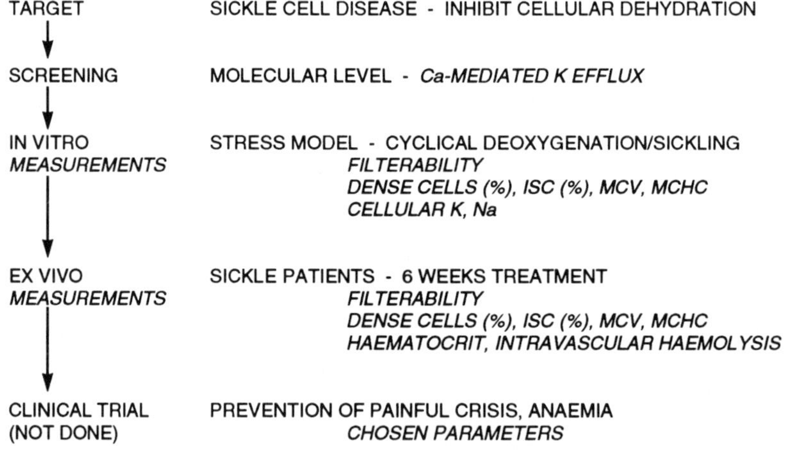

Figure 4. Schematic illustration of how a group of agents (Ca channel blockers) were screened (and found to inhibit Ca-mediated K efflux from red cells) and compared *in vitro* for rheological effects [41, 42]. The most potent (nitrendipine) was tested for efficacy in a group of patients with sickle cell disease [43]. A large-scale clinical trial was not attempted, because the *ex vivo* testing in patients did not reproduce the rheological effects observed during *in vitro* studies. The parameters measured are in italics; ISC = irreversible sickle cells; dense cells = cells with density outside the normal range; MCV = mean cell volume; MCHC = mean cell haemoglobin concentration

References

1. Matrai A, Whittington RB, Skalak R. Biophysics. In: Chien S, Dormandy J, Ernst E, Matrai A (eds), Clinical Haemorheology. Dordrecht: Martinus Nijhoff, 1987; 125–164.
2. Chien S. Physiological and pathophysiological significance of hemorheology. In: Chien S, Dormandy J, Ernst E, Matrai A (eds), Clinical Haemorheology. Dordrecht: Martinus Nijhoff, 1987; 125–164.
3. Harkness J. The viscosity of human blood plasma: its measurement in health and disease. Biorheology 1971; 8: 171–193.
4. Klose HJ, Volger E, Brechtelsbauer H, Heinich L, Schmid-Schonbein H. Microrheology and light transmission of blood. Pflugers Arch 1972; 333: 126–139.
5. Sigel B, Machi J, Beitler JC, Justin JR, Coelho JC. Variable ultrasound echogenicity in flowing blood. Science 1982; 218: 1321–1323.
6. Stuart J, Nash GB. Technological advances in blood rheology. Crit Rev Clin Lab Sci 1990; 28: 61–93.
7. Dacie JV, Lewis SM. Practical Haematology (4th edn). London: J & A Churchill, 1968; Ch 17.
8. Nash GB, Dormandy JA. The involvement of red cell aggregation and blood cell rigidity in impaired microcirculatory efficiency and oxygen delivery. In: Fleming JS (ed), Drugs and the Delivery of Oxygen to Tissue. Boca Raton: CRC Press, 1990; 227–252.
9. Pecsvarady Z, Fisher TC, Fabok A, Coates TD, Meiselman HJ. Kinetics of granulocyte deformability following exposure to chemotactic stimulus. Blood Cells 1992; 18: 333–352.
10. Nash GB. White blood cell rheology and atherosclerotic ischemic disease. Clin Hemorheol 1992; 12 (Suppl 1): 57–69.
11. Udeinya IJ, Schmidt JA, Aikawa M, Miller LH, Green I. Falciparum malaria-infected erythrocytes specifically bind to cultured human endothelial cells. Science 1981; 213: 555–557.
12. Hebbel RP, Yamada O, Moldow CF, Jacob HS, White JG, Eaton JW. Abnormal adherence of sickle erythrocytes to cultured vascular endothelium. J Clin Invest 1980; 65: 154–160.
13. Wautier J-L, Paton RC, Wautier M-P et al. Increased adhesion of erythrocytes to endothelial cells in diabetes mellitus and its relation to vascular complications. N Engl J Med 1981; 305: 237–242.
14. Zimmerman GA, Prescott SM, McIntyre TM. Endothelial cell interactions with granulocytes: tethering and signalling molecules. Immunol Today 1992; 13: 93–100.
15. Craddock PR, Hammerschmidt DE, White JG, Dalmasso AP, Jacob HS. Complement (C5a)-induced granulocyte aggregation in vitro: a possible mechanism for complement-mediated leukostasis and leukopenia. J Clin Invest 1977; 60: 260–264.
16. Expert Panel on Blood Rheology, International Committee for Standardization in Haematology. Guidelines for measurement of blood viscosity and erythrocyte deformability. Clin Hemorheol 1986; 6: 439–453.
17. Nash GB, Jones JG, Mikita J, Christopher B, Dormandy JA. Effects of preparative procedures and of cell activation on flow of white cells through micropore filters. Br J Haematol 1988; 70: 171–176.
18. Evans S-A, Jones JG, Wardrop CAJ, Lane I. Leukocyte filterability in peripheral vascular disease. Clin Hemorheol 1993; 13: 73–81.
19. Paulitschke M, Nash GB. Micropipette methods for analysing blood cell rheology and their application to clinical research. Clin Haemorheol 1993; 13: 407–434.

20. Perry I, Buttrum SM, Nash GB. Effect of activation on the adhesion of flowing neutrophils to cultured endothelium: time course and inhibition by a calcium channel blocker, nitrendipine. Br J Pharmacol 1993; 110: 1630–1634.
21. Fisher TC, Belch JJF, Barbenel JC, Fisher AC. Human whole-blood granulocyte aggregation *in vitro*. Clin Sci 1989; 76: 183–189.
22. Maeda T, Fisher AC, Nash GB. Modulation of platelet-induced granulocyte aggregation by pharmacological agents. Clin Haemorheol 1992; 12: 857–865.
23. Mohandas N, Chasis JA. Red blood cell deformability, membrane material properties and shape: regulation by transmembrane, skeletal and cytosolic proteins and lipids. Semin Hematol 1993; 30: 171–192.
24. Stuart J, Ellory JC. Effects of cation and water flux on erythrocyte rheology in clinical disorders. Clin Hemorheol 1987; 7: 827–851.
25. Bateman J, Parida SK, Nash GB. Neutrophil integrin assay for clinical studies. Cell Biochem Funct 1993; 11: 87–91.
26. Vedder NB, Harlan JM. Increased surface expression of CD11b/CD18 (Mac-1) is not required for stimulated neutrophil adherence to cultured endothelium. Blood 1988; 81: 676–682.
27. Arnaout MA. Structure and function of the leukocyte adhesion molecules CD11/CD18. Blood 1990; 75: 1037–1050.
28. Strieter RM, Remick DG, Ward PA et al. Cellular and molecular regulation of tumor necrosis factor-alpha production by pentoxifylline. Biochem Biophys Res Commun 1988; 155: 1230–1236.
29. Ernst E. Hemorheological treatment. In: Chien S, Dormandy J, Ernst E, Matrai A (eds), Clinical Haemorheology. Dordrecht: Martinus Nijhoff, 1987; 329–373.
30. Ward A, Clissold SP. Pentoxifylline: a review of its pharmacodynamic and pharmacokinetic properties, and its therapeutic efficacy. Drugs 1987; 34: 50–97.
31. Schmalzer EA, Chien S. Filterability of subpopulations of leukocytes: effect of pentoxifylline. Blood 1984; 64: 542–546.
32. Hammerschmidt DE, Kotasek D, McCarthy T, Huh P-W, Freyburger G, Vercellotti GM. Pentoxyfylline inhibits granulocyte and platelet function, including granulocyte priming by platelet activating factor. J Lab Clin Med 1988; 112: 254–263.
33. Weill D, Setiadi H, Wautier MP, Guillausseau PJ, Liote F, Wautier JL. Pharmacological modulation of monocyte adhesion to endothelial cells. Clin Hemorheol 1992; 12: 713–724.
34. Matrai A, Ernst E. Pentoxifylline improves white cell rheology in claudicants. Clin Hemorheol 1985; 5: 483–491.
35. Rao KM, Simel DL, Cohen HJ, Crawford J, Currie MS. Effects of pentoxyfylline administration on blood viscosity and leukocyte cytoskeletal function in patients with intermittent claudication. J Lab Clin Med 1990; 115: 738–744.
36. Nash GB, Loosemore T, Thomas PRS, Dormandy JA. Effects of acute Trental infusion on white blood cell rheology in patients with critical leg ischaemia. Clin Hemorheol 1991; 11: 309–315.
37. PACK Trial Group. Prevention of atherosclerotic complications: controlled trial of ketanserin. Br Med J 1989; 298: 424–431.
38. Bogar L, Matrai A, Flute PT, Dormandy JA. Haemorheological effects of a 5-HT receptor antagonist (ketanserin). Clin Hemorheol 1985; 5: 115–121.
39. Nash G, Dormandy J, Juhan-Vague I et al. Haemorheological results in a large multicentre study of claudicants treated with ketanserin. Clin Hemorheol 1990; 10: 321–327.
40. Stone PCW, Nash GB, Stuart J. Substituted benzaldehydes (12C79 and 589C80)

that stabilize oxyhaemoglobin protect sickle cells against Ca-mediated dehydration. Br J Haematol 1992; 81: 419–423.

41. Nash GB, Boghossian S, Parmar J, Dormandy JA, Bevan D. Alteration of the mechanical properties of sickle cells by repetitive deoxygenation: role of calcium and the effects of calcium blockers. Br J Haematol 1989; 72: 260–264.

42. Ellory JC, Nash GB, Stone PCW, Culliford SJ, Horowitz E, Stuart J. Mode of action and comparative efficacy of pharmacological agents that inhibit calcium-dependent dehydration of sickle cells. Br J Pharmacol 1992; 106: 972–977.

43. Nash GB, Millar B, Al Saady N, Bennett ED, Evans J, Bevan DH. Effects of nitrendipine on blood rheology and circulation in patients with sickle cell disease. Br J Haematol 1991; 78: 588–589.

44. Altman RD. Neutrophil activation: an alternative to prostaglandin inhibition as the mechanism of action of NSAIDs. Semin Arthritis Rheum 1990; 19 (Suppl 2): 1–5.

45. Neumann FJ, Waas W, Diehm W et al. Activation and decreased deformability of neutrophils after intermittent claudication. Circulation 1990; 82: 922–929.

46. Hickey NC, Gosling P, Baar S, Shearman CP, Simms MH. Effect of surgery on the systemic inflammatory response to intermittent claudication. Br J Surg 1990; 77: 1121–1124.

47. McCarthy DA, Bernhagen J, Liu Y-C, Perry JD. A rapid preparation method for leucocytes. J Microsc 1990; 158: 63–72.

7 PLATELET FUNCTION TESTS

Peter J. Wyld
Inveresk Clinical Research, Riccarton, Edinburgh, UK

Introduction

The methodologies of platelet function tests have been reviewed recently [1,2], as have antiplatelet drugs [3,4]. In this chapter, I shall attempt to associate appropriate clinical and laboratory tests with pathophysiological functions of the platelet, their relation to disease and also to disease prevention.

In any discussion of surrogate measures of drug evaluation, platelet function tests are relevant. It is not the function of the platelet or any pharmacological effect on the platelet which is important. The effect of the drug in modifying the risk of thrombosis is the primary aim of therapy. For example, 'the ultimate aim of thrombolysis is not to secure coronary artery patency—no patient will be grateful to his doctor for improvement in angiographic appearances—but to improve post-infarction morbidity and especially mortality' [5]. The bleeding time and its prolongation by drugs may be an indicator of efficacy but it is used most frequently for its ability to assess safety.

Structure

The platelet consists of an outer bilaminar membrane which contains many receptors, essential to its function. There is a submembrane filamentous system which helps maintain the shape of the cell and provide a contractile system involved in shape change. An open canalicular system links interior and exterior and this is the route by which release reaction products leave the platelet. The dense tubular system is the site where calcium is sequestered and where enzymes involved in prostaglandin biosynthesis are localised. Thus the membrane complexes serve a major regulatory function in platelet contractile physiology.

Clinical Measurement in Drug Evaluation. Edited by W. S. Nimmo and G. T. Tucker
© 1995 John Wiley & Sons Ltd

Physiological function

The physiological function of platelets may be summarised by two main features:

- Platelets adhere to a damaged vessel wall and form aggregates. This activity is the first stage in the formation of the haemostatic plug which results in arrest of haemorrhage.
- Platelet constituents are released subsequently. These constituents comprise proteins, mainly present in the α-granules and enzymes from lysosomes.

While all the secreted components have important roles, it is the familiar proteins such as von Willebrand factor (VWF), fibrinogen and factor V, all present in high concentrations in the platelet, whose activities are best known. The presence of specific receptors on the platelet surface for these proteins means their role in formation of the haemostatic plug has been defined most clearly.

Fibronectin—a protein involved in the adherence of cells to the extracellular matrix—is present in platelets in the α-granules. Specific fibronectin receptors (glycoprotein Ic/IIa) on the platelet surface are exposed following thrombin stimulation of the platelet.

Platelet membrane proteins

Recently a family of adhesion proteins—integrins—present on the platelet surface membrane and proteins in the granule membranes, including P-selectin, CD63, granulophysin and GHP-33, have been identified. Several integrins are present on the platelet surface and include receptors for fibrinogen binding, vitronectin, collagen, fibronectin and laminin. The granule membrane proteins include P-selectin, which functions in platelet–neutrophil and platelet–platelet interactions [6].

Platelet-specific α-granule proteins

These proteins are present either exclusively or predominantly in the α-granules of the platelet. They are of interest because they have activity in haemostasis and tissue repair as well as atherosclerosis and malignant disease.

PLATELET FACTOR 4

Platelet factor 4 (PF4) is the most abundant peptide released by platelets. While a heparin-neutralising activity has been identified, its more important physiological role is in interacting with cells which depend on the binding of glycosaminoglycans on the cell surface; for example, in the binding of an inhibitor of smooth muscle proliferation—heparan sulphate—through interaction with endothelial cells.

Other important actions include the modification of platelet aggregation and as a chemoattractant for fibroblasts and monocytes. It is a potent inducer of immunosuppression in mice.

β-THROMBOGLOBULIN-LIKE PROTEINS

β-Thromboglobulin (β-TG) is a platelet-specific protein and is a degradation product of two other immunologically identical species [7], present in the platelet in two identifiable fractions. β-TG has potent chemotactic activity for fibroblasts.

THROMBOSPONDIN

Thrombospondin is an α-granule constituent which becomes associated with platelet membranes after its release. An important interaction with fibrinogen occurs which is calcium dependent. There are also interactions between thrombospondin and platelet surface bound fibronectin and collagen. These suggest that platelet adhesion may be influenced by this interaction as well as tumour cells in pathological situations [8].

DISEASE STATES

The concentrations of all these proteins are reduced in the platelets of patients with the gray platelet syndrome. Platelets from these patients show impaired aggregation responses to standard agonists and the patients have a bleeding tendency from birth.

Increased concentrations of PF4 and β-TG in plasma have been reported in a number of thrombotic or pre-thrombotic conditions, including venous thrombosis, myocardial infarction, Disseminated Intravascular Coagulation (DIC), diabetes and cancer.

Chronic renal failure results in an increase in β-TG antigen in plasma, whereas the concentration of PF4 remains normal. Estimates of PF4 and β-TG show significant inter-laboratory variation. As platelet activation may occur as a result of sample handling, great care is necessary when processing these blood samples.

In vivo activation of platelets

Platelets may be activated *in vivo* by a number of events; most of these involve biochemical reactions and some may be initiated by contact with exposed collagen, for example after intimal endothelial injury. The first reaction is with a receptor on the platelet. Platelets possess external receptors to collagen, thromboxane A_2, platelet activating factor (PAF), ADP, vasopressin, thrombin and lysophosphatidic acid. A number of events occur, including the trigger of a series of biochemical reactions and physical changes in the platelet. The so-called shape change involves a change from the normal discoid shape to a more plate-like structure and the production of pseudopods, resulting in an increase in surface area of the platelet.

Platelets adhere to each other, forming aggregates, and this is the trigger for the final stages of platelet granule constituent secretion resulting in local activation of the coagulation system and leading to the development of the irreversible platelet aggregate.

Platelet–vessel wall interaction [10]

Platelets first adhere to an injured vessel and the resultant thrombi may effect an arrest of haemorrhage or, if more superficial injury occurs, begin the development of atherosclerotic disease or even vascular occlusion. Adhesion proteins are present in the plasma, platelet α-granules and the vessel wall, with receptors expressed on the platelet membrane. Blood flow and blood vessel size determine the shear rates which apply in different areas of the vasculature. These rheological factors influence the relative importance of plasma factors, mainly cellular, which may then determine the clinical effects in disease states.

If red cell numbers are reduced, there is an increased tendency to haemorrhagic phenomena. This is because the numbers of platelets near the endothelial surface are reduced owing to the reduction in red cell influence. On the other hand, decreased red cell deformability, as is seen in sickle cell disease, increases platelet transport to near the endothelial surface and with it the risk and frequency of thrombosis.

Plasma viscosity may also influence platelet adhesion. As plasma viscosity increases up to a value of 0.95 mPa s there is a decrease in adhesion. Further increases in viscosity beyond this level result in an increase in platelet adhesion. This supports the clinical observations of both haemorrhagic and thrombotic events which may be seen in patients with raised plasma viscosity [11].

Platelet-adhesive proteins

VWF is a multimeric protein present in the platelet, subendothelium and plasma, with repeating epitopes for its receptor glycoprotein Ib. It is this interaction which compensates for the high shear forces exerted on the cell in the circulation. For the vessel wall, different proteins may be accessible to the platelet and at low shear rates, for example, some proteins may exert more influence than others. For example, fibronectin is important in the interaction between platelets and subendothelium.

Glycoprotein IIb/IIIa is the most abundant glycoprotein complex on platelets and has important effects as the fibrinogen receptor. It undergoes a conformational change on activation of the platelet. This allows binding of fibrinogen and local activation of the coagulation system.

Measurement of VWF activity and fibrinogen in plasma are both readily available assays [12,13]. Determination of platelet receptor protein complexes has been performed for many platelet agonists [14–16]. Deficiency of VWF may result in significant bleeding tendency. Reduced fibrinogen (>60 g/l) concentrations can also result in bleeding. In Glanzmann's thrombasthenia, glycoprotein IIb/IIIa deficiency is present and this results in prolonged bleeding, absent platelet aggregation responses and defective clot retraction. The role of the platelet membrane glycoproteins in platelet vessel wall interactions has been reviewed by Nuerden and Nuerden [17].

Platelet function tests

The variety and types of tests of platelet function are indicated in Table 1. This shows the types of activities and functional components which may be subject to quantitative or qualitative analysis.

PLATELET COUNTING

The number and appearance of platelets on a blood film may provide important information and provide an indication of the cause of any clinical problem. Both the number and size (volume) of the platelet may be measured by automated haematology analysers. The importance of total platelet mass (number × volume) has been explained, particularly in relation to thrombosis. For example, Steen and Martin [18] have shown a direct association between the degree of shortened bleeding time,

Table 1. Examples of platelet function tests

Platelet size and distribution
Platelet structure
Bleeding time
Platelet aggregation
Platelet release reaction
Platelet coagulant activity
Platelet survival
Platelet glycoproteins
Prostaglandin metabolism
Platelet activation

myocardial infarction and raised platelet volume. Modification of bleeding time in thrombocytopenia may be determined by the disease state. In immune thrombocytopenic states where there is peripheral destruction and increased production of platelets and thus the risk of haemorrhage, the bleeding time may be little affected until a marked drop in counts occurs. Compare this with aplastic anaemia where haemorrhagic manifestations may occur with relatively high numbers of platelets in the peripheral blood and where both quantitative and qualitative defects may be present.

BLEEDING TIME

The bleeding time, when conducted by one of a number of standard methods, has become a valuable tool for assessing normal haemostasis in an individual. The bleeding time is the time from incision, most frequently a standardised incision, to the time of cessation of bleeding. Different methods of measurement produce different durations of bleeding time. This intra-method variability is manifest by longer bleeding times resulting from a greater trauma. Most frequently the Ivy technique or some modification of it is used [19,20].

The bleeding time by the Ivy method using three punctures and Simplate II (a commercial device which causes two standard incisions) has been compared by a number of authors, including Sramek and colleagues [21]. These investigators have shown equal sensitivity of the test by either method, though the results by the Ivy method were on the whole shorter (mean 3.2 min) than Simplate (mean 7.5 min) (Table 2). Horizontal incisions on the forearm using Simplate were also associated with longer bleeding times than vertical incisions using the same technique. Both of these methods can be used to determine changes in bleeding time in response to anticoagulant or aspirin, though the patient's preference was for the least traumatic and shortest technique (the Ivy method using a lancet) (Table 3).

The bleeding time is prolonged in thrombocytopenia when the platelet count falls below $100 \times 10^9/l$ and in familial disorders such as von Willebrand's disease or Glanzmann's thrombasthenia. That is when plasma factors, e.g. factor VIII, VWF or platelet factors, such as the VWF receptor

Table 2. Comparisons of bleeding time results

	IVY (min)	Simplate II vertical (min)	Simplate II horizontal (min)
Mean	3.2	7.5	8.2
Ref. range	1.6–4.75	3–12.0	4.6–15.0

Table 3. Patient preference for bleeding time techniques

48% preferred IVY
10% preferred one/both Simplate I I techniques
Simplate I I horizontal least popular

are absent or reduced. Some drugs such as aspirin and ticlopidine may prolong bleeding time by a number of different effects.

The results of studies such as those reported by Sramek indicate that some methods of bleeding time may be more valuable because of acceptability to patients. They also indicate the potential benefits of short bleeding times, particularly in the conduct of phase I trials where the time available for making a measurement may be limited.

PLATELET AGGREGATION

Platelet aggregation, usually using light transmission (Born technique) through platelet-rich plasma [22,23], measures platelet–platelet adhesion which is metabolically dependent. Its measurement has proved most helpful in defining hypofunction rather than hyperfunction of platelets. It is an ideal technique to use in the assessment of antiplatelet drugs.

Many agents will cause platelets to aggregate. This effect may be modified by other factors such as calcium ion concentration and centrifugation speed used in preparation of platelet-rich plasma. Final platelet concentration or pH may determine response to agonists as well as the temperature and speed of stirring. It is important that these procedures and conditions are standardised when performing aggregometry.

Normal responses to commonly used agonists in the investigation of antiplatelet drugs in clinical practice from our laboratories are shown in Table 4. This shows examples of responses to two different concentrations of two commonly used agonists: ADP and collagen. There is considerable variability in response seen particularly with low concentrations of agonists. It is important to consider these variations when determining arbitrary criteria for entry of normal subjects to clinical trials.

Studies in platelet-rich plasma (PRP) mean that it is necessary to separate the platelets from the other blood components. Even with the slow centrifugation speeds normally adopted, large, dense platelets are selected out from the PRP. Any effect of selection by this procedure must be considered as it may affect the results of aggregation studies.

Whole blood aggregometers have been developed more recently and this technique may be used instead. These instruments measure the change in resistance between two electrodes. Cardinal and Flower described the

Table 4. Platelet aggregation reference ranges for normal human male subjects: per cent maximum aggregation induced by ADP and collagen at typical concentrations

	0.2 µmol ADP	10 µmol ADP	0.5 µg/ml collagen	1.0 µg/ml collagen
Mean	53.32	73.86	65.52	74.40
SD	24.27	10.77	18.65	13.29
Range	12–87	54–91	19–93	50–93
Number	100	100	100	100

whole blood aggregometer [24] as a means of assessing the combined activities of all blood cells without loss of 'heavy' platelets during the centrifugation step in the preparation of PRP. In the same way as with the Born technique, response in maximal platelet aggregation is directly proportional to the log of the dose of agonist. The technique produces aggregation traces which are similar to those obtained for PRP. This may suggest that the loss of dense platelets previously referred to has little effect. Whole blood aggregometry is performed immediately after sampling although its performance takes considerably more technical time than using PRP.

Another approach to platelet aggregation is to quantify the number of single platelets within the blood after addition of agonist [25]. This may help distinguish between the inhibition of aggregation and the enhancement of disaggregation which can be seen with some drugs with antiplatelet activity.

Despite these potential advantages, investigation of platelet aggregation in most laboratories relies on the use of the Born technique. Results are expressed mainly as the percentage of maximum aggregation.

SPECIFIC RECEPTORS

With the increasing recognition of specific platelet receptors, highly specific antagonists have been developed. The following section is a discussion of the use of platelet aggregation tests in the evaluation of antagonists to two specific receptors.

PAF receptor

The PAF receptor is present on platelets and many other cells in man, including macrophages, bronchial epithelial cells, endothelial and myocardial cells. It has been possible to use the presence of the platelet receptor to PAF to evaluate the activity of specific antagonists by using platelet aggregation as a surrogate measure [26,27]. This may be of general safety interest but may also provide specific guidance to dose and duration of action in therapy. Currently the main therapeutic areas under consideration are asthma, allergy, endotoxic shock and inflammatory disorders.

In such clinical disorders it can be difficult to define or measure clinical benefit and such tests of a compound's activity may provide a means for comparison with other similar agents.

5-HT$_2$ receptor

5-HT$_2$ receptors have been identified in rat and human central nervous system as well as human platelets and vascular smooth muscle, where they mediate some serotonin-excitatory activities. It has been possible to evaluate the activities of antagonists to 5-HT$_2$ receptors using platelet aggregation in platelet-rich plasma from individuals who have received oral doses of ICI 170 809 [28]. PRP was prepared from blood samples taken at intervals after oral dosing. Different concentrations of serotonin were added to the PRP and the extent of aggregation measured in a Payton aggregometer, using the Born technique. The results showed dose-related effects on the inhibition of aggregation after dosing compared with placebo.

Antagonism of 5-HT$_2$ receptor of the platelet has also been used to monitor efficacy in patients with Raynaud's phenomenon and this has proved valuable in determining dose frequency in relation to clinical efficacy [29].

Overall platelet aggregation tests usually using the Born technique have proved to be one of the most valuable laboratory measures in regular use in the evaluation of drugs with antiplatelet activity. They are valuable because they are relatively simple to perform on blood samples, which are straightforward to acquire. Their performance does not demand a high level of technical expertise and aggregometers are available which will generate reproducible responses, provided conditions such as citrate concentrations are kept standard.

PLATELET ADHESION

The most widely used test of platelet adhesion is the simple passage of whole blood through a glass bead column. There are commercially available columns of fixed length and diameter containing glass beads of a constant size. Platelet retention is measured by counting platelets before and after passage through the tube.

While the test may be useful in defining hypoadhesive states, because much of the retention results from VWF activity and fibrinogen, direct measurement of these specific factors is preferable. Problems with quality control of commercial tubes and the effects of haematocrit may make these procedures difficult to interpret.

PLATELET SURVIVAL

The normal life-span of a platelet is 7–10 days. Demonstration of a change in life-span of a platelet is possible using cohort labelling with indium-111. There are a number of unusual situations where reductions in life-span of the platelet occurs, such as in polycythaemia, diabetes and patients with replacement heart valves.

The benefits of antiplatelet therapy can be measured using this technique as well as determination of the life of transfused platelets after storage. This may be valuable for the assessment of new methods of collecting and storing human cells for transfusion purposes.

PLATELET ACTIVATION

The products of platelet activation, induced by a number of agonists, collagen and adrenaline in particular, require amplification by a positive feedback loop through the production of thromboxane A_2. A cyclooxygenase enzyme converts arachidonic acid to cyclic endoperoxide. This, in turn, is then transformed to the potent platelet agonist thromboxane A_2. This is converted rapidly in the plasma to thromboxane B_2 (TxB_2) and it is in the plasma and following urinary excretion that it may be measured by radioimmunoassay.

Levels of urinary TxB_2 are increased in patients with venous thrombosis, with a higher sensitivity (72%) in patients not taking aspirin than in patients taking aspirin (64%) [30].

PLATELET SECRETION

A number of proteins are secreted from platelet granules. The α-granule proteins have been found to be most specific for platelets, and both PF4 and β-thromboglobulin (β-TG) have been measured frequently in a variety of clinical situations [31].

PLATELET FACTOR 4

PF4 has heparin-binding properties and after secretion binds to heparin-like molecules on the endothelial surface. Its concentration in plasma increases following heparin administration as a result of its displacement. Platelet concentrations of PF4 and β-TG are similar but β-TG concentrations in plasma are consistently higher because of the endothelial cell binding of PF4. Measurement of both proteins may be valuable in assessing the quality of venepuncture.

β-THROMBOGLOBULIN

β-TG is secreted also by the platelets and there may be some advantages in its measurement compared with PF4 as a marker of release, as it has a longer half-life in plasma. It is secreted by the kidney, thus concentrations are elevated in patients with renal impairment in the absence of platelet activation. Plasma concentrations may be raised in patients with proven thrombosis though they do not appear to predict venous thrombosis patients after surgery. Urinary β-TG is elevated for a few days after leg scans have shown the presence of deep vein thrombosis. In this case sensitivity of urinary β-TG may be low (37%) but specificity may be 100% of suspected patients [32]. Raised plasma β-TG and PF4 are not specific for venous thrombosis as raised concentrations have been reported in a wide range of disorders.

THROMBOSPONDIN

Thrombospondin is produced by endothelial and other cells as well as being secreted from the platelet α-granules. Whether the other sources of thrombospondin secrete into plasma is not clear. Sensitive and specific radioimmunoassays are available and the fact that thrombospondin is not cleared by the kidney suggests it may be more valuable than β-TG.

In practice when considering a number of diseases, including myeloproliferative disorders, leukaemia, diabetes or total hip replacement, β-TG is the most sensitive of the protein assays except in patients with renal failure or those receiving heparin for haemodialysis, where thrombospondin is preferable. No assay is satisfactory for estimation of platelet release in liver disease.

The direct platelet assays, numerical, size and tests of platelet aggregation, are repeatable, reproducible and relatively simple to perform. They may be taken as valuable means of assessing safety and dynamic measurements in relation to platelet function. In the evaluation of antiplatelet drugs they may prove to be valuable in predicting the dose and frequency of dosing of a drug with antiplatelet activity.

New initiatives in thrombosis with antiplatelet activities

Aspirin remains the most important drug with antiplatelet activity because of its proven ability to prevent clinical thrombosis. The search for more potent compounds continues and review of the mechanisms involved in platelet activation, amplification loops and final pathways of aggregation may suggest ways in which this search may continue logically.

The realisation that natural inhibitors of adhesion exist in the form of nitric oxide, cytokines (by acting on endothelial cells) and of course prostacyclin is important. The identification of adhesion receptors, including the integrins, is invaluable to a complete understanding of function.

Thrombin is not only important as a coagulation pathway activator but also as a potent agonist of platelet aggregation. Specific thrombin inhibitors may prove invaluable in the selection of optimal antithrombotics. In this regard, monoclonal antibodies, hirudin and competitive thrombin inhibitors may prove to be extremely valuable therapeutic agents in future.

CLINICAL TRIALS

'Proving efficacy of antiplatelet drugs is hard work.' It demands huge resources if the types of collaborative studies performed with aspirin are to be followed by developers of new antiplatelet drugs. It is unlikely that platelet function tests alone will provide any regulatory body with sufficient information to obviate the need for large clinical studies. They can and will, however, point investigators in the right direction for therapeutic activity, whether it be in venous or arterial thrombosis and in which specific clinical situations one might expect activity. For example, the antithrombotic value of dipyridamole has been demonstrated in haemodialysis. Dipyridamole acts at least in part by impeding the reuptake of adenosine by red cells; its effect may then be best seen where adenosine is generated locally by prosthetic surface-mediated red cell damage.

The clinical trial is undoubtedly the ultimate test but the path to the appropriate study may be clarified by judicious use and proper interpretation of tests of platelet function.

References

1. Ludlum CA. Assessment of platelet function. In: Bloom AC, Thomas DP (eds), Haemostasis and Thrombosis. Edinburgh: Churchill Livingstone, 1987; 933–952.
2. Haemostasis Thrombosis Task Force. Platelet function testing. J Clin Pathol 1988; 41: 1322–1330.
3. Vermylen J, Deckmyn H. Antiplatelet agents: pharmacology and clinical use. In: Poller L (ed), Recent Advances in Blood Coagulation. Edinburgh: Churchill Livingstone, 1993; 125–144.
4. Kelton JG, Hirsch J. Antiplatelet agents: rationale and results. In: Bloom AC, Thomas DP (eds), Haemostasis and Thrombosis. Edinburgh: Churchill Livingstone, 1982; 886–901.
5. Anon. Surrogate measures in clinical trials. Lancet, 1990; i: 261–262.
6. McNicol A, Israel SJ, Gerrard JM. Platelets. In: Poller L (ed), Recent Advances in Blood Coagulation. Edinburgh: Churchill Livingstone, 1993; 17–49.

7. Niewiarowski S, Walz DA, James P, Rucinski B, Kneppers F. Identification and separation of secreted platelet proteins by electric focusing: evidence that low affinity platelet factor 4 is converted to β-thromboglobulin by limited proteolysis. Blood 1980; 55: 453–456.

8. Tuszynski GP, Gasic TB, Rothman VL et al. Thrombospondin, a potentiator of tumor cell metastases. Cancer Res 1987; 47: 4130–4133.

9. Levy-Toledano S, Caen JP, Breton-Gorius J et al. Gray platelet syndrome: granule deficiency, 1b influence on platelet function. J Lab Clin Med 1981; 98: 831–848.

10. de Groot PG, Sixma JJ. Platelet–vessel wall interaction. Vascular Med Rev 1993; 4: 145–155.

11. Van Breyel HHFI, de Groot PhG, Sixma JJ. The role of plasma viscosity in platelet adhesion. Blood 1992; 80: 953–959.

12. Greaves M, Preston FE. The laboratory investigation of acquired and congenital platelet disorders. In: Thomson JM (ed), Blood Coagulation and Haemostasis: A Practical Guide (3rd edn). Edinburgh: Churchill Livingstone, 1985; 56–134.

13. Emer T, Burridge J, Power P, Rickard KA. An evaluation of currently available methods for plasma fibrinogen. J Clin Pathol 1979, 71: 521.

14. Colman RW. Platelet activation: role of an ADP receptor. Semin Hematol 1986; 23: 119.

15. De Clerck F, Xhonneux B, Leysen J, Janssen DAJ. Evidence for functional 5HT$_2$ receptor sites on human blood platelets. Biochem Pharmacol 1984; 33: 2807.

16. Thibonmier M, Roberts JM. Characterisation of human platelet vasopressin receptors. J Clin Invest 1985; 76: 1857.

17. Nuerden A, Nuerden P. A review of the role of platelet membrane glycoproteins in the platelet–vessel wall interaction. In: Caen JP, Tobelem JP (eds), Clinical Haematology vol 6.3. London: Bailliere Tindal, 1993: 653–690.

18. Steen DK, Martin JF. Platelet heterogenicity and coronary artery thrombosis. Platelets 1991; 2: 11–17.

19. Borchgrevink CF, Waller BA. The secondary bleeding time: a new method for differentiation of haemorrhagic diseases. Acta Med Scand 1958; 162: 361–374.

20. Meikle CH. The template bleeding time, technical evaluation and comparison to other methods in normal adults. In: Fay HJ, Holmsen H, Zucher MB (eds), Platelet Function Testing. US Department of Health Education and Welfare, 1978; 13–20.

21. Sramek R, Sramek A, Kester T, Briet E, Rosenbauch FR. A randomised and blinded comparison of three bleeding time techniques: the Ivy method and the Simplate II method in two directions. Thromb Haemost 1992; 67 (5): 514–518.

22. Born GVR. Aggregation of blood platelets by adenosine D1 phosphate and its reversal. Nature 1962; 194: 927.

23. O'Brien JR. Platelet aggregation I: some effects of adenosine phosphate, thrombin and cocaine upon platelet adhesiveness. J Clin Pathol 1967; 15: 556.

24. Cardinal DC, Flower RJ. The electronic aggregometer: a device for assessing platelet behaviour in blood. J Pharmacol Methods 1980; 3: 135–158.

25. Lewis SM, Wardle J, Cousins S, Skelly JV. Platelet counting—development of a reference method and a reference preparation. Clinical and Laboratory Haematology 1979; 1: 227.

26. Herbert JM, Bernat A, Valette G, Gigo V, Lale A et al. Biochemical and pharmacological activities of SR27417, a highly potent, long acting platelet-activating factor receptor antagonist. J Pharmacol Exp Ther 1991; 259 (1): 44–51.

27. Coras-Stenzel Muacevic G, Weber KH. Pharmacological actions of WEB-2086, a

new specific antagonist of platelet activating factor. J Pharmacol Exp Ther 1987; 241: 974–981.

28. Millson DS, Jessup CL, Swaisland A, Howarth S, Rushton A, Harry JD. The effects of a selective 5HT$_2$ receptor antagonist (ICI 170.809) on platelet aggregation and pupillary responses in healthy volunteers. Br J Clin Pharmacol 1992; 33: 281–288.

29. Menarini B, Brodini ML, Mollica B. Effect of chronic ketanserin treatment of serotonin induced platelet aggregation in patients with Raynaud's phenomenon. Eur J Ther 1990; 39: 289–290.

30. Preston FE, Cooke KB, Foster ME, Winfield DA, Lee D. Myclomatosis and the hyperviscosity syndrome. Br J Haematol 1978; 38: 517.

31. Klotz TA, Cohn LS, Zipser RP. Urinary excretion of thromboxane B$_2$ in patients with various thromboembolic disease. Client, 1984; 85: 329–335.

32. Kaplan KL, Owen J. Blood tests in the diagnosis of various thrombosis. In: Hirsh J (ed), Venous Thrombosis and Pulmonary Embolism, Common Diagnostic Methods, Edinburgh: Churchill Livingstone, 1987: 77–102.

8 ASSESSMENT OF THE EFFECTS OF DRUGS ON THE PERIPHERAL VASCULATURE

David J. Webb and Malcolm F. Hand
University of Edinburgh, Western General Hospital, Edinburgh, UK

Introduction

Forearm plethysmography has an established place in the study of vascular physiology in man. Its additional value in studying vascular pharmacology and physiology when combined with intra-arterial drug administration is now also appreciated widely, and the complementary development of externally applied strain gauges and computerised analysis of blood flows has increased greatly the utility of this technique. Over recent years, forearm plethysmography has been employed to study the function of blood vessels in health and disease; and specific pharmacological probes have been employed to examine physiological mechanisms, including the role of the newly discovered local hormones such as nitric oxide and endothelin. Such techniques have been used to show whether new physiological mechanisms discovered in animals are also important *in vivo* in humans and to characterise the vascular properties of new drugs. The wide range of potential uses of forearm plethysmography is the subject of this review.

Measurement of forearm blood flow

Plethysmography—that is, measurement of variation in volume of part of the body—was used in humans as early as 1875 [1]. It was first shown to be suitable for measuring forearm blood flow and venous compliance by Hewlett and van Zwaluwenburg in 1909 [2]. Their technique, known as

Clinical Measurement in Drug Evaluation. Edited by W. S. Nimmo and G. T. Tucker
© 1995 John Wiley & Sons Ltd

venous occlusion plethysmography, involves rapid inflation of a cuff applied around the upper arm, to well above venous pressure but below diastolic pressure. Until venous pressure rises sufficient for blood to pass the cuff, arterial blood can flow into the arm but cannot escape. The linear rate at which the volume of the forearm distal to the cuff increases during this early period represents the blood flow to the limb. This principle is still used today, in the same manner, for measurement of blood flow in the upper or lower limbs. Measurements of flow can be made at intervals, although sufficient time must be allowed between measurements to allow venous emptying.

The majority of the blood flow in the hand is to the skin. Blood flow to skin varies more markedly with temperature and emotion than blood flow to forearm muscle [3], and it can behave differently to drugs. Also, the tissues of the hand cannot stretch in the same way as those of the forearm, and inclusion of the hand during forearm blood flow measurement can result in non-linear and unmeasurable flows. Therefore, hand flow must be excluded by wrist cuffs inflated to above systolic pressure during measurements. It has been shown that flow only stabilises after 60 s of wrist cuff inflation [4], so the wrist cuff must be inflated for this time before, and then during, the period of measurement. The associated hand ischaemia and subsequent paraesthesia limit the maximum time of any one period of measurement to around 10 min. Even with hand exclusion, forearm blood flow is a composite measure of skin and muscle blood flow. Anatomical studies have shown that forearm muscle provides the greatest tissue mass (64%), while bone (14%), skin (9%), fat (8%) and tendons (6%) contribute to a lesser extent [5]. Of these, only skin makes an important contribution to blood flow. By iontophoresing adrenaline across the skin, skin blood flow can be halted briefly, and its contribution to total blood flow determined. With this technique, skeletal muscle appears to account for around 75% of forearm blood flow with flows of less than 6 ml/100 ml per minute, and for around 50% with greater flows [5]. This has been confirmed, using the same technique, by other workers [6].

Originally, air, and then water, plethysmographs were used. A major advance was the development of an easily calibrated device for external application, using mercury-in-rubber or silastic, as one limb of a Wheatstone bridge [7]. Changes in arm circumference, and hence arm volume, are detected as a change in electrical resistance of the strain gauge. The mathematical principles underlying this technique have been reviewed elsewhere [7,8]. Its reliability compared with other methods for measuring blood flow [9], and its repeatability in individual subjects [10], with a coefficient of variation of around 10%, appear satisfactory compared with other non-invasive methods. For good results it is important that forearm blood flow is measured in a quiet, draught-free environment maintained at a constant temperature of between 22 and 26 °C, with the subject in a comfortable position—usually supine—where the arms can be maintained in a rested state above heart level with venous emptying unimpeded.

Use of plethysmography with systemic drug administration

ASSESSMENT OF FOREARM VASCULAR RESISTANCE

Measurement of forearm blood flow during systemic drug administration has been used to assess the effects of drugs on vascular tone and regional blood flow [11,12]. However, because the effects of a drug on the forearm are of little direct clinical significance, these responses are generally being assessed as a surrogate for drug effects on peripheral vascular resistance (where forearm vascular resistance = arterial pressure/forearm blood flow). For this purpose, a combination of non-invasive measurement of cardiac output, using bioimpedance techniques, and arterial pressure may be of more direct value (peripheral vascular resistance = arterial pressure/ cardiac output) [13,14].

During systemic drug administration, changes in forearm blood flow and vascular resistance do not denote a direct effect of the drug on blood vessels, but are the synthesis of drug effects on the arterial and venous blood vessels, the kidneys, heart, brain and other organs, and neuro-hormonal influences either directly mediated by the drug or occurring as a response to alteration of arterial pressure. Where it is important to know whether a drug has direct effects on blood vessel function—for instance, whether a drug relaxes vascular smooth muscle—local intra-arterial techniques have major advantages over the systemic approach (see later).

ASSESSMENT OF VASCULAR HYPERTROPHY USING MINIMUM VASCULAR RESISTANCE

An increase in limb blood flow can be induced by exercise, limb warming or in the period immediately following limb ischaemia—the last known as reactive hyperaemia. Following limb ischaemia, hyperaemia reaches a maximum soon after release of the cuff and blood flow then returns gradually to its basal value. The time for which blood flow remains raised increases with the duration of ischaemia, and the area under the curve for excess blood flow with time shows an essentially linear relationship with duration of ischaemia [15]. However, the maximum blood flow occurring shortly after ischaemia is reproducible and, with prolonged ischaemia [16,17] which may need to last 13 min, reaches a maximum which cannot be exceeded.

The minimum vascular resistance associated with maximal blood flow following ischaemia is unaltered by increased sympathetic activity [16], or by acute administration of vasoconstrictors or vasodilators [17]. There appears to be no tone in the blood vessels in this state, and vascular resistance appears to represent a measure of the underlying structure of the resistance vessels. Indeed, an increase in minimum vascular resistance occurs in established human hypertension [18–20], indicating the development of vascular hypertrophy, and is consistent with studies in animals. Increased minimum vascular resistance has been described also in patients with borderline and 'white-coat' hypertension [21] (Chapter 3), and in people with a familial predisposition to develop hypertension [16].

Studies have shown that the elevated minimum vascular resistance in patients with established hypertension can be reduced with anti-hypertensive treatment [20,22], implying that the structural changes are reversible. It remains to be established whether patients with substantial vascular hypertrophy prove to be at higher risk of vascular events—a reasonable supposition since these vascular changes might be expected to lead to an increase in cardiac work, particularly on exercise. It also remains to be seen whether some antihypertensive treatments are superior to others in reversing its development, as may be the case for cardiac hypertrophy [23].

Use of plethysmography with local intra-arterial drug administration

METHODOLOGY

The first descriptions of arterial cannulation as a means to assess responses of skeletal muscle to local drug administration—in this case adrenaline given into the femoral artery—were provided by Barcroft [24,25], though most workers now use the brachial artery route. This technique is now employed widely and has been responsible for establishing several fundamental mechanisms in human vascular physiology.

Allen [24] noted the major advantage of the technique over systemic administration, which is that it can be used to examine the direct effects of a drug on the resistance vessels without eliciting effects mediated through actions on other organs or by stimulation of neurohumoral reflexes. These unwanted effects can be avoided during local infusion studies by giving doses that do not have systemic actions. This is feasible because the blood flow to resting muscle is low, with forearm blood flow around 50 ml/min compared with a cardiac output of 5000 ml/min. Hence doses 100-fold lower than active systemically are effective within the upper limb circulation. Assuming that drugs are used for short periods, or are short-lived, effects are restricted to the infused limb. Also, where there are no systemic effects, the opposite arm can act as a contemporaneous control for the experimental arm receiving drug [26]. This then takes account of any minute-to-minute changes in blood flow that affect both arms, as a result of emotion or minor changes in basal state, for example [27]. Although results can be shown as absolute flows (Figure 1A), they are provided usually in the form of the percentage change in flow in the infused arm with drug adjusted for concurrent flows in the control arm (Figure 1B).

Some researchers use cannulae of a size large enough to allow direct measurement of arterial blood pressure. However, this is not usually necessary because intermittent non-invasive measurement of arterial pressure, either at the brachial or digital artery, is sufficient to exclude, or assess, any systemic haemodynamic effect. If direct pressure measurements are not made, cannulae as fine as 27 SWG can be used. These can be used repeatedly—as frequently as weekly in a study with several phases—are very well tolerated, and are associated with minimal trauma. Such needles have been used for more than 20 years in the UK without complications. In our personal experience at St George's Medical School and in Edinburgh, more than 1000 cannulations have been performed with 27 SWG needles inserted under local anaesthesia and the discomfort is no greater than with insertion of intravenous cannulae.

LOCAL ACTIONS OF DRUGS AND HORMONES

Because the effects of the infused drug are generally restricted to the forearm, it is possible to construct full dose–response relationships for the effects of drugs on forearm blood flow, for instance to vasoconstrictors such as angiotensin II (Figure 1A) [26] and vasodilators such as atrial natriuretic peptide (Figure 1B). Most agents produce a log-linear dose–response relationship across a wide range of doses, allowing alteration of dose–response relationships to be examined. Although there may be a contribution from skin blood flow to the effect of a drug on forearm blood flow this is not assessed easily in a quantitative manner. Nevertheless, it is possible to determine whether a locally infused vasodilator drug has an effect on skin blood flow using laser Doppler velocimetry, because this technique is not influenced by the blood flow of underlying skeletal muscle [28]. This technique has been used to show, for instance, that atrial natriuretic peptide increases both skin and muscle blood flow in a dose-dependent manner [29] (Figure 1c).

It is important to note that when drugs are given systemically, there may be greater effects on some vascular beds, such as the splanchnic circulation, than on others. With some drugs causing vasoconstriction, for instance angiotensin II, the effect of the increase in arterial pressure may even be to increase forearm blood flow [14]. However, when drugs are infused locally into the forearm circulation, the effects are usually predictive of those to be found in the major resistance beds.

A good example of an alteration in the dose–response relationship is

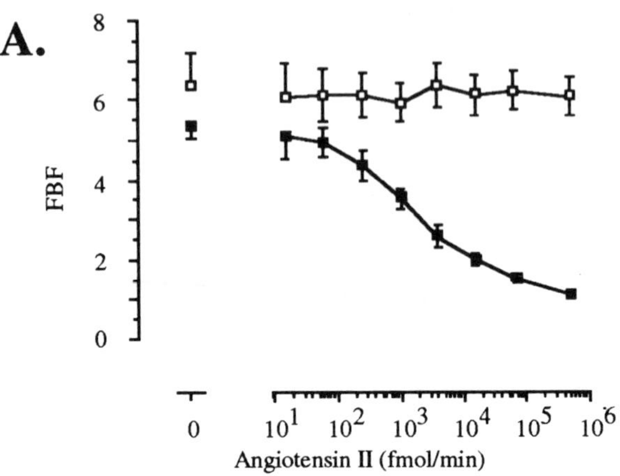
A.
FBF
8
6
4
2
0
0
10^1 10^2 10^3 10^4 10^5 10^6
Angiotensin II (fmol/min)

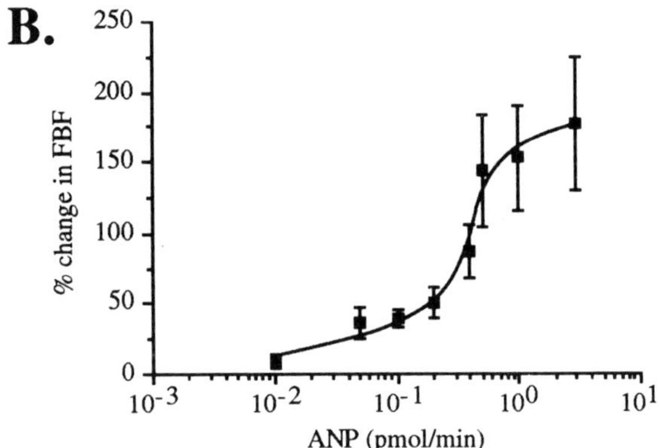
B.
250
200
150
100
50
0
% change in FBF
10^-3 10^-2 10^-1 10^0 10^1
ANP (pmol/min)

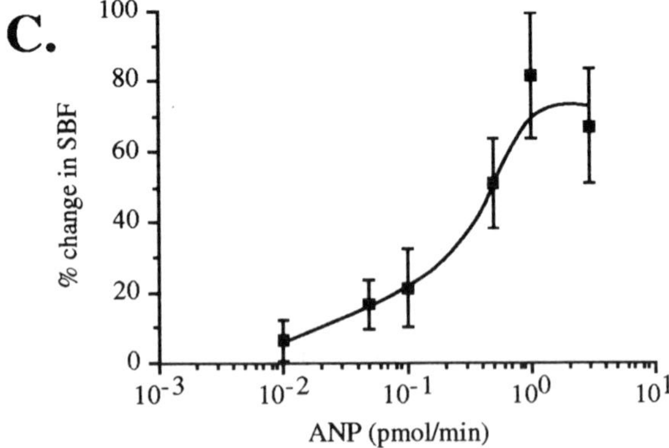
C.
100
80
60
40
20
0
% change in SBF
10^-3 10^-2 10^-1 10^0 10^1
ANP (pmol/min)

provided by the effects of the oral angiotensin converting enzyme (ACE) inhibitor, enalapril, and intra-arterial infusion of its active metabolite, enalaprilat, on responses to angiotensin I and II. A rightward shift of the vasoconstriction in response to intra-arterial angiotensin I but not angiotensin II can be shown during local co-administration of enalaprilat [26] and following oral administration of enalapril [30] (Figure 2). As expected, a rightward shift of the response to intra-arterial infusion of both angiotensin I and angiotensin II is found following systemic administration of losartan [30]. These studies can be performed without the unacceptable effects on arterial pressure that would occur with equivalent systemic dosing with the angiotensins.

Similarly, the vascular responses to the potent vasoconstrictor, endothelin, have now been characterised in the forearm [31,32] and can be used as the basis for dose-ranging studies with orally active endothelin receptor antagonists. An effective oral or intravenous dose of endothelin antagonist should produce a clear rightward shift of the response to intra-arterial endothelin. This strategy avoids the potential risks associated with systemic administration of the endothelins, and allows systemic dose-ranging studies to be performed under circumstances in which the maximum tolerated dose of antagonist might otherwise be the only available endpoint, causing unnecessarily high doses of antagonist to be developed. It should be noted here, that where pharmacological considerations have been taken into account, vasoconstrictors have proved safe in the forearm, avoiding the risks associated with systemic administration. Although critical closure is theoretically possible in resistance vessels maintaining constant transmural pressure in the face of an increasing tension secondary to administration of a vasoconstrictor agent [33], this has not been observed in practice even with major reduction in local blood flow with the potent vasoconstrictors angiotensin II [26] and endothelin-1 [32]. Local oedema has been seen in one study with endothelin [34], but in this case large systemic, rather than local, doses of endothelin were administered by the intra-arterial route.

This technique has also been used to assess the sensitivity to constrictor mediators potentially causing hypertension, such as angiotensin II or endothelin-1. Studies are performed in hypertensive patients and responses

---

Figure 1. (A) The effects of arterial infusion of angiotensin II on forearm blood flow (FBF) in the infused (■) and non-infused forearm (□). Redrawn from Benjamin *et al.* [26] with permission. (B) The effect of atrial natriuretic peptide (ANP) on forearm blood flow (FBF), given as the percentage change in flow with ANP corrected for flow in the non-infused arm. Redrawn from Webb *et al.* [29] with permission. (C) The effect of atrial natriuretic peptide (ANP) on skin blood flow (SBF), given as the percentage change in flow with ANP in the infused arm. Redrawn from Webb *et al.* [29] with permission

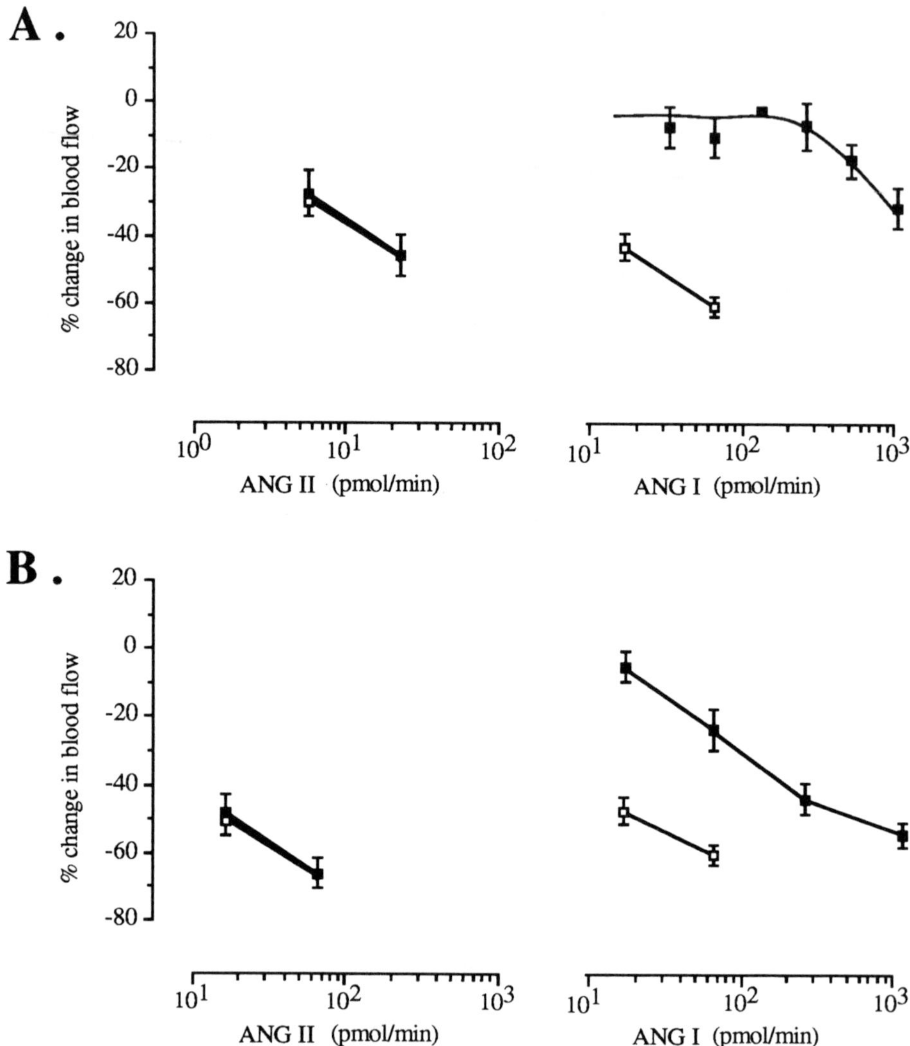

Figure 2. The effects of arterial infusions of angiotensin I (ANG I) and angiotensin II (ANG II) on blood flow in the forearm in the presence (■) and absence of ACE inhibitor (□). (A) The effects of intra-arterial co-infusion of enalaprilat (10 μg/min). Redrawn from Benjamin *et al.* [26] with permission. (B) The effects of treatment with oral enalapril (10 mg) 4 h previously. Redrawn from Cockcroft *et al.* [30] with permission.

compared with those in a normotensive control group. Here, caution is required in interpretation for two reasons: first, the baseline alters whether changes in absolute flow or calculated vascular resistance are used [35]; and second, with constant rate infusion, the drug concentration and its effect on blood flow will depend on the prevailing forearm blood flow. In addition, hypertension is associated with enhanced sensitivity to a broad range of locally infused vasoconstrictors [36], probably through development of vascular hypertrophy. One way to handle this issue is to find doses of two or more drugs that have an equivalent effect on blood flow in normotensive subjects, and show whether this relationship changes in hypertensive patients [37]. Difficulties arise also if studies are performed in normotensive subjects in whom arterial pressure alters in a consistent manner between different phases of the study. Studies in hand veins may be helpful here, though the assumption is made that any altered sensitivity in hypertension is shared by the arterial and venous systems.

Another problem arises with the use of vasodilator drugs to examine vasoconstrictor mechanisms. It might be assumed that, if intra-arterial infusion of the dihydropyridine calcium antagonist, nicardipine, reversed the vasoconstriction produced by intra-arterial endothelin-1, vasoconstriction to endothelin-1 involves dihydropyridine-sensitive calcium channels. However, when nicardipine is given in this manner it causes an increase of forearm blood flow to values substantially above basal [31]. This implies that at least some, and perhaps all, of the effect of nicardipine is mediated against basal arteriolar tone, rather than specifically against vasoconstriction to endothelin-1. A lack of specificity against endothelin-1 is also supported by the observation that nicardipine causes greater reversal of forearm vasoconstriction induced by angiotensin II [31]. Other workers have used an alternative approach to overcome the problem of basal tone, by eliciting maximum vasodilatation to intra-arterial calcium antagonists before administration of endothelin-1 [38]. However, this by no means removes all of the underlying tone, as the maximum forearm blood flow during post-ischaemia hyperaemia is substantially greater than that achieved using calcium antagonists. Also, in the prolonged studies needed to examine the effects of endothelin-1, the doses of vasodilators used intra-arterially are close to those exerting systemic effects with potential for stimulation of reflex responses. Many of these difficulties can be overcome by examining vascular sensitivity in the dorsal hand veins since they have no basal tone, and any drug-induced dilatation of venoconstriction is more likely to be specific [39].

LOCAL INHIBITION OF VASCULAR ENZYMES

By giving angiotensin I and II by brachial arterial infusion, with and without co-infusion of the ACE inhibitor enalaprilat, it has been possible to show that angiotensin I is a vasoconstrictor in forearm resistance vessels only after conversion to angiotensin II [26] (Figure 2). The rate of conversion of angiotensin I in the forearm, at around 40%, is similar to that across the pulmonary circulation, suggesting that the lung does not have a central role in angiotensin I conversion. Interestingly, the effects of locally infused enalaprilat on responses to angiotensin I far outlast the time for which it is being infused, even though there is no evidence of systemic ACE inhibition. Because the circulation time within the forearm is less than 15 s, and the local effect of enalaprilat lasts over 20 min, these studies show that angiotensin I conversion is a function of tissue ACE within the blood vessel wall rather than of ACE circulating in blood [26,40]. Inhibition of vascular ACE also produces a leftward shift of the dose response to bradykinin, confirming that ACE is responsible for the metabolism of this dilator substance *in vivo* [26]. ACE is not, however, responsible for metabolism of substance P [41] or atrial natriuretic peptide [42] in the human forearm.

It has been shown recently that the vascular endothelium produces many potent vasoactive substances with important actions on the underlying vascular smooth muscle. One such endothelial mediator is the vasodilator nitric oxide (NO), generated from L-arginine by the action of the NO synthase enzyme, the so-called L-arginine–NO pathway. A specific substrate analogue inhibitor of NO synthase, N^G-monomethyl-L-arginine (L-NMMA), has been employed in arterial studies in healthy subjects [43] to examine the role of NO in regulation of vascular tone. Because L-NMMA produces around a 50% reduction in resting blood flow, it is clear that basal production of NO plays a major role in opposing vasoconstrictor influences in the forearm. That this is important in regulation of arterial pressure has recently been confirmed in systemic studies with L-NMMA [44]. Another important local mediator is the vasoconstrictor endothelin, generated from a prohormone, big-endothelin, by the action of a unique 'endothelin converting enzyme' (ECE). Arterial studies have recently been performed using phosphoramidon, a weak inhibitor of neutral endopeptidase 25.11 (NEP 25.11), but a substantially more potent inhibitor of ECE. Phosphoramidon increases forearm blood flow but potent inhibitors of NEP 25.11 do not. Therefore, it appears that endothelin, like NO, may play an important part in maintenance of basal vascular tone [45]. Such studies serve to emphasise the importance of the endothelium in regulation of the function of underlying vascular smooth muscle.

ASSESSMENT OF ENDOTHELIAL FUNCTION

The importance of the endothelium in regulation of vascular function has been reviewed widely [46–48]. Impaired endothelial function has been described in hypertension, atherosclerosis, hyperlipidaemia and diabetes mellitus; all of which are associated with an increased risk of vascular events, particularly stroke and heart attack. Because NO is a potent vasodilator and inhibits platelet adhesion and aggregation, reduced NO production may contribute to cardiovascular risk. Most of the patient studies of endothelial function have used arterial infusion of the muscarinic agonist acetylcholine to stimulate production of NO-mediated vasodilatation (via the NO synthase enzyme), and sodium nitroprusside to generate NO spontaneously (independent of the NO synthase enzyme). It is important to choose the muscarinic agonist carefully because some agents, such as methacholine, appear to cause vasodilatation that is not NO-mediated [49].

Generally, patient studies have shown selective impairment of the responses to acetylcholine, and their findings, at least in hypertension, have subsequently been confirmed using the NO synthase inhibitor L-NMMA [37]. Recently, ACE inhibitors have been shown to improve endothelial function in patients with hypertension [50], and cholesterol-lowering drugs have been shown to improve endothelial function in patients with hypercholesterolaemia [51]. In view of the major significance of the L-arginine–NO pathway in regulation of blood vessel and platelet function, studies designated to examine whether drugs have beneficial effects on endothelial function are likely to become more widespread.

ASSESSMENT OF SYMPATHETIC FUNCTION AND MEDIATOR RELEASE

Application of a small degree of negative pressure to the lower body (10–15 mmHg) causes retention of venous blood within the legs, leading to unloading of low-pressure cardiopulmonary baroreceptors and around a 20% reduction in the blood flow of both forearms [52]. Forearm vasoconstriction occurs through a local increase in sympathetic nerve activity without affecting arterial pressure or heart rate [52].

Coupled with intra-arterial drug administration, low doses of angiotensin II, without direct effects on blood flow [52], markedly and selectively enhance sympathetic vasoconstriction, approximately doubling the reduction in blood flow in the infused arm. Further confirmation of these findings has been provided in a study in which bilateral antecubital vein sampling showed increased noradrenaline overflow during angiotensin II infusion [53]. These effects are specific to agents which enhance sympathetic function and can be used to screen for peripheral sympathetic facilitation. These effects are not found non-specifically with other vasoconstrictor mediators such as neuropeptide Y, noradrenaline or endothelin.

ASSESSMENT OF ARTERIOVENOUS SELECTIVITY

Several methods exist for studying venous responses in the upper limb [54]. It is possible to study compliance in deep forearm veins using venous occlusion plethysmography and such studies can be performed during intra-arterial infusion to assess simultaneously the effects of drugs on the arteries and veins. More widely used, and perhaps of greater utility, is the assessment of venous compliance in a single dorsal hand vein, particularly when used with the technique described by Aellig [55], which has superseded earlier methods. One limitation of this method is that the vein has to be pre-constricted to study dilator agents, and responses may depend on the constrictor agent chosen; noradrenaline is preferred generally, being the endogenous mediator of sympathetic tone [56]. There may well be differences between responses in the deep and superficial veins. Because the deep veins do not participate in the venomotor reflexes [57], and the hand veins are easier to study, these are generally used in preference to the deep veins.

Studies in forearm resistance vessels and hand veins have generated important evidence concerning the arterioselectivity of many drugs [58], identifying the relatively venoselective agents like the organic nitrates, the mixed acting agents like prazosin and verapamil, and the arterioselective agents like hydralazine and nifedipine. More recently, the same technique has been used to show that the potassium channel opener cromakalim is arterioselective [59]. Because venodilatation may be of benefit, for instance in congestive heart failure, such studies may be important to determining the likely clinical profile of a drug.

Summary

The measurement of forearm blood flow by venous occlusion plethysmography using lightweight externally applied strain gauges provides a relatively simple means to assess the effects of drugs on vascular structure and function. When coupled with local drug infusion through the brachial artery of one arm, measurement of blood flow in both forearms allows very precise assessment of drug effects on vascular smooth muscle *in vivo*, with the non-infused arm acting as a contemporaneous control.

Intra-arterial drug infusion allows the use of very small drug doses and avoids their influence on arterial pressure and neurohumoral reflexes and on other organs such as the heart and kidney. Full dose responses to vasoconstrictors and dilators can then be studied, including alterations in sensitivity caused by drugs or disease. The arterial technique has been widely applied to examine whether the function of blood vessels differs in health and disease and, during local drug infusion, responses in the forearm tend to reflect those of the major resistance beds. This technique has also been used to assess the effects of drugs on sympathetic and endothelial function, local mediator release and *ex vivo* platelet aggregation. Furthermore, evidence of inhibition of an arterially administered vasoconstrictor, such as endothelin, can be established using a systemically administered antagonist in dose-ranging studies that might not readily be considered using systemic administration of this potent vasoconstrictor peptide. Coupled with venous studies, brachial artery studies have also provided the basis for assessing the relative arterioselectivity of many drugs. Used appropriately, these techniques provide extremely valuable and powerful tools in the evaluation of drugs during their early clinical development.

References

1. Mosso A. I movimenti dei vasi sanguigni. Atti R Accad Sci Torino, Classe di scienze fisiche e matematiche 1875/6; 11: 21–81.
2. Hewlett AW, van Zwaluwenburg JG. The rate of blood flow in the arm. Heart 1909; 1: 87–97.
3. Abramson DI, Ferris EB Jr. Responses of blood vessels in the resting hand and forearm to various stimuli. Am Heart J 1940; 19: 541–553.
4. Kerslake DMcK. The effect of the application of an arterial occlusion cuff to the wrist on the blood flow in the human forearm. J Physiol (Lond) 1949; 108: 451–457.
5. Cooper KE, Edholm OG, Mottram RF. The blood flow in skin and muscle of the human forearm. J Physiol (Lond) 1955; 128: 258–267.
6. Zelis R, Mason DT, Braunwald E. Partition of blood flow to the cutaneous and muscular beds of the forearm at rest and during leg exercise in normal subjects and in patients with heart failure. Circ Res 1969; 24: 799–806.
7. Whitney RJ. The measurement of volume changes in human limbs. J Physiol (Lond) 1953; 121: 1–27.
8. Ensink FBM, Hellige G. History and principle of strain-gauge plethysmography. In: Jageneau AHM (ed), Noninvasive Methods on Cardiovascular Haemodynamics. Amsterdam: Elsevier/North Holland, 1981; 169–183.
9. Ensink FBM, Baller D, Wolpers HG, Zipfel J, Hellige G. The reliability of venous capacity and blood flow determination by plethysmography. In: Jageneau AHM (ed), Noninvasive Methods on Cardiovascular Haemodynamics. Amsterdam: Elsevier/North Holland, 1981; 215–226.
10. Roberts DH, Tsao Y, Breckenridge AM. The reproducibility of limb flow measurements in human volunteers at rest and after exercise by using mercury in Silastic strain gauge plethysmography under standardised conditions. Clin Sci 1986; 70: 635–638.
11. Fox JS, Whitehead EM, Shanks RG. Cardiovascular effects of cromakalim (BRL 34915) in healthy volunteers. Br J Clin Pharmacol 1991; 32: 45–49.
12. Scott RA, Woods KL, Barnett DB. The effects of flosequinan on regional blood flow in normal man. Br J Clin Pharmacol 1991; 31: 41–46.
13. Thomas SHL, Clark KL, Allen R, Smith SE. A comparison of the cardiovascular effects of phenylpropanolamine and phenylephrine containing cold remedies. Br J Clin Pharmacol 1991; 32: 705–711.
14. Motwani JG, Struthers AD. Dose–response study of the redistribution of intravascular volume by angiotensin II in man. Clin Sci 1992; 82: 397–405.

15. Patterson GC, Whelan RF. Reactive hyperaemia in the human forearm. Clin Sci 1955; 14: 197–211.
16. Takeshita A, Mark AL. Decreased vasodilator capacity of forearm resistance vessels in borderline hypertension. Hypertension 1980; 2: 610–616.
17. Pedrinelli R, Spessot M, Salvetti A. Reactive hyperemia during short-term blood flow and pressure changes in the hypertensive forearm. J Hypertens 1990; 8: 467–471.
18. Conway J. A vascular abnormality in hypertension: a study of blood flow in the forearm. Circulation 1963; 27: 520–529.
19. Folkow B. Physiological aspects of primary hypertension. Physiol Rev 1982; 62: 347–504.
20. Sivertsson R, Hansson L. Effects of blood pressure reduction on the structural vascular abnormality in skin and muscle vascular beds in human essential hypertension. Clin Sci Mol Med 1976; 51: 77s–79s.
21. Julius S, Mejia A, Jones K, Krause L et al. 'White coat' versus 'sustained' borderline hypertension in Tecumseh, Michigan. Hypertension 1990; 16: 617–623.
22. Agabiti-Rosei E, Muiesan ML, Rizzoni D, Romanelli G, Beschi M, Castellano M. Regression of cardiovascular structural changes after long-term antihypertensive treatment with the calcium antagonist nitrendipine. J Cardiovasc Pharmacol 1991; 18 (Suppl 5): S5–S9.
23. Dahlöf B. Regression of left ventricular hypertrophy: are there differences between antihypertensive agents. Cardiology 1992; 81: 307–315.
24. Allen WJ, Barcroft H, Edholm OG. On the action of adrenaline on the blood vessels in human skeletal muscle. J Physiol (Lond) 1946; 105: 255–267.
25. Barcroft H, Konzett H. On the actions of noradrenaline, adrenaline and isopropyl noradrenaline on the arterial blood pressure, heart rate and muscle blood flow in man. J Physiol (Lond) 1949; 110: 194–204.
26. Benjamin N, Cockcroft JR, Collier JG, Dollery CD, Ritter JM, Webb DJ. Local inhibition of converting enzyme and vascular responses to angiotensin and bradykinin in the human forearm. J Physiol (Lond) 1989; 412: 543–555.
27. Greenfield ADM, Patterson GC. Reactions of the blood vessels of the human forearm to increases in transmural pressure. J Physiol (Lond) 1954; 125: 508–524.
28. Saumet JL, Kellogg DL Jr, Taylor WF, Johnson JM. Cutaneous laser-Doppler flowmetry: influence of underlying muscle blood flow. J Appl Physiol 1988; 65: 478–481.
29. Webb DJ, Benjamin N, Allen MJ, Brown J, O'Flynn M, Cockcroft JR. Vascular responses to local atrial natriuretic peptide infusion in man. Br J Clin Pharmacol 1988; 26: 245–252.
30. Cockcroft JR, Sciberras DG, Goldberg MR, Ritter JM. Comparison of angiotensin-converting enzyme inhibition with angiotensin II receptor antagonism in the human forearm. J Cardiovasc Pharmacol 1993; 22: 579–584.
31. Clarke JG, Benjamin N, Larkin SW et al. Endothelin is a potent long-lasting vasoconstrictor in men. Am J Physiol 1989; 257 (Heart Circ Physiol 26): H2033–2035.
32. Haynes WG, Clarke J, Cockcroft J, Webb DJ. Pharmacology of endothelin-1 in vivo in man. J Cardiovasc Pharmacol 1991; 17 (Suppl 7): S284–S286.
33. Ashton H. Peripheral circulation in man: critical closure in human limbs. Br Med Bull 1963; 19: 149–154.
34. Dahlöf B, Gustafsson D, Hedner T, Jern S, Hansson L. Regional haemodynamic effects of endothelin-1 in rat and man: unexpected adverse reactions. J Hypertens 1990; 8: 811–817.

35. Robinson BF. Assessment of responses to drugs in forearm resistance vessels and hand veins of man: techniques and problems. In: Kuhlmann J, Wingender WW (eds), Dose–Response Relationship of Drugs. München: Zuckswerdt Verlag, 1990; 40–43.
36. Doyle AE, Fraser JRE, Marshall RJ. Reactivity of forearm vessels to vasoconstrictor substances in hypertensive and normotensive subjects. Clin Sci 1959; 18: 441–454.
37. Calver A, Collier J, Moncada S, Vallance P. Effect of intra-arterial N^G-monomethyl-L-arginine in patients with hypertension: the nitric oxide mechanism appears abnormal. J Hypertens 1992; 10: 1025–1031.
38. Kiowski W, Lüscher TF, Linder L, Bühler FR. Endothelin-1 induced vasoconstriction in humans: reversal by calcium channel blockade but not by nitrovasodilators or endothelium derived relaxing factor. Circulation 1991; 83: 468–475.
39. Haynes WG, Webb DG. Venoconstriction to endothelin-1 in humans: the role of calcium and potassium channels. Am J Physiol 1993; 265 (Heart Circ Physiol 34): H1676–H1681.
40. Webb DJ, Collier JG. Vascular angiotensin conversion in humans. J Cardiovasc Pharmacol 1986; 8 (Suppl 10): S40–S45.
41. Benjamin N, Webb DJ. The effect of local converting enzyme inhibition on the dilator response to substance P in the human forearm. Br J Clin Pharmacol 1990; 29: 774–776.
42. Cockcroft JR, Allen MJ, Benjamin N, Webb DJ. The effect of local angiotensin converting enzyme inhibition on the action of atrial natriuretic peptide in the human forearm. J Hum Hypertens 1989; 3: 49–52.
43. Vallance P, Collier J, Moncada S. Effects of endothelium-derived nitric oxide on peripheral arteriolar tone in man. Lancet 1989; ii: 977–999.
44. Haynes WG, Noon JP, Walker BR, Webb DJ. L-NMMA increases blood pressure in man. Lancet 1993; ii: 931–932.
45. Haynes WG, Webb DJ. Contribution of endogenous enthothelin-1 to basal vascular tone in man. Lancet 1994; 344: 852–854.
46. Henderson AH. Endothelium in control. Br Heart J 1991; 65: 116–125.
47. Bassenge E. Clinical relevance of endothelium-derived relaxing factor (ERDF). Br J Clin Pharmacol 1992; 34: 37S–42S.
48. Lüscher TF. Heterogeneity of endothelial dysfunction in hypertension. Eur Heart J 1992; 13 (Suppl D): 50–55.
49. Chowienczyk PJ, Cockcroft JR, Ritter JM. Differential inhibition by N^G-monomethyl-L-arginine of vasodilator effects of acetylcholine and methacholine in human forearm vasculature. Br J Pharmacol 1993; 110: 736–738.
50. Hirooka Y, Imaizumi T, Masaki H et al. Captopril improves impaired endothelium-dependent vasodilation in hypertensive patients. Hypertension 1992; 20: 175–180.
51. Leung W-H, Lau C-P, Wong C-K. Beneficial effect of cholesterol-lowering therapy on coronary endothelium-dependent relaxation in hypercholesterolaemic patients. Lancet 1993; i: 1496–1500.
52. Seidelin PH, Collier JG, Struthers AD, Webb DJ. Angiotensin II augments sympathetically mediated arteriolar constriction in man. Clin Sci 1991; 81: 261–266.
53. Taddei S, Favilla S, Duranti P, Simonini N, Salvetti A. Vascular renin–angiotensin system and neurotransmission in hypertensive persons. Hypertension 1991; 18: 266–277.
54. Robinson BF. Assessment of the effect of drugs on the venous system in man. Br J Clin Pharmacol 1978; 6: 381–386.

55. Aellig WH. A new technique for recording compliance of human hand veins. Br J Clin Pharmacol 1981; 11: 237–243.
56. Benjamin N, Collier JG, Webb DJ. Angiotensin II augments sympathetically induced venoconstriction in man. Clin Sci 1988; 75: 337–340.
57. Zelis R, Mason DT. Comparison of the reflex reactivity of skin and muscle veins in the human forearm. J Clin Invest 1969; 48: 1870–1877.
58. Robinson BF, Collier JG. Vascular smooth muscle: correlations between basic properties and responses of human blood-vessels. Br Med Bull 1979; 35: 305–312.
59. Webb DJ, Benjamin N, Vallance P. The potassium channel opening drug cromakalim produces arterioselective vasodilatation in the upper limbs of normal volunteers. Br J Clin Pharmacol 1989; 27: 757–761.

9 WHAT ARE THE VALID MEASUREMENTS OF DRUG EFFICACY IN PATIENTS WITH INTERMITTENT CLAUDICATION?

P. Demol and T. R. Weihrauch
Bayer AG, Research Centre, Wuppertal, Germany

Introduction

In Europe, many drugs are available to treat chronic peripheral arterial occlusive disease [1]. Unfortunately, their real clinical efficacy and utility have not been substantiated by well-controlled clinical trials. Moreover, no dose-finding trial has been realised in this field, which means that the proposed dosage could be totally irrelevant.

Although the treadmill exercise test is considered as the gold standard to test the efficacy of a new drug, several other technologies have been proposed as potential surrogates. Recently precise guidelines have been proposed from different health authorities but they are somewhat contradictory.

The aim of this presentation is to review the validity of the assessment techniques and their potential use in clinical trials.

DEFINITION

Intermittent claudication (IC), which is a consequence of chronic occlusive peripheral arterial disease of the legs, is defined as pain usually in the calfs, that develops with muscle exercise. Pain must come as a muscle cramp in the thigh or calf after the patient has walked a predictable dis-

Clinical Measurement in Drug Evaluation. Edited by W. S. Nimmo and G. T. Tucker
© 1995 John Wiley & Sons Ltd

tance; it must be relieved after a predictable period of time and should recur after walking a similar distance again [2].

PHYSIOPATHOLOGICAL FACTORS

Resistance at the level of an arterial stenosis results in a lower potential energy distal to the stenosis and a decrease in distal mean pressure and pulse pressure [2]. Pain during exercise is the result of an imbalance between metabolic needs of the muscle and the capacity of the vascular system to bring enough blood to this muscle as a result of stenosis.

INCIDENCE AND RISK FACTORS

Peripheral arterial occlusive disease (PAOD) is common as it affects more than 5% of the population and increases steadily with age [3–5]. The incidence of new cases has a male to female ratio of 2 : 1 and follows a similar pattern to that for angina, but occurring a decade later. Major risk factors are cigarette smoking (which increases the risk two- to four-fold both in men and women), hypertension (two-fold increased risk) and diabetes (vascular disease of extremities occurs 20 times more frequently compared to non-diabetics). The role of lipids is less clear.

In terms of *local* disease, IC runs a relatively benign course: symptoms remain stable or improve in around 70% of patients and amputation is required for less than 10% of cases [6]. However, compared with the general population of similar age, the mortality of men with chronic leg ischaemia is more than three times higher after 10 years [7]. The average life expectancy is decreased by 10 years, principally because of associated atherosclerotic cardiac and brain disease, with 75% of deaths being of cardiovascular origin.

In other words: 'All patients with peripheral vascular disease should be considered to be at life long risk for fatal and non-fatal cardiac events and should undergo appropriate clinical and laboratory evaluation and be treated appropriately' [8].

Diagnosis of intermittent claudication

HISTORY AND CLINICAL EVALUATION

Detailed clinical interview and physical examination remain essential. Interview can be assessed by the WHO/Rose Questionnaire [9]. This questionnaire has a high specificity (96%) but a low sensitivity (only around 55% for large-vessel peripheral arterial disease [10]). More recently, Leng and Fowkes [11] proposed a modified improved questionnaire—the Edinburgh Claudication Questionnaire—which they showed had the same specificity as the Rose Questionnaire (99.3%) but a much better sensitivity (91.3%).

NON-INVASIVE VASCULAR DIAGNOSTIC ASSESSMENT METHODS

Non-invasive diagnostic assessment techniques are assuming an increasingly important role in the management of patients with PAOD [12]. These non-invasive techniques should be used in clinical trials also whenever possible.

The two principal non-invasive techniques for vascular assessment are ultrasound and plethysmography. With improvements in both direct real-time B-mode ultrasonic imaging, Doppler ultrasonic detection of flow and colour Doppler flow mapping, plethysmography and other indirect techniques are assuming a more limited role in vascular management and clinical trials. The Doppler ultrasonic detector is the most simple, versatile and widespread method available for screening and follow-up of vascular disease: it has the virtue of simplicity and low cost to measure peripheral arterial pressure and the ankle brachial pressure index (ratio of systolic pressure of ankle to arm) or ABI.

Real-time B mode associated with Doppler spectral analysis (duplex scanning) and Doppler colour flow (DCF) mapping offers the most accurate method to detect, quantify and follow the course of PAOD [12].

In a prospective study, DCF has been shown to diagnose accurately iliac and femoropopliteal disease (correlation factor of around 0.8 with the gold standard, angiography) [13]. DCF is a useful screening procedure that could prevent unnecessary angiography in clinical trials [14–16]. More recently, more sophisticated techniques, like the electro-magnetic flow meter, have made it possible to analyse the muscle pulsatile arterial flow, which is considered to be the most relevant measurement for PAOD [17].

Measurements

Ultrasonic and plethysmographic instruments provide the clinician with four measurements that are of value in evaluating vascular disease: arterial pressure, blood velocity, pulse waveforms, and vascular imaging.

Arterial pressure

The measurement of arterial pressure at the ankle allows detection of haemodynamically significant arterial stenosis: a diameter reduction of $>50\%$ in a major leg artery will cause the systolic pressure to drop below the arm value [18].

The ABI is the best indicator of the presence or absence of 'haemodyna-mically significant' arterial occlusive disease [19].

Normal subjects have an ABI of >0.97 [20]. Typically patients with IC have an ABI of <0.95 and >0.5. Patients with later stages of disease have usually an ABI of <0.5 or an absolute systolic pressure of <50 mmHg. Studies have confirmed a good correlation between ABI and the percen-tage stenosis by angiogram [21] and 95% sensitivity for ABI of <0.9 for detecting angiographically proven disease [22]. The ABI is a non-invasive marker of diffuse atherosclerosis: an ABI of <0.9 is associated with a two-fold increase in risk of prevalent cardiovascular disease [23].

ABI is also an independent predictor of mortality and there is a direct correlation between the level of ABI and survival [24].

To quantify further the functional impairment of patients with claudica-tion, the response of ankle pressure to treadmill exercise may be deter-mined [25–27]. In healthy persons the ankle pressure will not fall in the minutes following exercise, whereas legs with claudication will show a drop by an amount and duration (for up 30 min) that is proportional to the severity of the arterial disease (Figure 1). A drop of more than 10% is used as inclusion criteria in drug trials. The ABI is very useful for screen-ing patients for entry in clinical trials. However, it is too insensitive a therapy to be useful for analysing efficacy. A change of at least 0.15 has to be observed before it can be considered significant, i.e. indicative of

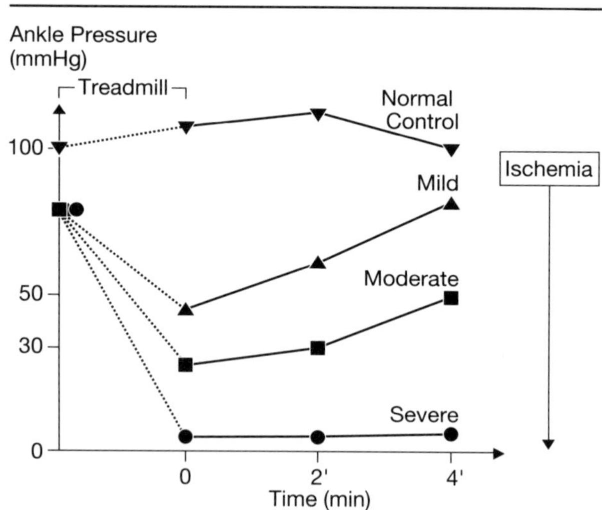

Figure 1. Changes in ankle pressure in the minutes following the treadmill exer-cise. While in normal controls no significant change is observed, the drop of arterial pressure in claudicants is related to the severity of the ischaemia (severity of arter-ial disease). Adapted from Boccalon [17]

changed haemodynamics [28]. Moreover, as ABI is 'poorly correlated' to the walking distance measured by treadmill [29], it cannot be used as a substitute efficacy parameter.

Blood velocity

Spectral analysis of the pulsed Doppler data offer the possibility of localising vascular stenosis.

Pulse waveform analysis

In conjunction with plethysmography this is useful in the case of a diabetic patient with calcified extremities which preclude accurate ultrasound pressure measurements [12].

Arterial flow

Arterial flow is more relevant to vascular disease than pressure. Recent new technology, electromagnetic flowmetry [17] and NMR (nuclear magnetic resonance) flowmetry, have made it possible to measure the *pulsatile* arterial flow, which is already abnormal in Fontaine stage I, contrary to the mean arterial flow. However, these techniques are not available for large clinical trials. They could be used in small pilot phase IIa studies to obtain a pharmacodynamic profile in relation to the kinetic profile of new drugs. To our knowledge no such trial has been published.

INVASIVE VASCULAR DIAGNOSIS

Arteriography remains the diagnostic standard for PAOD diagnosis. However, it has two major limitations [12]:

- The cost, discomfort and risks pre-empt the routine use of angiography for screening and follow-up procedures in clinical studies.
- The morphological methods are not directly (well) correlated with the haemodynamic impairment. Arteriography is only indicated when a surgical intervention is planned.

Recently introduced magnetic resonance imaging techniques allow the investigator to analyse more precisely than arteriography all the aspects of atherosclerosis: size, shape and lipid content of atheroma plaques, arterial compliance, pulse-wave velocity and pattern of flow can be studied [30]. This non-invasive technique could become an important tool in studying the effect of drugs in interventional trials.

Relevance for clinical trials

The European Guidelines for clinical trials [31] strongly suggest that arteriography should be available for patients included in clinical trials. However, today arteriography is only considered necessary for patients awaiting surgery. The newly published Guidelines of the German Society of Angiology [32] suggest that either arteriography or duplex scanning should be available for each patient in pivotal trials. However, as a practical approach in clinical trials, segmental pressures realised with Doppler ultrascanning can provide a good idea of the location of vascular lesions and differentiate between lesions at thigh and calf level.

Treatment

Drugs of various classes are prescribed widely for IC, although their clinical efficiency has not been proven adequately. The major classes are: rheological agents (e.g., pentoxifylline), vasodilators (e.g., nifedipine), antiplatelet drugs (e.g., aspirin), anticoagulants (e.g., warfarin), prostanoids (e.g., Iloprost) and metabolic enhancers (e.g., derivates of L-carnitine) [1].

Around three-quarters of all trials of drug therapy for IC published between 1965 and 1985 were found to have serious flaws of design [33]. The main problems were lack of a placebo control group, failure to use a double-blind randomised design, inadequate sample size (no statistical power calculation), no objective measurement of claudication distance, too short a duration of treatment and no dose finding. Surprisingly, no dose finding has been published in the field even with the most tested drug, pentoxifylline: the trial realised by Lindgärde *et al.* [34] according to European Guidelines has compared only one dose of pentoxifylline to placebo. In view of these deficiencies guidelines for design have been proposed [31,32,33].

Guidelines for assessment of drug efficacy

Clinical trials of new drugs in IC should be realised according to general rules of clinical methodology and also according to specific guidelines proposed by different health authorities. The most important guidelines for trials in IC are as follows:

- Absolute necessity of a precise definition of the principal objective. The main objective is to increase the walking distance (WD) analysed with the treadmill test. According to the German Guidelines the WD observed at the end of treatment should be 50–60% higher than the baseline value and at least 30% better than the placebo value [32]. Determination of the WD with the treadmill should be realised under standardised conditions (see below).

- Specification of entry criteria:

  - History of more than six months stable claudication.
  - Confirmation of the diagnosis, type of occlusion and its location, if possible by angiography [31] or colour Doppler flow mapping [32].
  - Resting ABI between 0.9 and 0.5 or post-treadmill decrease of ABI of more than 10%. Absolute value of ankle systolic pressure not below 60 mmHg at both ankles and in both the dorsalis pedis and the posterior tibial arteries.
  - Stable WD measured by treadmill during the run-in phase (less than 25% change between two successive measurements).
  - Absolute WD between 100 and 300 m [32] or initial claudication distance between 50 and 200 m [34] as assessed by standardised treadmill.

Patients with concurrent diseases interfering with treadmill testing or with later stages of Fontaine (stages III and IV) should be excluded from a trial.

- A placebo-controlled group is essential because untreated claudication improves spontaneously. Walking time may increase by 30% after one year [35]. Comparative trials should be realised only once the drug has been shown to be more effective than a placebo because no drug is accepted as a standard reference drug. For NDA (New Drug Application) submission a comparative trial is not necessary. Comparative trials, however, can be useful for price negotiation and could include a cost-effectiveness analysis.
- Studies should be double-blind and randomised because suggestion appears to have significant effects on claudication distance [36].
- Concomitant therapy which could interfere with the interpretation of the results should be avoided as well as intensive exercise training, which has a potent positive effect on walking capacity [37].
- Necessity of statistical power: sample size must be adequately based on primary objectives and defined in the trial protocol.
- Study duration: according to most experts, an effective drug should already show some signs of efficacy during the first month of therapy. However, the duration of pivotal studies should be at least eight weeks [38]. The EC Guidelines [31] request at least six months therapy because the effect of drugs can fluctuate in time, as was observed in the decisive pentoxifylline trial [39] (Figure 2). Moreover, certain drugs like carnitine derivates can show a short-term (three weeks) strongly

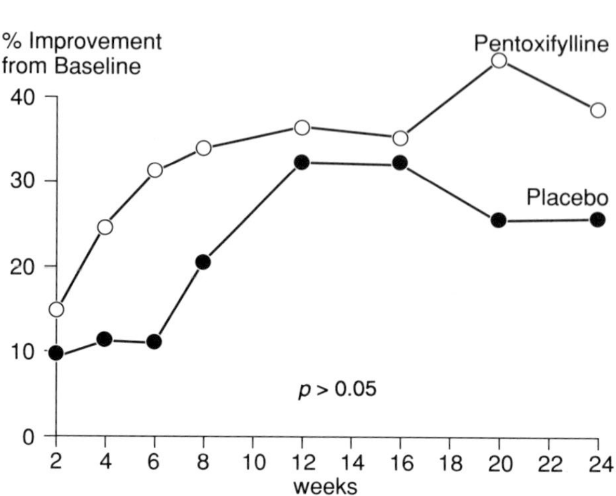

Figure 2. Although statistically significant the percentage increase of the AWD induced by Pentoxifylline in comparison to placebo is not impressive and fluctuates with time. This study demonstrates the necessity of a placebo arm as the spontaneous improvement reaches around 25% after six months. Reproduced from Porter *et al.* [39]

positive effect [40], which was not confirmed in a larger six-month trial [41].

The placebo-controlled treatment period should be preceded by a run-in phase of 2 to 4 weeks during which the stability of the WD is tested by repeated treadmill.

- Necessity of dose-finding trials: at least two doses (ideally three) should be compared with a placebo in pivotal trials (this has never been realised in this field, and it is impossible to know whether higher doses of drugs on the market would show higher efficacy). Ideally the integration of pharmacokinetic and pharmacodynamic analyses, i.e. interrelating concentration and drug action, should be investigated in phase I–II trials [42]. This assessment is a great help in accelerating the clinical development of new drugs, as stated recently by Judy Weissinger from the US Food and Drug Administration (FDA) [43]: 'Development of pharmaceuticals without incorporating kinetic and dynamic information is currently associated with more costly, more time consuming, less utilisable knowledge and subsequent studies are often needed to explain anomalous results.'

Technical assessment of drug efficacy

TREADMILL EXERCISE

Treadmill exercise is the gold standard of assessing response to treatment because it is easily standardised, which is absolutely essential for multi-centre trials.

Official guidelines recommend a slope between 10% and 12% and a speed around 3–3.2 km/h (around 2 miles/h). The absolute WD and pain-free (claudication) WD are to be measured. However, this single-stage 'constant load work' treadmill is characterised by a large inter-individual variability [44], which means the necessity of a large number of patients to demonstrate superiority over a placebo (the coefficient of variation (CV) is between 30% and 45%). Several authors [20,45–47] have analysed the variability of WD when patients are submitted to two different treadmill conditions: a classical single-stage treadmill (constant speed of 2 km/h and a fixed slope of 10%), and a progressive treadmill (same speed but progressive increase in slope of 2–3.5% every 2 min). The progressive treadmill protocols more than halved (from around 40% to less than 20%) the CV of both initial and maximal WD. The major advantage of this progressive (adaptative) protocol is to reduce the number of patients necessary for clinical trials. However, until now this procedure has not been included in official guidelines. Moreover, Bollinger (Zürich) doubts that such protocols which last up to 15 min are applicable to patients who often have heart problems (personal communication).

Gardner *et al.* [46] have analysed also the effect of handrail support during treadmill test on the reliability during single-stage and progressive protocols (Table 1). They confirmed that the progressive protocol

Table 1. Reliability of claudication responses during repeated walking test [46]

	CV (%)	
Protocol	ICD	ACD
Single stage		
Handrail	31	28
No handrail	22	20
Progressive		
Handrail	33	17
No handrail	22	11

ICD, claudication pain distance; CV, coefficient of variation; ACD, maximal walking distance.

decreased significantly the CV of ACD when realised with a handrail (17% v. 28% respectively), although no difference was seen for the ICD (31% v. 33%). Interestingly the absence of handrail significantly reduced the CV of ACD during the single-stage protocol (20% v. 28%) and the progressive protocol (11% v. 17%). The lowest CV was observed for the ACD obtained with the progressive protocol without the handrail (11%).

The conclusion of the study is that handrail support should not be allowed unless balance cannot otherwise be maintained.

Baker and Dix [28] have measured the variability of ankle pressures, branchial–ankle pressure gradient and ABI at rest. The CV was the lowest with ABI. Ten repeated measurements in one patient showed a CV between 11% and 13% for right and left index. These authors recommend use of the ABI instead of the gradient. They showed also that the ABI had to change at least 0.15 before it could be considered significant.

Post-exercise measurements of ABI do not show an improvement in CV in comparison with resting ABI (Table 2). However, resting or post-exercise changes in ankle systolic pressure and ABI are insensitive to drug treatment and exercise training and cannot be used in clinical trials to assess drug efficacy [20,35]. Recently Feinberg et al. [48] proposed the concept of 'ischaemic window', which is the area under the curve of the post-exercise reduction of ankle pressure and its recovery over time (Figure 3). They showed that a 12-week intensive exercise therapy induced a significant (around 59%) reduction of the ischaemic window which was correlated with a strong increase in absolute WD (more than 600%). Absolute resting ankle pressure and ABI were unchanged in this study. The sensitivity to drug treatment of this ischaemic window has, however, not been tested until now.

Reactive hyperaemia (realised with 4 min cuff occlusion of the thigh) does not increase the diagnostic accuracy of PAOD compared with ABI [49]. Moreover it is tolerated poorly [20].

Other techniques

Several techniques to analyse drug efficacy in IC have been proposed either to serve as surrogate to the treadmill test or to provide complementary information on the mechanism of drug effect.

ACHILLES REFLEX: HALF-RELAXATION TIME

In 1970, Grüntzig and Bollinger [50] proposed a simple technique to analyse the direct effects of blood flow impairment on muscle functioning: photomotography of the Achilles reflex. The half-relaxation time (HRT) of the Achilles reflex had been used since the 1950s to diagnose thyroid diseases. The test may be done directly after the treadmill. The photocell of the apparatus allows the registration of a contraction and relaxation curve after induction of the reflex.

In normal controls the HRT lies around 100.2 ± 22.9 ms (SD). This value increases to 180.9 ± 52.7 ms with claudicant legs ($p < 0.001$), with no change in normal legs. The evolution in time after treadmill of percentage change of HRT is shown in Figure 4. The HRT is clearly increased during the first 2 min in claudicating legs. Taking 15% as threshold increase, there were no false positives (specificity = 100%).

The sensitivity of the technique was not determined precisely and depends on the severity and location of the atherosclerotic process. This technique was used in a small eight-week double-blind placebo-controlled study to analyse the effect of pentoxifylline (600 mg/d) [51]. In this study, pentoxifylline induced a 208% increase of mean walking time (WD) versus baseline, while placebo induced an increase of only 52%. However, the baseline WD was lower in the placebo group. The mean of HRT after treadmill exercise decreased from 95 ms to 55 ms in the treatment group, with no changes observed in the placebo group. However, the baseline value was very different between the two groups (nearly 20 ms difference). Although interesting, these results should be confirmed by a larger trial.

MUSCLE TISSUE OXYGEN PRESSURE

In order to assess directly the nutritive flow to the muscles during exercise, Schroeder [52] and Ehrly [53] proposed to introduce thin microplatin needle electrodes into the muscle and to measure muscle pO_2 at rest and immediately after exercise with a special pneumatic pedal ergometer specifically developed for it.

In two small controlled studies it was demonstrated that an intravenous injection of one dose of buflomedil or pentoxifylline [54,55] induced a small but significant increase of muscle pO_2 after exercise. This technique seems attractive but its sensitivity and specificity have not been analysed and its variability is large. It could be used for determining a dose range of new drugs before embarking on long and difficult phase II dose-finding trials (Ehrly, personal communication). However, no dose finding has been published.

TRANSCUTANEOUS OXYGEN TENSION

Methodological aspects

Recently Scheffler and Rieger [56] published an interesting critical review of the clinical interest and limitations of transcutaneous oximetry in peripheral arterial diagnosis and assessment of drug efficacy.

Table 2. Variability and validity of techniques to measure drug efficacy in PAOD

Technique	Variability—reproducibility	Sensitivity to drug treatment	Advantages	Disadvantages
1. Treadmill exercise – Standard single stage – Progressive	CV 30–45% [44,45] CV for ICD of 22–33% [46,47] CV for ACD of 9–17% [46,47]	Clin. relevant change > 80 m or > 30–40% v. placebo	Reference gold standard	Time-consuming Expensive Hazardous if co-existing coronary disease
2. ABI Resting ABI	CV: 9.5% [49] to 11% [28,47]	Insensitive to drug and exercise therapy	Effective, accurate simple diagnostic test Sensitivity: 97% [49] Specific: 100% [49] (v. Angiography)	Needs Doppler probe Insensitive to treatment
Post-treadmill ABI Single stage Progressive	CV: 16% [49] CV: 12–17% [47]	No advantage over resting ABI		
3. Achilles reflex half-relaxation time (after treadmill)	CV: 29%	Not tested in dose-finding studies Spec.: 100% Sens.: function of disease localisation	Simple technique	Needs a photomotograph Not yet tested in dose-finding studies

4. Muscle tissue oxygen pressure	Intra-ind.: not tested Inter-indiv.: CV [53] Baseline: 25% After exercise: 40–50%	Max. effect: +50%	Direct analysis of muscle oxygen supply Surrogate parameter? Analysis of acute effects of drugs	Necessity of electrodes and pedal ergometer Risk of muscular bleeding? No dose-finding Validity not proven
5. TcPO$_2$	Resting TcPO$_2$: good reproducibility (CV: around 20%) [73,74]	Int. claudication: Resting TcPO$_2$: insensitive Post-exercise: sensitive to drug (1/2 time to basal) CLI: dose-related increases with prostanoid [73,74]	Objective measurement	Needs oxygen sensor Resting TcPO$_2$: no value Hyperbolic relation to flow Post-exercise changes needs treadmill exercise Very useful in CLI = > diagnosis and prognosis Pharmacodynamic dose titration
6. Post-exercise increase in urinary alb./creat. ratio [72]	Variability large	Not tested to drug therapy Significant decrease with surgery	Very easy—cheap	Unspecific Not yet validated Large variability
7. ^{31}P-NMR	Conflicting data in volunteers	One study with buflomedil: no change	Analysis of metabolic effect of drugs Potential use in healthy volunteers	Expensive—complicated

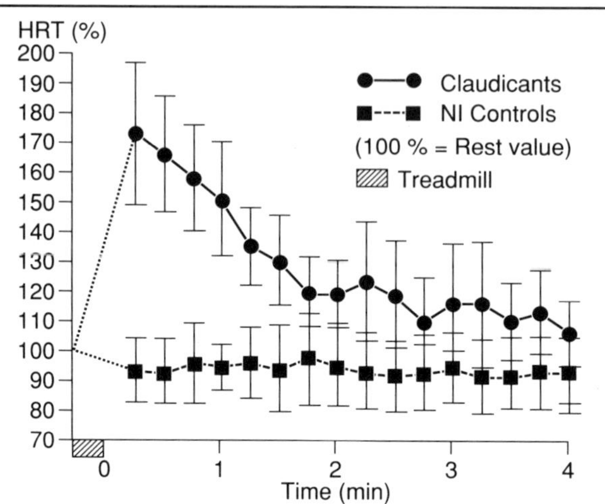

Figure 3. The half-relaxation time (HRT) of the Achilles reflex (expressed as a percentage of the basal value) is significantly increased in claudicating legs during the minutes following the end of exercise. Adapted from Grüntzig and Bollinger [50]

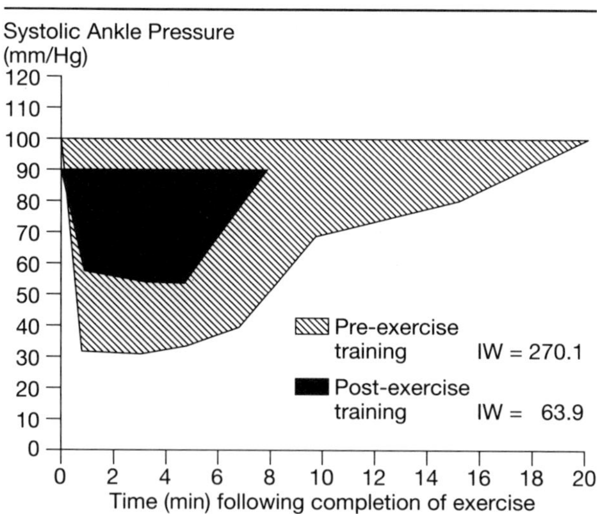

Figure 4. The area under the curve of the drop of ankle systolic pressure in relation to time after treadmill represents the 'ischaemic window' (IW) in one patient with intermittent claudication. This ischaemic window is significantly reduced by 12 weeks intensive training (by more than 75%). Reproduced from Feinberg *et al.* [48]

The major limitations of this technique are the non-linear (hyperbolic) relationship between transcutaneous oxygen tension ($TcPO_2$) and the ankle arterial pressure and the existence of a flow-insensitive range (under a blood pressure of 30 mmHg). This insensitive range can be reduced by provocational measures like measuring $TcPO_2$ in sitting position or after exercise. The reproducibility varies between 5 and 10 mmHg for single supine $TcPO_2$ readings and the scatter is largest for a $TcPO_2$ between 10 and 40 mmHg (flow hyperbola). To eliminate cardiorespiratory influences, limb (per.) $TcPO_2$ has been normalized to chest values, i.e. $TcPO_2$ per./$TcPO_2$ chest [57]. $TcPO_2$ is not useful for making the diagnosis of stage I or II (too much overlap with normal values). However, Schmidt *et al.* [57] found that $TcPO_2$ index in per cent (foot/ thorax) after exercise differentiated patients with claudication from normal controls with 100% sensitivity and specificity. Moreover, they found a good correlation ($R = +0.61$, $p < 0.001$) between $TcPO_2$ index and pain-free WD. Holdrich *et al.* [58] also found that the $TcPO_2$ drop after exercise is a relevant, reliable and accurate test to quantify intermittent claudication. Larson *et al.* [59] propose to use the slope of $TcPO_2$ exercise profile as an indirect measure of a 'metabolically critical stenosis' which might be used as an objective variable to quantify intermittent claudication. The best differentiation between groups of decreasing walking capacity was the 1 min post-exercise slope: the patients with the lowest exercise capacity had the most pronounced relative decrease of $TcPO_2$.

Supine resting $TcPO_2$ measurement can be useful for confirming critical leg ischaemia [60].

Use of TcPO₂ in clinical trials

Sensitivity and reliability of $TcPO_2$ measurements should be increased by measuring more than one site, and using provocational measures (post-exercise, leg dependency). The $TcPO_2$ method has frequently been applied to evaluate pharmacological effects in claudicant patients [61,62]. However, in Fontaine stage II, resting $TcPO_2$ did not change after six months intensive exercise training, although WD increased by 90% [61]. The post-exercise-induced drop of $TcPO_2$ has been found to be reduced after vasodilator therapy [62]. Moreover, no validity study or dose finding has been realized with this technique in IC. $TcPO_2$ could be used in analysing the clinical efficacy of drugs in critical leg ischaemia.

However, in the French 'Iloprost Lower Limb Ischaemia Study', Iloprost, although improving resting pain in 50% of patients versus 19% in the placebo group, did not significantly change the $TcPO_2$ after 120 days therapy [63].

In conclusion, 'the $TcPO_2$ method should be applied to pharmaceutical investigations only with caution' [56].

NUCLEAR MAGNETIC RESONANCE OF THE MUSCLE WITH PHOSPHORUS-31

Nuclear magnetic resonance (NMR) spectrometry could allow the investigator to analyse non-traumatically and repeatedly muscle metabolism after exercise [64,65]. The changes of three waves of ATP can be analysed very precisely in time. During exercise there is a drop of phosphocreatine (P_{cr}) and an increase of inorganic phosphate (P_i). A recuperation time of at least 80% of the initial $P_{cr}/P_{cr} + P_i$ ratio is significantly longer in claudicant legs than in control legs and there is a correlation between this time in seconds and the angiographic lesions [65]. Keller *et al.* [64] found that the recovery speed of P_{cr} values was different in patients compared with controls only after ischaemic (tourniquet) exercise. As a direct correlation between the $t_{1/2}$ of P_{cr} recovery and vascular lesions (analysed by Doppler and angiography) was observed it was postulated that delay in recovery was not a result of a biochemical abnormality but of the impaired increase in blood flow after ischaemic exercise. Surprisingly, no correlation was found between P_{cr} recovery and the claudication score (analysed by a stepping exercise at 75 min^{-1} for 3 min). A recent paper [66] assessed the effect of one-week intravenous therapy with a 'vasodilator' drug (buflomedil) in six patients with a light intermittent claudication (WD around 350 m). The recovery rate in seconds of the P_{cr} index ($P_{cr}/P_{cr} + P_i$) after exercise with provoked ischaemia (blood pressure cuff around the mid-thigh) was analysed. Anaerobic exercise duration was improved after treatment (78.9 $\pm$ 18.8 v. 51.4 $\pm$ 5.5 s). On the other hand, the recovery process of P_{cr} and P_i was not significantly improved after exercise (0.019 $\pm$ 0.003 v. 0.013 $\pm$ 0.002 s^{-1}) and neither was the resting blood flow obtained through plethysmography. The inter-individual variability of this technique has been found too high in volunteers [67]. This technique after validation could eventually be used to analyse the pharmacodynamic effect of new drugs on cellular metabolism of muscle. However, it is a sophisticated and expensive method and is available only in certain university centres.

BIOCHEMICAL ASPECTS OF PERIPHERAL ARTERIAL OCCLUSIVE DISEASE

Clinical studies have suggested strongly that leucocytes could play a major role in ischaemia of the leg [68,69].

Leucocytes, which are more than 1000 times more viscous than red cells, can hinder flow in microvessels by adhering to endothelial cells [70]. This adhesion induces the release of several inflammatory factors like oxygen-derived free radicals. Recently Shearman *et al.* [71] have demonstrated a significant increase in urinary albumin (measured by radioimmunoassay) in patients with claudication after exercise, accompanied by a significant increase in serum lysozyme. These effects disappeared after successful vascular surgery. These results suggest that exercise-induced ischaemia in patients with Fontaine stage II is accompanied by a general increase in permeability which could be explained by factor released during leucocyte adhesion and activation. The analysis of urinary albumin–creatinine ratio could be used as an induced and easy screening test to test the effects of drugs in intermittent claudication [72]. The variability and sensitivity to drug treatment of this essay technique have yet to be analysed.

Conclusion

The treadmill test remains the gold standard for analysing the efficacy of a drug in IC. It could be possible to reduce its variability by using graded, better patient protocols.

- Distal pressure and ABI are to be used for diagnosis and as inclusion criteria but are not sensitive enough to be used for drug efficacy.
- Other techniques like muscle oximetry, Achilles reflex, HRT, ^{31}P-NMR and biochemical variables could give some indications on the mechanism of drug effect but cannot replace the treadmill test.
- Capillaroscopy and $TcPO_2$ are useful for analysing the effect of drugs on the microcirculation and are to be used in testing drug efficacy in later stages (III and IV) of the disease.

Table 2 summarises the variability, sensitivity to treatment, advantages and disadvantages of the different techniques.

References

1. Bevan EG, Waller PC, Ramsay LE. Pharmacological approaches to the treatment of intermittent claudication. Drugs Aging 1992; 2 (2): 125–136.
2. Criado E, Ramadan F, Keagy BA et al. Intermittent claudication. Surgery 1991; 173: 165–170.
3. Kannel WB, Skinner JJ, Schwartz MJ et al. Intermittent claudication: incidence in the Framingham study. Circulation 1970; 41: 875–883.
4. Kannel WB, McGhee DL. Update on some epidemiological features of intermittent claudication: the Framingham study. J Am Geriatr Soc 1984; 33: 13–18.
5. Criqui MH, Fronek A, Klauber MR et al. The prevalence of peripheral arterial disease in a defined population. Circulation 1985; 71: 510–515.
6. Dormandy J, Mahir M, Ascady G et al. Fate of the patients with chronic leg ischaemia. J Cardiovasc Surg 1989; 30: 50–57.
7. Criqui MH, Langer RD, Fronek A et al. Mortality over a period of 10 years in patients with peripheral arterial disease. N Engl J Med 1992; 326: 381–386.
8. Gersh BJ, Rihal CS, Rooke TW et al. Evaluation and management of patients with both peripheral vascular and coronary artery disease. J Am Coll Cardiol 1991; 18: 203–214.

9. Rose GA. The diagnosis of ischaemic heart pain and intermittent claudication in field surveys. J Prev Soc Med 1977; 31: 42–48.

10. Criqui MH, Fronek A, Klauber MR et al. The sensitivity, specificity, and predictive value of traditional clinical evaluation of peripheral arterial disease: results from non-invasive testing in a defined population. Circulation 1985; 71: 516–522.

11. Leng GC, Fowkes RGR. The Edinburgh Claudication Questionnaire: an improved version of the WHO/ROSE Questionnaire for use in epidemiological surveys. J Clin Epidemiol 1992; 45 (10): 1101–1109.

12. Barnes B. Non-invasive diagnostic assessment of peripheral vascular disease. Circulation 1991; 83 (Suppl 1): 1-20–1-27.

13. Whyman MR, Gillespie I, Ruckley CV et al. Screening patients with claudication from femoropopliteal disease before angioplasty using Doppler colour flow imaging. Br J Surg 1992; 79: 907–909.

14. Cossman DV, Ellison JE, Wagner WH et al. Comparison of contrast arteriography to arterial mapping with color-flow duplex imaging in the lower extremities. J Vasc Surg 1989; 10: 522–529.

15. Legemate DA, Teeuwen C, Hoeneveld H et al. The potential of duplex scanning to replace aorto-iliac and femoropopliteal angiography. Eur J Vasc Surg 1989; 3: 49–54.

16. Baxter GM, Polak JF. Lower limb colour flow imaging: a comparison with ankle: brachial measurements and angiography. Clin Radiol 1993; 47: 91–95.

17. Boccalon H. The measurement of the pulsatile arterial flow is necessary to assess the effects of vasoactive drug on lower limbs. Acta Chir Scand 1988; (Suppl 546): 63.

18. Carter SA. Response of ankle systolic pressure to leg exercise in mild or questionable arterial disease. N Engl J Med 1972; 272: 578–582.

19. Fronek A, Johansen KH, Dilley RB et al. Noninvasive physiologic tests in the diagnosis and characterization of peripheral arterial occlusive disease. Am J Surg 1973; 126: 205–214.

20. Hiatt WR, Jones DN. The role of hemodynamics and duplex ultrasound in the diagnosis of peripheral arterial disease. Curr Opinion Cardiol 1992; 7: 805–810.

21. Kiekara O, Riekkinen H, Soimalkallio S et al. Correlation of angiographically determined reduction of vascular lumen with lower-limb systolic pressures. Acta Chir Scand 1985; 151: 437–440.

22. Laing S, Greenhalgh RM. The detection and progression of asymptomatic peripheral arterial disease. Br J Surg 1983; 70: 628–630.

23. Newman AB, Siscovick DS, Manolio TA et al. Ankle–arm index as a marker of atherosclerosis in the cardiovascular health study. Circulation 1993; 88: 837–845.

24. Vasli LR, Larsen S. The predictive value of noninvasive testing in intermittent claudication. Vasc Surg 1991; 25: 396–404.

25. Strandness DE, Bell JW. An evaluation of the hemodynamic response of the claudicating extremity to exercise. Surg Gynecol Obstet 1964; 19: 1237–1242.

26. Carter SA. Indirect systolic pressures and pulse waves in arterial occlusive disease of the lower extremities. Circulation 1968; 37: 624–638.

27. Laing S, Greenhalgh RM. The detection and progression of asymptomatic peripheral arterial disease. Br J Surg 1983; 70: 628–630.

28. Baker JD, Dix D. Variability of Doppler ankle pressures with arterial occlusive disease: an evaluation of ankle index and brachial–ankle pressure gradient. Surgery 1981; 89: 134–138.

29. Arfvidsson B, Wennmalm A, Gelin AG et al. Co-variation between walking

ability and circulatory alterations in patients with intermittent claudication. Eur J Vasc Surg 1992; 6: 642–646.

30. Underwood SR, Mohiaddin RH. Magnetic resonance imaging. In: Fowkes FRG (ed), Epidemiology of Peripheral Vascular Disease. London: Springer-Verlag, 1991; 55–66.

31. EC Guidelines. Clinical investigation of drugs for the treatment of chronic peripheral arterial diseases. 87/19 EEC–75/318 EEC.

32. Heidrich H, Allenberg J, Cachovan M et al. Guidelines for therapeutic studies on peripheral arterial occlusive disease in Fontaine stages II–IV. VASA 1992; 21 (4): 339–343.

33. Cameron HA, Waller PC, Ramsay LE. Drug treatment of intermittent claudication: a critical analysis of the methods and findings of published clinical trials, 1965–1985. Br J Clin Pharmacol 1988; 26: 569–576.

34. Lindgärde F, Jelnes R, Bjorkman H et al. Conservative drug treatment in patients with moderately severe chronic occlusive peripheral arterial disease: Scandinavian Study Group. Circulation 1989; 80 (6): 1549–1556.

35. PACK Claudication Substudy. Randomized placebo-controlled double-blind trial of ketanserin in claudicants: changes in claudication distance and ankle systolic pressure. Circulation 1989; 80 (6): 1544–1548.

36. Waller PC, Solomon SA, Ramsey LE. The acute effects of cigarette smoking on treadmill exercise distance in patients with stable intermittent claudication. Angiology 1989; 40: 164–169.

37. Mannarino E, Pasqualini L, Menna M et al. Effect of physical training on peripheral vascular disease: a controlled study. Angiology 1989; 40: 5–10.

38. FDA Guidelines for the study of drugs in the treatment of patients suffering from intermittent claudication (lameness/limping). FDA Guidelines 1973.

39. Porter JM, Lee BS, Reich T et al. Pentoxifylline efficacy in the treatment of intermittent claudication: multicentre controlled double-blind trial with objective assessment of chronic occlusive arterial disease patients. Am Heart J 1982; 104: 66–72.

40. Brevetti G, Chiariello M, Ferulano G et al. Increases in walking distance in patients with peripheral vascular disease treated with L-carnitine: a double-blind, cross-over study. Circulation 1988; 77 (4): 767–773.

41. Coto V, D'Alessandro L, Grattarola G et al. Evaluation of the therapeutic efficacy and tolerability of levocarnitine propionyl in the treatment of chronic obstructive arteriopathies of the lower extremities: a multicentre controlled study vs. placebo. Drugs Exp Clin Res 1992; XVIII (1): 9–16.

42. Yasuda SU, Schwartz SL, Wellstein A et al. The integration of pharmacodynamics and pharmacokinetics in rational drug development. In: Yacobi A, Skelly JP, Shah VP, Benet LZ (eds), Integration of Pharmacokinetics, Pharmacodynamics and Toxicokinetics in Rational Drug Development. New York: Plenum, 1993; 225–238.

43. Weissinger J. Utility of kinetic, dynamic, and metabolic data in nonclinical pharmacology/toxicology studies. In: Yacobi A, Skelly JP, Shah VP, Benet LZ (eds), Integration of Pharmacokinetics, Pharmacodynamics and Toxicokinetics in Rational Drug Development. New York: Plenum, 1993; 15–22.

44. Clyne CAC, Tripolitis A, Jamieson CW et al. The reproducibility of the treadmill walking test for claudication. Surg Gynecol Obstet 1979; 149: 727–728.

45. Gardner AW, Skinner JS, Cantwell BW et al. Progressive vs single-stage treadmill tests for evaluation of claudication. Med Sci Sports Exerc 1991; 23 (4): 402–408.

46. Gardner AW, Skinner JS, Cantwell BW et al. Effects of handrail support on

claudication and hemodynamic responses to single-stage and progressive treadmill protocols in peripheral vascular occlusive disease. Am J Cardiol 1991; 68: 99–105.

47. Hiatt WR, Nawaz D, Regensteiner JG et al. The evaluation of exercise performance in patients with peripheral vascular disease. J Cardiopulmonary Rehabil 1988; 12: 525–532.

48. Feinberg RL, Gregory RT, Wheeler JR et al. The ischemic window: a method for the objective quantitation of the training effect in exercise therapy for intermittent claudication. J Vasc Surg 1992; 16: 244–250.

49. Ouriel K, McDonnel AE, Metz CE et al. A critical evaluation of stress testing in the diagnosis of peripheral vascular disease. Surgery 1982; 91: 686–693.

50. Grüntzig A, Bollinger A. Die Veränderung des Achillessehnenreflexes nach Arbeit als Parameter der Muskelischämie bei Claudicatio Intermittens. Z Kreislaufforsch 1970; 60: 247–260.

51. Bollinger A, Frei Ch. Double-blind study of pentoxifylline against placebo in patients with intermittent claudication. Pharmatherapeutica 1977; 1: 557–562.

52. Schroeder W. Die Messung des Sauerstoffdruckes in der Skelettmuskulatur: eine quantitative Methode zur Kontrolle der Sauerstoffversorgung und der Funktion der terminalen Muskelstrombahn. Herz/Kreisl 1978; 10 (3): 146–153.

53. Ehrly AM, Dehn R. Verhalten des Muskelgewebesauerstoffpartialdruckes (pO_2) bei Gesunden und Patienten mit Claudicatio Intermittents nach Definierter Fussergometrischer Belastung. VASA 1986; (Suppl 14): 1.

54. Ehrly AM, Saeger-Lorenz K. Influence of pentoxifylline on muscle tissue oxygen tension (pO_2) of patients with intermittent claudication before and after pedal ergometer exercise. Angiology 1987; 38 (2): 93.

55. Ehrly AM, Saeger-Lorenz K. Exercise-induced variations in muscle tissue oxygen pressure in claudicants: effects of buflomedil. Blood Vessels 1991; 28: 27–32.

56. Scheffler A, Rieger H. Clinical information content of transcutaneous oxymetry ($tcpO_2$) in peripheral arterial occlusive disease (a review of the methodological and clinical literature with a special reference to critical limb ischaemia). VASA 1992; 21: 111–126.

57. Schmidt JA, Bracht C, Leyhe A et al. Transcutaneous measurement of oxygen and carbon dioxide tension ($TcPO_2$ and $TcPCO_2$) during treadmill exercise in patients with arterial occlusive disease (AOD): stages I and II. Angiology 1990; 547–552.

58. Holdrich TAH, Reddy PJ, Walker RT et al. Transcutaneous oxygen tension during exercise in patients with claudication. Br Med J 1986; 292: 1625.

59. Larson JF, Christensen KS, Egeblad K. Assessment of intermittent claudication by means of the transcutaneous oxygen tension exercise profile. Eur J Vasc Surg 1990; 4: 409–412.

60. Second European Consensus Document on Chronic Critical Leg Ischemia. Circulation 1991; (Suppl), 84 (4): IV-1–IV-26.

61. Mannarino E, Pasqualini L, Innocente S et al. Physical training and antiplatelet treatment in stage II peripheral arterial occlusive disease: alone or combined? Angiology 1991; 42 (7): 513–521.

62. Caillard P, Mouren X, Bailliart O et al. Evaluation of ifenprodil efficacy on exercise-induced tissue ischemia in stage II arteriopathy by measurement of transcutaneous oxygen tension during a standard treadmill test: double-blind study of injectable ifenprodil versus placebo. Angiology 1993; 44: 552–560.

63. Guilmot J-L, Diot E. Treatment of lower limb ischaemia due to atherosclerosis

in diabetic and nondiabetic patients with Iloprost, a stable analogue of prostacyclin: results of a French multicentre trial. Drug Invest 1991; 3 (5): 351–359.
64. Keller U, Oberhänsli R, Huber P et al. Phosphocreatine content and intracellular pH of calf muscle measured by phosphorus NMR spectroscopy in occlusive arterial disease of the legs. Eur J Clin Invest 1985; 15: 382–388.
65. Le Bas JF, Reutenauer H, Franco A et al. Spectrométrie RMN du Phospore 31 au niveau du muscle du mollet chez le claudicant artériel. J Maladies Vasc 1987; 12: 70–77.
66. Wahl D, Simon JP, Escanye JM et al. Assessment of the efficacy of vasodilator drugs in peripheral vascular disease through a study of skeletal muscle metabolism using ^{31}P nuclear magnetic resonance (NMR) spectroscopy. Therapie 1992; 47 (2): 125–126.
67. Hoffman H, Windeck P, Labs K-H et al. Was leistet die ^{31}Posphor-Kernspinspektroskopie? Eine Validierung an gesunden Probanden. VASA 1991; Suppl 33: 316 (Abstract).
68. Nash GB, Thomas PRS, Dormandy JA. Abnormal flow properties of white blood cells in patients with severe ischaemia of the leg. Br Med J 1988; 296: 1699.
69. Ciuffetti G, Mercuri M, Lombardini R et al. Leucocyte behaviour in controlled ischaemia of the calves. J Clin Pathol 1989; 42: 1083–1087.
70. Ricevuti G, Mazzone A, Pasotti D et al. Role of granulocytes in endothelial injury in coronary heart disease in humans. Atherosclerosis 1991; 91: 1–14.
71. Shearman CP, Gosling P, Gwynn BR et al. Systemic effects associated with intermittent claudication: a model to study biochemical aspects of vascular disease. Eur J Vasc Surg 1988; 2: 401–404.
72. Hickey NC, Shearman CP, Gosling P et al. Assessment of intermittent claudication by quantitation of exercise induced microalbuminuria. Eur J Vasc Surg 1990; 4: 603–606.
73. Creutzig A, Caspary L, Alexander K. Zur Reproduzierbarkeit des transcutanen Sauerstoffdruckes bei fortlaufender Registrierung. VASA 1992; Suppl 35: 32–33.
74. Creutzig A, Caspary L, Alexander K. Doppelblinde placebokontrollierte Studie zum Verhalten des $TcPO_2$ während intravenöser Infusion von Prostaglandin E_1 bei Patienten mit schwerer AVK. VASA 1992; Suppl 35: 36–38.

PART III
PRECISION, VALIDITY AND REPRODUCIBILITY OF MEASUREMENT

10 BIAS AND CONFOUNDING IN CLINICAL STUDIES

David R. Jones
Epidemiology and Public Health, University of Leicester,
Leicester, UK

Random and systematic errors

Several types of clinical study are represented in a typical programme of investigation and development of a new treatment or intervention. The detailed objectives of each study will depend on its design, its place in the broader programme, and the therapeutic area concerned. Broadly, however, all such studies will be intended to investigate the effects of the intervention, be they primary therapeutic effects or side-effects. As far as possible the emphasis should be on *estimation* of the magnitude of such effects [1,2] in view of the direct clinical and pharmacological relevance of the size of effects in many cases. The measure of which an estimate is sought will vary according to the phase of the investigation; in early studies, evidence of a response following treatment may be the objective, followed by investigation of dose–response relationships in dose-finding studies. In later phases, estimates of comparative treatment efficacy and of the incidence of side-effects and adverse reactions will become the focus.

At any stage in the programme, inaccurate estimates may prove to be costly, either in financial terms to a sponsor who as a result wrongly continues or fails to continue development, or in generalised cost terms to patients and health authorities inappropriately using or failing to use a new product. Consideration of the sources of inaccuracy or, more fundamentally, of what is meant by 'inaccuracy', is thus of great practical importance, and a potentially major step towards choice of study design, conduct and analysis options to minimise its occurrence. Unfortunately, the meaning of the term 'accuracy' varies between users; to some it is synonymous with precision, or the extent of the spread of a set of measurements ascribable to *random* (chance) mechanisms, while to others it

Clinical Measurement in Drug Evaluation. Edited by W. S. Nimmo and G. T. Tucker
© 1995 John Wiley & Sons Ltd

embodies ideas of both precision and unbiasedness, where the latter refers to lack of *systematic* errors [3,4].

In clinical studies, random errors may result from biological variability, namely inter- or intra-subject variations, or from technical measurement errors, resulting, say, from varying estimations by observers of values between calibrations on the scale of interest. Not all measurement error should, however, be assumed to be random in nature; perhaps the best-known example of systematic measurement biases are the digit preferences reported in the measurement of blood pressure [5]. As we shall see shortly, there are many other possible sources of systematic error—both other measurement errors and other types of systematic error.

A final dimension which must be mentioned concerns the degree to which the error is intentional. The issue of fraudulent execution of or reporting of results from studies has received special attention elsewhere [6] recently. It will be assumed hereafter that the occurrence of errors in clinical studies is unintentional, although the degree of negligence on the part of investigators through poor study design, conduct and analysis practice will often be debatable.

Bias

Bias may be variously defined as a *systematically wrong estimate* of a parameter of interest, the *amount by which* an estimate differs from the true value, or any process tending to lead to results differing *systematically* from the truth. In the present context of clinical studies, the last of these three definitions is the most pertinent. Possible sources of bias are legion and they can arise in most areas of study design, conduct and analysis. Sackett [7], for example, lists 56 types of bias, 35 of them drawn from the areas of selection and measurement, in the particular context of case–control studies. Selection biases, measurement biases and confounding are commonly identified subsets of biases, but there is no standard taxonomy and little in the way of standard terminology in this area. Most textbooks dealing with methods in epidemiology, clinical trials or clinical studies in general include a list of sources and types of bias [8,9]. Rather than present a detailed compilation of the contents of such lists here, broad classes of bias will be considered. Detailed lists are, however, valuable as checklists to be consulted during all stages of a study, from design onwards, as an aid to ensuring that a full range of potentially important sources of bias is considered.

The existence of long lists of potential biases is not an argument for giving up attempts to design, conduct and analyse studies adequately, or for accepting serious bias as inevitable. More emphasis should be given to 'responsible' and quantitative consideration of each source. A competent critic can find some weaknesses in any study; it is important then go on to ask 'Does it matter?' or 'How much difference does it make?' and attempt to estimate the answers to the questions as far as possible. In some situations this may require only a simple recalculation of results in a 2×2 table—to check the effect of misclassification of disease category in the table on the odds ratio or treatment difference, say—but in others substantial reanalysis of the study under new assumptions, and possibly an extensive sensitivity analysis, will be necessary.

Although some details of Sackett's list may be inappropriate in (mainly experimental) clinical studies, it provides an invaluable outline structure, shown in Table 1. We shall find below that it needs to be supplemented with fuller consideration of confounding.

All of the stages in Sackett's scheme may be regarded as aspects of measurement in the general sense of being part of the effort to obtain an appropriately accurate estimate of treatment-related outcome in a clinical study. The quality of a study, or of the results it yields, is thus limited by the weakest link in the design–conduct–analysis chain. There is little point in wasting resources on elaborate analysis of a fundamentally poorly designed or poorly conducted study. It is appropriate, therefore, that a good deal of the emphasis of Good Clinical Practice (GCP) [10] is concerned with obtaining good quality data from well-conducted studies; these issues are addressed in more detail in Chapter 11. The forthcoming biostatistical guidelines [11] supplement GCP in the areas of study design, analysis, interpretation and reporting. This is essential to restore balance since, for example, a well-designed and conducted study can be spoilt by inadequate analysis, although if the problem is recognised it is at least amenable to solution by appropriate reanalysis. The Biostatistical Guidelines refer principally to the circumstances of phase III, comparative efficacy trials, but the relevance of many of the issues and recommendations to studies in other phases is explicitly noted.

The outline of the methodology of a phase III trial shown in Table 2 provides us with a familiar framework in which to consider important examples of bias in clinical studies, and approaches to tackling them. The principal sources of error in comparative trials will be familiar to most practitioners in the field, as will the usual approaches to their avoidance or

Table 1. Stages of research in which bias may occur

Literature
Study sample selection
Conduct of study/intervention
Measurement of exposures, outcomes (and covariates)
Analysis
Interpretation (and dissemination)

Table 2. Outline of phase III trial to compare treatments A and B

Obtain	comparable groups of patients, G_A and G_B
Allocate	G_A to be given treatment A
	G_B to be given treatment B
Maintain	comparability of G_A and G_B
Assess	using same criteria of outcome in G_A and G_B
Estimate	difference in outcomes in two groups G_A, G_B
Interpret	attribution of difference to treatments

minimisation. These are now briefly reviewed, following the structure shown in Table 1. Although there is much in common with studies in other phases, there are some important differences to be considered as well.

Selection bias

Bias may enter in several ways during the selection of the overall sample of subjects for the trial and their allocation to groups to receive the various treatment interventions to be compared. Each stage in moving from a population to which the treatments are relevant (and to which it will be wished to generalise the results of a trial) to the samples who actually receive the treatments to be compared offers the opportunity for introduction of bias [12].

Most obviously, the nature of the inclusion/exclusion criteria may not match the target population. For example, certain subgroups such as the elderly may be excluded from the set of trial subjects despite being a legitimate part of the target population, or the source of subjects may be inappropriately restricted—as exemplified in the classical Berkson (hospital-based) bias. The samples investigated in the study then become unrepresentative of the target population and so may yield estimates of treatment efficacy (or differences between efficacies of two or more treatments) differing systematically from those which would have been obtained in the whole population. As Smith [13] notes, recognition of the importance of selection effects for inference and interpretation of data sets affected by them is now on the increase, and some more formal statistical responses to the issue are beginning to emerge. However, perhaps the most important prerequisite for monitoring selection biases in the conduct of clinical studies is to keep a complete log of all patients who could conceivably enter the study [14] with details of their baseline characteristics and the reasons for their exclusion or withdrawal. While this is possible for later phase studies, it is entirely impractical for early healthy volunteer studies.

Indeed, selection biases are almost certain to occur by design in the studies characteristic of earlier phases in the programme of drug development, where the most that can be hoped is that the characteristics of volunteer groups are relevant to but not representative of potential target populations. However, bias in individual studies at this stage need not be a fatal deficiency from the viewpoint of the development programme as a whole, if, for example, assumptions about uniformity of treatment effects across population subgroups are supported in a suitable range of studies at a later stage in the programme [11,15]. Unfortunately, similar problems are also evident in phase IV and safety studies in general, where the remedy is more difficult.

Returning to the phase III study paradigm, selection bias can be introduced at the next stage in 'refinement' of the study sample, by exclusion (in the terminology of Peto *et al.* [16,17]) of some of the group who have satisfied the study entry criteria but who are not actually allocated to treatment group (usually by randomisation). This renders hazardous any generalisation of the results obtained in the groups actually compared.

Confounding

Bias is of course also a clear possibility if the allocation procedure is systematic. Whatever the basis for the allocation—perhaps hospital number, date of presentation, or surname—if any prognostic factors are associated with the allocation criterion the possibility that the treatment groups will differ in respect of these factors arises. Differences in response or outcome between the treatment groups may then occur as a result of the differing patterns of prognostic factors represented in each group as well as or instead of as a result of differences in efficacy of the treatments. This is known as *confounding* [18,19] (Table 3), although clear and precise definitions are scarce. Bias in estimation of the treatment effect or treatment difference may result from it. For example, if age is a prognostic factor for a particular disease and the allocation method is such that the distribution of age in the group allocated to one treatment is materially different from

Table 3. Confounding

A confounding factor is:

1. associated with treatment
              and
2. correlated with outcome

Exposure (treatment)
$\updownarrow$
Confounder
$\updownarrow$
Disease (outcome)

that in another, then we would expect the outcome of disease in the two groups to differ, even in the absence of any difference between the effects of the treatments *per se*. Ignoring this will lead us systematically to ascribe incorrect estimates of differences of outcome between groups to differences of treatment efficacy.

This is widely recognised to be a problem of early-phase investigations in which for practical and ethical reasons a comparison group is missing and comparisons are effectively made with the experience in previous groups of subjects. Although inferences are thus potentially hazardous at this stage, the evidence provided by well-controlled later studies should overcome this problem. Hence, avoidance of allocation biases in these later studies is of paramount importance, and randomisation has for some time been recognised as the key to avoidance of biases which may result from use of historical or some other form of non-randomised control group [20].

Although randomisation as a method of allocation to treatment group does indeed have much to recommend it [20,21], it is unwise to assume that all of the problems associated with confounding of treatment effects with those of some other factor are solved by it. Randomisation is an unbiased *method of allocation*, so resultant groups do not differ *systematically*. It avoids allocation biases on the part of clinicians or patients, since it denies them the opportunity to select a treatment for a particular patient; the allocation is independent of patient characteristics. Through its use, balance of both identified and unidentified prognostic factors between treatment groups may be achieved (whereas it is in the nature of any systematic allocation method which attempts to achieve balance by some form of matching of the characteristics of subjects allocated to each group that this can only be achieved, at best, for those factors identified as important enough to be so dealt with).

However, the balance of factors between groups may differ by chance in any particular study. Recognition of this possibility is indicated by the widespread importance attached to demonstrating that the balance between the baseline characteristics of the groups is satisfactory, which is often approached illogically through hypothesis testing methods [22]. To ignore a baseline imbalance is to confuse the long-run properties of the randomisation approach to allocation with the need adequately to analyse and interpret the results obtained in the data set in hand.

If imbalance on a potentially prognostic factor may result in confounding, how should it be avoided? The first prerequisite is that potential confounding factors should have been identified at the design stage, and efforts made to ensure that they are measured carefully. This provides the basis for avoidance of confounding either at the design or the analysis stage. The effects of some confounding factors can be avoided by choice of a suitable restricted or blocked randomisation method [23], or perhaps an alternative such as a 'minimisation' technique [24], which aims to limit the degree of imbalance possible in respect of the factors dealt with in this way. Some residual imbalance may remain even if such methods are used and, more importantly, there will almost certainly be other factors it is not possible to incorporate into the restricted randomisation design if undue complexity is to be avoided. Thus, recourse must be made to allowing for the effects of potential confounding factors in the analysis.

The simplest approach is to analyse results separately in strata defined by level of confounding variable, but integration of these analyses is usually required, so that the final approach is to model variation of results with confounding factors as well as the dependence on treatment, in some kind of regression analysis or analysis of covariance. A corrected or adjusted estimate of, say, the difference in efficacy between treatments is obtained; if all relevant confounding factors have been properly modelled, confounding should no longer be a problem, but in practice this is difficult to achieve, and even more difficult to demonstrate. There will often be some scepticism about the adequacy of the analysis performed, and especially so if the essence of the study results depends upon such analyses [25].

Interestingly, consideration of modelling of and adjustment for confounders leads us back to an operational definition of a confounding factor [26] as a factor which affects the estimate of interest (here, the treatment difference) when allowance is made for it in a suitable analysis. This brings to mind Gertrude Stein's maxim that 'A difference is only a difference if it makes a difference', and reminds us that only adjustment for potential confounding factors—those in imbalance and of potential prognostic value—is necessary, and thus, on grounds of simplicity, desirable.

Attrition biases

We have naturally moved on from problems of allocation bias to methods of analysis intended to respond to them. We now need to return to other sources of bias which may occur later in the conduct of a study than allocation. However good the balance of characteristics in the treatment groups achieved by the allocation procedure, drop-outs from the groups before the intervention is complete or losses to follow-up subsequently may endanger unbiased estimation of treatment effects, and at very least lead to problematical 'missing values' in the outcome data set.

These missing values may be replaced with imputed values, but any such manoeuvre requires assumptions about the mechanism of drop-out or loss; for example, many classical methods assume that losses occur (completely) at random, unrelated to the treatment received or the outcome [27,28], although less restricted statistical models are now under development [29]. Practitioners of clinical studies will, on the contrary, be able to suggest many reasons for drop-out or loss which directly relate to treatment or outcome. For example, either subject or clinician may not like or approve of the random allocation of treatment received, if this is known, and so may decide to absent the subject from the study after allocation but before treatment commences. This could clearly bias the assessment of efficacy if, for example, 'good-risk' patients were differentially removed from the new (experimental) treatment group. Fortunately, problems of this kind are well recognised, and so is a desirable solution, namely blinding (masking) both subjects and treating clinicians to the identity of the allocated treatment. This will not, however, always be possible, in the case of invasive techniques or interventions with characteristic side-effects, for example. More subtly, selection biases may result from the very process of randomisation, combined with the obligation to obtain the informed consent of subjects to randomised allocation [30], since some subjects will withdraw as a result of finding that the treatment they are to receive is to be decided by a chance mechanism.

In general terms, avoidance of biases due to drop-outs and losses must rest in the first instance on prevention by tight study design and conduct, attempting to ensure that all participants know, understand and accept the 'rules of the game' and that these, and the criteria for exclusion and so on, are clearly specified beforehand in the study protocol. Some drop-outs and losses are, however, almost inevitable, and approaches to analysis must recognise this and attempt to cope with the consequences. The first requirement of an adequate analysis is simply that it accounts clearly for the progress of all subjects through the study, so that it is clear when drop-outs etc. occurred and, as far as possible, for what reason.

Another familiar strand of attempts to maintain the possibility of unbiased analyses is the use of the 'intention-to-treat' (ITT) approach to definition of the groups to be compared [20]. In its simplest form this follows the rule 'once randomised, always analysed' and demands inclusion of all subjects in the group to which they were allocated, regardless of whether they receive the treatment specified in the study protocol or not. This has the merit of avoiding biases due to selection of a subset for treatment, but the disadvantage that some investigators regard with incredulity the inclusion of subjects known *not* to have received the specified treatment [12]! In the now infamous example from the Coronary Drug Project trial of clofibrate [31] even compliance in the *placebo* arm was associated with a very substantial reduction in mortality, perhaps implying a role for control by the subject over choice of his or her treatment as a prognostic factor. Non-compliance with treatment regimens as specified in study protocols is thus an important source of bias, which continues to receive much theoretical and practical attention [28,32,33].

However, intention-to-treat analysis does not resolve entirely the problems of drop-outs and losses if outcome measurements are not available for some lost subjects. Here Gould [34] offers some formalisation of commonsense approaches avoiding the need simply to omit from analyses those patients for whom the outcome data are unobserved or to assume that the latest observation which is available on each patient may be 'carried forward' as an unbiased assessment of outcome. Either approach, although common, may lead to biased estimates if the reasons for withdrawal are related to treatment, such as those resulting from unpleasant side-effects. Gould's method involves allocating each withdrawal to one of several categories (withdrawal because cured, because of intolerance, because of lack of therapeutic effect, etc.) which may be put in order in some reasonable way, allowing non-parametric analysis of the outcome measure.

Since none of these methods can entirely resolve the uncertainty about the circumstances of drop-outs or losses and the possible resultant biases, investigation of the sensitivity of conclusions drawn from analyses based on them to the detailed assumptions made seems a wise step, towards both understanding the results of a study and convincing others, including regulatory authorities, of their worth [12,35].

There are, of course, many other points in the analysis of results from clinical studies at which biased estimates of treatment effects may be obtained by inappropriate choice or application of analysis methods. In some cases, such as the problems arising from there being several events of interest in studies of survival times, the correct approach has been clearly identified [36]; in other cases, such as that of cross-over trials in which differential carryover of treatment effects from period to period may occur, the most appropriate approach is debatable [37–40]. Other well-known problems include those associated with repeated inspection of accruing data [41] where formal solutions of the problem are available, and those emanating from other aspects of multiplicity, such as use of multiple endpoints [42] or subgroup analyses, where solutions are less clear cut.

Measurement biases

Moving on through the stages set out in Table 1 we now reach the assessment of outcome, and hence need to consider measurement biases as they relate to outcome measures. In fact, most of the considerations also relate in general terms to the measurement of the intervention and of variables describing other characteristics of the subjects and their experiences, including any potential confounding factors.

Table 4 outlines desirable properties of any measurement, although it is usually necessary to trade these properties off against each other to some extent in respect of any particular measure. For example, ethical constraints on the invasiveness of any investigation, restricted resources for measurement, or consideration of the problems resulting from missing

Table 4. Desirable properties of
measurement scales

A good measurement is:
Valid
Reliable (repeatable)
Responsive (sensitive)
Practical

outcome data, may convince us of the importance of practicality as a
criterion in choice of measurement. The shortest, cheapest and most acceptable measure may, however, not be as valid, reliable or sensitive as other
choices.

Sensitivity (or responsiveness)—the ability of the measurement scale to
discriminate differences or changes of importance in the study—is vital. So
too are the validity of a measure—broadly speaking, measuring what it is
intended to measure—and its reliability—doing so repeatably or repro-
ducibly—although clear evaluation of these characteristics of measurements in practice is rarer than the vast literature of these metrological
issues may suggest. For example, the traditional clinical measurement of
blood pressure may have obvious validity and responsiveness properties
and reasonable acceptability (to subjects), but repeatability appears to be
an issue [5]. Rather less traditional measures such as those in the rapidly
developing field of health-related quality-of-life assessment may be more
open to doubt on all counts [43]. The controversy concerning the use of
surrogate markers, particularly in AIDS studies [44], stems from a conflict
between practicality (wanting early indicators of later outcomes) and
validity (doubt whether the indicators really do predict later outcome on a
'valid' scale such as mortality).

Measurement bias could materialise through failure of the measurement
against any of the criteria, but most attention is usually paid to problems of
validity and reliability. For example, outcome measurements requiring subjective assessment or judgement on the part of the assessor (who may be
the treating clinician, an independent clinical professional, or the subject)
may yield inconsistent values on inter-rater comparisons. Validity may also
be questioned if the assessment may be affected by knowledge of the treatment or perhaps some other patient characteristic; blinding (masking) of
the assessor, whoever that may be, to the identity of the treatment received
in a comparative study is thus desirable if possible. Choice of an 'objective'
measure is sometimes proposed as an alternative; in practice very few if
any unambiguously objective measures exist. Even establishment of the
time and event of death is open to some inter-observer variation, and certi-
fication of the cause of death even more so, but in any case the validity of
this outcome measure in many clinical contexts is doubtful.

Interpretation biases

Finally, we need to consider biases which may arise during interpretation of study results. As far as possible, the analyses should have been carried out by a statistician who is blind to the identity of the treatment groups being compared, but this blindness will almost inevitably be broken at some stage as the pattern of responses becomes apparent; in the case of non-comparative studies, blindness is hardly ever feasible. Thus subjective and judgemental biases may easily enter at this final stage of a clinical study, where analysis feeds into interpretation and presentation of results.

Biases resulting from confusion of statistical significance of results with their clinical importance, or of correlation with causation, are unfortunately still quite common. So too is the drawing of conclusions which are not supported by the results and/or analysis of the study. In interpreting study results as evidence that an apparent association between a treatment (or other clinical intervention) and an outcome measure is a causal one, we should not only assess the possible role of chance in bringing about the association, but also consider whether it could be (wholly or partially) artefactual, due to measurement, selection or other biases, or indirect, due to confounding [45].

Summary

Potential sources of bias in clinical studies are all-pervasive, and a vigilant and multi-faceted approach to avoiding them wherever possible, and allowing for their effects as necessary, must be adopted. To do so we must, as far as is feasible:

- Use valid, reliable and practical measures.
- Consult checklists of biases and quantify their possible effects.
- Randomise allocation to treatment.
- Conduct and analyse studies blind.
- Adjust for confounding factors in analysis.
- Use intention-to-treat and related approaches.
- Perform sensitivity analyses.
- Report results with scrupulous integrity.

References

1. Langman MJS. Towards estimation and confidence intervals. Br Med J 1986; 292: 716.
2. Gardner MJ, Altman DG (eds). Statistics with Confidence. London: British Medical Journal, 1989.
3. Chatfield C. Statistics for Technology (2nd edn). London: Chapman & Hall, 1978.

4. Last JM (ed). A Dictionary of Epidemiology (2nd edn). Oxford: Oxford University Press, 1988.
5. Rose GA, Holland WW, Crowley EA. A sphygmomanometer for epidemiologists. Lancet 1964; i: 296–300.
6. Lock SP, Wells FO (eds). Fraud and Malpractice in Medical Research. London: British Medical Journal, 1993.
7. Sackett DL. Bias in analytic research. J Chronic Dis 1979; 32: 51–63.
8. Rothman KJ. Modern Epidemiology. Boston: Little, Brown & Co., 1986.
9. Feinstein AR. Clinical Epidemiology. Philadelphia: Saunders, 1985.
10. European Commission. Good Clinical Practice for Trials on Medicinal Products in the European Community. In The Rules governing Medicinal Products in the European Community. Volume III. Guidelines on the quality, safety and efficacy of medicinal products for human use. Addendum 57–98. Brussels: Commission of the European Communities, 1990.
11. European Community. Note for Guidance: Biostatistical methodology in clinical trials, in applications for marketing authorizations for medicinal products. European Community (in preparation).
12. Gillings D, Koch G. The application of the principle of intention-to-treat to the analysis of clinical trials. Drug Inf J 1991; 25: 411–424.
13. Smith TMF. Populations and selection: limitations of statistics. J R Statist Soc A 1993; 156: 145–166.
14. Armitage P. Exclusions, losses to follow-up, and withdrawals in clinical trials. In: Shapiro SH, Louis TA (eds), Clinical Trials. New York: Marcel Dekker, 1983.
15. Jones DR, Lewis JA. Meta-analysis in the regulation of medicines. Pharm Med 1992; 6: 195–205.
16. Peto R, Pike MC, Armitage P et al. The design and analysis of randomised controlled trials requiring prolonged observation of each patient. I. Introduction and design. Br J Cancer 1976; 34: 585–612.
17. Peto R, Pike MC, Armitage P et al. The design and analysis of randomised controlled trials requiring prolonged observation of each patient. II: Analysis. Br J Cancer 1977; 35: 1–39.
18. Stone R. The assumptions on which causal inferences rest. J R Statist Soc B 1993; 55: 455–466.
19. Miettinen OS, Cook EF. Confounding: essence and detection. Am J Epidemiol 1981; 114: 593–603.
20. Hill AB, Hill ID. Bradford Hill's Principles of Medical Statistics (12th edn). London: Edward Arnold, 1991.
21. Pocock SJ. Clinical Trials: A Practical Approach. Chichester: Wiley, 1983.
22. Altman DG, Dore CJ. Randomisation and baseline comparisons in clinical trials. Lancet 1990; 335: 149–153.
23. Friedman LM, Furberg CD, Demets DL. Fundamentals of Clinical Trials. Boston: John Wright/PSG, 1981.
24. Pocock SJ, Simon R. Sequential treatment assignment with balancing for prognostic factors in the controlled clinical trial. Biometrics 1975; 31: 103–115.
25. Bagenal FS, Easton DF, Harris E, Chilvers CED, McElwain TJ. Survival of patients with breast cancer attending Bristol Cancer Help Centre. Lancet 1990; 336: 606–610.
26. Hauck WW, Neuhaus JM, Kalbfleisch JD, Anderson S. A consequence of omitted covariates when estimating odds ratios. J Clin Epidemiol 1991; 44: 77–81.
27. Little RJA, Rubin DB. Statistical Analysis with Missing Data. New York: Wiley, 1987.

28. Sommer A, Zeger SL. On estimating efficacy from clinical trials. Statist Med 1991; 10: 45–52.
29. Diggle P, Kenward MG. Informative drop-out in longitudinal data analysis. Appl Statist 1994; 43: 49–93.
30. Simes RJ, Tattersall MHN, Coates AS, Raghavan D, Solomon HJ, Smartt H. Randomised comparison of procedures for obtaining informed consent in clinical trials of treatment for cancer. Br Med J 1986; 293: 1065–1068.
31. Coronary Drug Project Research Group. Influence of adherence to treatment and response of cholesterol on mortality in the Coronary Drug Project. N Engl J Med 1980; 303: 1038–1041.
32. Efron B, Feldman D. Compliance as an explanatory variable in clinical trials. J Am Statist Assoc 1991; 86: 9–21.
33. Peduzzi P, Wittes J, Detre K, Holford T. Analysis as-randomized and the problem of non-adherence: an example from the Veterans Affairs randomized trial of coronary artery bypass surgery. Statist Med 1993; 12: 1185–1195.
34. Gould AL. A new approach to the analysis of clinical drug trials with withdrawals. Biometrics 1980; 36: 721–727.
35. Jones DR. Improving statistics in licence applications: handle with sensitivity? Drug Inf J 1993; 27: 833–836.
36. Kay R, Schumacher M. Unbiased assessment of treatment effects on disease recurrence and survival in clinical trials. Statist Med 1983; 2: 41–58.
37. Freeman PR. The performance of the two-stage analysis of two-treatment, two-period crossover trials. Statist Med 1989; 8: 1421–1432.
38. Senn SJ. Is the 'simple carry-over' model useful? Statist Med 1992; 11: 715–726.
39. Greenfield AA. Crossing with caution. Pharm Med 1992; 6: 193–195.
40. Grieve AP. A Bayesian analysis of the two-period crossover clinical trial. Biometrics 1985; 42: 593–600.
41. Whitehead JR. The Design and Analysis of Sequential Clinical Trials (2nd edn). Chichester: Ellis Horwood, 1992.
42. Pocock SJ, Geller NL, Tsiatis AA. Analysis of multiple endpoints. Biometrics 1987; 43: 487–498.
43. Fitzpatrick R, Fletcher AE, Gore SM, Jones DR, Spiegelhalter DJ, Cox DR. Quality of life measures in health care. I: Applications and issues in assessment. Br Med J 1992; 305: 1074–1077.
44. Ellenberg SS. Surrogate endpoints in clinical trials. Br Med J 1991; 302: 63–64.
45. Elwood JM. Causal Relationships in Medicine. Oxford: Oxford University Press, 1988.

11 WHAT DOES GOOD CLINICAL PRACTICE HAVE TO SAY ABOUT CLINICAL MEASUREMENT?

Eigill F. Hvidberg
University Hospital, Copenhagen, Denmark

Introduction

The title of this presentation might well have read: what do drug regulatory authorities require concerning clinical measurement of drug effect? The reason for involving Good Clinical Practice (GCP) is probably its growing role in drug trial regulation. For clinical measurements the introduction of GCP—as a set of standards for clinical drug research—implies that this area in principle is covered by rigorous requirements. However, the guidance contained in the various GCP documents is of a more general nature; details are not specified. Such details are left to be given in special instructions, e.g. Standard Operating Procedures (SOP). In other words, it was never meant that GCP should detail experimental procedures, but only provide a framework and a philosophy for the performance of high-quality clinical drug trials. In essence, GCP says that all those involved must be responsible, careful, knowledgeable, experienced and honest.

The answer to the question raised in the title of this chapter could, therefore, be brief by stating that GCP does not provide details about clinical measurement. There can, however, be no doubt that indirectly GCP has considerable implications for the correct measurement of drug efficacy, as is the case for many other elements of drug testing. In fact, this is exactly the basic idea of GCP. It is in this context that the general problems will be discussed, particularly on basis of the EC GCP document [1].

Clinical Measurement in Drug Evaluation. Edited by W. S. Nimmo and G. T. Tucker
© 1995 John Wiley & Sons Ltd

Framework of clinical measurements

It might be worthwhile to recapitulate a few general points of particular relevance in order to interpret regulatory requirements correctly, including those stated in GCP. Thus, it should be appreciated that the clinical measurement of drug response is an essential part of the overall efficacy testing necessary for optimum safety/efficacy evaluation of any drug. However, the concept of drug efficacy is a very complex issue: first, because efficacy only becomes meaningful if related to safety; second, because efficacy can be measured as an absolute characteristic or as relative to the efficacy of other drugs; third, because the demonstration of efficacy relies on measurements of drug response performed according to strict scientific, clinical and ethical standards with a strong influence of drug regulation. Finally, various assessors and drug agencies, as within the EC, may evaluate the same data in different ways.

The theoretical basis for clinical measurements [2] of drug response includes, in a narrow sense, three consecutive elements: first, the selection of one or more appropriate variables; next the measurement itself, meaning the choice of methods and instruments and their intelligent application; and finally the outcome in the form of data and other information treated in an unbiased, relevant and meaningful way. The philosophy behind this process is that the measurement of drug effects in clinical trials means recording, classification and grading of observations according to a preconceived design. In the context of clinical drug development, measurement of response should not be considered as a voyage of discovery, but a tool for qualitative and quantitative estimation of the effect(s) [2], thereby being an important part of the safety/efficacy evaluation of the drug in question. This tool must, therefore, be relevant to the clinical problem, constructed according to detailed previous knowledge, and validated carefully. The last point—validation—is of utmost importance, and must be applied to all kinds of measurements, whether they concern true or surrogate endpoints, or whether they concern soft or hard variables.

Several of the problems concerning the measurement of drug effects and how proof of efficacy is provided have been discussed elsewhere [3,4]. All this has been in the back of the minds of those who constructed the requirements for GCP.

GCP requirements relevant to clinical measurement

Those involved in clinical trials must be familiar with GCP. Basically the GCP concept is a merger of philosophy and technical requirements that results in a set of standards and principles. If clinical drug studies are undertaken in accordance with such standards, they will provide documentation on the clinical qualities of the medicinal product in question and assure that such studies are designed, conducted, terminated, audited, analysed and reported to ensure that they are both scientifically and ethically sound, that the trial subjects are protected and that the data can be verified. This description is more elaborate than the definition used in the EC GCP document, but the meaning is the same.

The principle of GCP can be expanded further by looking at sections of the foreword to the EC GCP document, where it is stated that 'pre-established, systematic written procedures for the organisation, conduct, data collection, documentation and verification of clinical trials are necessary . . . to establish the credibility of data and to improve the ethical, scientific and technical quality of trials'. The background is the demand for optimal scientific performance and it is, therefore, important that the integration of scientific quality, ethical performance and the regulatory requirements is fully understood, also in the context of measuring drug effect.

Another aspect of EC GCP which is highly relevant to clinical measurement in general is the requirement for establishing a system of quality assurance, including auditing of the document (Chapter 5). For example, all observations and findings should be verifiable, which is particularly important for the credibility of generated data. Furthermore, the guideline includes requirements for statistical design and for handling of data—all relevant to clinical measurement in drug trials.

In this way, the general obligations advanced in the GCP guideline set the stage for how measurements must be performed. In the light of more recent developments it would have been useful if more details, for example about surrogate endpoints, could have been included. The similar WHO GCP guidelines [5], now being published, also do not specify such methodological details. However, in the various GCP guidelines, including the EC document, several requirements of a more specific nature are given, and it is particularly important that these requirements coincide with the appropriate scientific requirements.

In paragraph 2.5 point 1 of the EC GCP document it is stated that the investigator must 'collect, record and report data properly'. This seems like a very general and almost superfluous direction, but it should be understood in the context of other requirements in the GCP, first and foremost that SOPs must be established. According to the European GCP, it is a responsibility of the sponsor to develop such SOPs, but it is implied that the investigator must provide technical and clinical details in accordance with the specifications given in the protocol. In the Glossary, the SOP is defined as 'standard, detailed, written instructions for the management of clinical trials. They provide a general framework enabling the efficient implementation and performance of all the functions and activities for a particular trial . . .'. Thus, SOP occupies a central position important to the clinical measurement of drug response.

The other essential document in a clinical project is the trial protocol. In the Annex of the EC guideline a list of items to be included in the protocol is presented and, under paragraph 6.8, the following are required for 'Assessment of Efficacy':

(a) specification of the effect parameters to be used;
(b) description of how effects are measured and recorded;
(c) times and periods of effect recording;
(d) description of special analyses and/or tests to be carried out (pharmacokinetic, clinical, laboratory, radiological, etc.).

Furthermore, in item 6.12 on 'Evaluation' the following are required:

(a) a specified account for how the response is to be evaluated;
(b) methods for computation and calculation of effect;
(c) description of how to deal with and report subjects withdrawn from/ dropped out of the trial;
(d) quality control of methods and evaluation procedures.

It should be noted that these requirements are in accordance with those previously cited on the theoretical procedures for measuring drug response. Thus, unconditional demands are given for measuring and assessing drug effects correctly, and regulatory requirements follow scientific standards, not the other way around. Understood in this way, the EC GCP clearly requires details to be worked out for clinical measurement of drug effect, and that methods and assays must be validated if a trial shall be accepted as being performed according to GCP standards.

Other documents and legal implications

GCP is not the only official EC document to consult about instructions regarding efficacy measurements. The Directives may not be so interesting in this context, but the so-called Notice to Applicants [6] does contain requirements related to measuring clinical effect, although these are also quite general. Of much more significance are the many Notes for Guidance on specific areas and drug categories issued by CPMP. Furthermore, the EC guidance of how Clinical Study Reports should be arranged gives additional information. Some of these issues are now being elaborated on by ICH (International Conference Harmonisation) working parties.

It is necessary, therefore, to view GCP as an integral part of the entire spectrum of regulatory and scientific requirements for clinical trials and marketing authorisation. GCP does not exist in a vacuum, but integrates with other kinds of information and regulations. This may lead to the question of the legal status of some of these requirements in Europe. This is a complex issue which is not entirely agreed upon. The GCP document does not yet have the power of law. Only if built into a directive and subsequently implemented in the national legislations of the member states would regulatory requirements become obligatory in a legal sense. However, this is partly the case for GCP as some of the requirements have been included in Directive 91/507/EEC. This means that GCP is now on its way to achieving a higher legal status. Also, the fact that several states such as Italy, Spain and, outside the EC, Hungary, have incorporated GCP into their legislation is of significance. Nevertheless, it is difficult to imagine that non-binding requirements, as the GCP Notes for Guidance still are, will be ignored by those planning clinical trials at the present time, as these requirements are sensible and scientifically based. A potential future EC regulation on clinical trials in the form of a Directive, now being considered by the Commission, will probably not change this situation. Thus, such a regulatory document will not go into details on, for example, measurement of effects.

A final point is, as previously indicated, that it is now becoming apparent that the conception of GCP as well as the rate of its implementation may differ between member states. Whether or not this will influence the way measurement of clinical effects are carried out has yet to be seen. However, these problems, as well as the present systems for notification and approval of trial protocols by the national drug agencies, are bound to influence clinical drug trials [7]. The drug authorities have a shared responsibility with both investigators and sponsors regarding the details of clinical measurement.

Conclusion

The GCP document from the EC only addresses the problems of clinical measurement of drug effect in general. The text points indirectly to more detailed obligations and requires that all work must be scientifically based.

SOP must be developed to specify means and methods stated in the protocol. Furthermore, quality assurance and validation must be applied.

Used in the context of other documents and regulatory requirements, GCP has important implications for the clinical measurement of drug effect.

References

1. EEC Note for Guidance: Good Clinical Practice for Trials on Medicinal Products in the European Community. Committee on Propriety Medicinal Products (CPMP) 1990. Pharmacol Toxicol 1990; 67: 361–392.
2. Chaput de Saintonge DM, Vere DW (eds). Measurements. In: Current Problems in Clinical Trials. Oxford: Blackwell Scientific Publications, 1984; 13–21.

3. Spilker B. Guide to Clinical Trials. New York: Raven Press, 1991.
4. Garbe E, Röhmel J, Gundert-Remy U. Clinical and statistical issues in therapeutical equivalence trials. Eur J Clin Pharmacol 1993; 45: 1–7.
5. WHO Guidelines for Good Clinical Practice (GCP) for Trials on Pharmaceutical Products (Draft), Division of Management and Policies. Geneva: WHO, August 1993.
6. Notice to Applicants for Marketing Authorization for Medicinal for Human Use in the Member States of the European Community. III/3567/92. Rules governing Medicinal Products in the European Community, Vol IIA, 1993.
7. Hvidberg EF. Regulatory implications of Good Clinical Practice: towards harmonization. Drugs 1993; 45: 171–176.

12 MEASUREMENT OF BIOEQUIVALENCE AND ITS RELEVANCE TO THE CLINICAL SITUATION

Tomas Salmonson
SmithKline Beecham Pharmaceuticals, Harlow, UK
Formerly: Medical Products Agency, Uppsala, Sweden

Introduction

In many situations it is important to transfer clinical efficacy and safety data from one dosage form to another in an easy way without having to repeat large clinical trials. These situations include cases when it is necessary to document:

- A final versus a clinical trial formulation.
- A new versus an old approved dosage form.
- A major change in the manufacturing process.
- A generic versus an innovator product.

In fact, clinical efficacy and safety have been shown for only a minority of all dosage forms on the market today. The approval of all other products have relied on data obtained with other formulations. Hence, the problem of transferring data from one dosage form to another is not something that only concerns the generic drug industry. On the contrary, the majority of all bioequivalence studies submitted to the regulatory agencies are performed by so-called 'innovator' companies.

Simple ways of establishing therapeutic equivalence between two formulations are preferable from many points of view compared with repeating large clinical trials. In some cases, this can be done with *in vitro* studies but in other cases *in vivo* human data are required.

In vivo methods used to demonstrate that data are transferable to the new dosage form must be reliable and valid to the clinical situation. For

Clinical Measurement in Drug Evaluation. Edited by W. S. Nimmo and G. T. Tucker
© 1995 John Wiley & Sons Ltd

oral formulations of drugs with systemic therapeutic effects, bioequivalence between two dosage forms, i.e. similar blood concentration–time curves, is the most common *in vivo* method of demonstrating therapeutic equivalence. This method assumes that identical concentration–time curves in a group of patients result in similar efficacy and safety. Once the drug is absorbed into the systemic circulation, the dosage form can no longer influence the fate of the drug and the clinical response should then be formulation independent.

The aim of this presentation is to highlight the assumptions behind the conventional bioequivalence study design and to present briefly the current regulatory guidelines. The validity of the design of a conventional bioequivalence study to the clinical situation will also be discussed.

Methods of comparing concentration–time curves

Two products with similar concentration–time curves may be considered to be bioequivalent. This is defined in the EC Note for Guidance *Investigation of Bioavailability and Bioequivalence* as:

> Two products are bioequivalent if they are pharmaceutical equivalents or alternatives and if their bioavailabilities (rate and extent) after administration in the same molar dose are similar to such degree that their effects, with respect to both safety and efficacy, will be essentially the same.

How does one compare two curves and conclude that they are identical or similar? In theory this could be done in several ways. One way would be to compare the measured concentration at selected time points. If the concentrations at these time points are similar it seems reasonable to conclude that the entire curves are similar. However, this method is connected with statistical and regulatory difficulties and it has not been used frequently in the past. A simple, alternative approach would be to put one concentration–time curve above the other (both obtained in the same subject) and cut away the parts of the bottom curve which are not covered by the top one. The two curves could then be switched and the procedure repeated. If, for example, more than 20% of the area is cut away from more than 10% of the subjects, the two products could be regarded to be bioinequivalent.

The currently preferred way of making this comparison is to describe first the obtained concentration–time curves with some resulting variables and then compare these measurements in one or several statistical tests. Philosophically, there are two ways of looking at this: a non-pharmacokinetic and a pharmacokinetic approach. However, the two approaches may result in identical variables.

NON-PHARMACOKINETIC APPROACH

A curve can be defined by its size and shape. The size can be measured relatively easily. Assuming that once the drug is absorbed the fate of the drug is formulation independent (i.e., the dosage form cannot influence the distribution of the drug), only one or two relatively early shape factors during the absorption phase are needed to define the curve. The peak concentration (C_{max}) and sometimes the time to the peak concentration (T_{max}) are the most commonly used shape factors.

PHARMACOKINETIC APPROACH

Let us assume that drug concentration follows a one-compartment model with first-order absorption, i.e. the drug is absorbed and eliminated by two first-order processes. The concentration at any given time point, C_t, is then determined by the equation:

$$C_t = A \exp^{(-kt)} - A \exp^{(-k_a t)},$$
$$A = k_a F \text{ dose}/V(k_a - K) \tag{1}$$

Systemic variables such as clearance (Cl), apparent volume of distribution (V_d) and elimination rate constant (K) are again assumed to be formulation independent. Similar values of the percentage of the dose absorbed (F) and the absorption rate constant (k_a) would therefore result in similar concentration–time curves.

By integrating and rearranging equation (1), it can be shown that F is directly proportional to the total area under the concentration–time curve, AUC, and the amount excreted unchanged, A_e.

$$\text{AUC} = F \text{ dose}/Cl \tag{2}$$
$$A_e = F \text{ dose } Cl_R/Cl \tag{3}$$

Hence, both these variables can be used to obtain a relative estimate of the bioavailability from one formulation to the other ($\text{AUC}_1/\text{AUC}_2$ or A_{e_1}/A_{e_2}) but it is important to recognise that the assumptions are slightly different. When using AUC, total clearance is assumed to be dosage independent and should change as little as possible between the two test periods to reduce the variability. Using A_e assumes that the ratio of renal clearance over total clearance is formulation independent. For a drug which is mainly excreted unchanged in urine the variability in the ratio is probably lower, as a change in renal clearance from one test period to the other will result in a corresponding change in total clearance. The ratio therefore stays relatively unchanged while the absolute value of total clearance changes.

The rate of absorption could be characterised by T_{max}. However, as can be seen in the equation below, T_{max} is a relatively insensitive measurement of absorption rate. C_{max} is dependent on F as well as the rate of absorption. In many situations C_{max} is as sensitive as AUC to changes in F, but it is generally very insensitive to changes in the absorption rate constant.

$$T_{max} = 2.3 \, \log(k_a/K)/(k_a - K) \tag{4}$$

$$C_{max} = F \, \text{dose}/V \, \exp^{(-KT_{max})} \tag{5}$$

Identical or not too different?

Most bioequivalence studies conducted today have a randomised, two-period cross-over design. The concentration–time curves of the test and the reference preparation are determined and compared within each subject. However, two concentration–time curves obtained in one subject are never identical in its true meaning. To conclude bioequivalence we therefore have to set criteria which define that two products are no more different than the difference lacks clinical importance.

The problem can be illustrated with an example from sports. A number of years ago, thousandths of a second were used to determine who won a swimming competition. With the technology available today, even smaller differences could probably be measured. However, the swimming organisations decided that only hundreds of a second should be used. Smaller differences are neglected and two swimmers with the same time within one-hundredth of a second are considered to be equally fast despite the fact that there always exists a difference.

In bioequivalence testing, the acceptance range used should ideally be based on knowledge of the relationship between changes in the concentration and changes in clinical efficacy/safety. Regardless of where the true relative bioavailability of the test formulation falls within the acceptance range, this should lack clinical importance. The definition of bioequivalence above is based on this idea.

However, for many drugs, information on the relationship between plasma concentration and effect is poor and even lacking. That is one reason why the regulatory requirements on bioequivalence are the same for most drugs.

The current EC guidelines in Europe, *Investigation of Bioavailability and Bioequivalence*, came into operation in 1992. These were preceded by at least two European, multinational guidelines: the earlier EC guideline *Investigation of Bioavailability* and the Nordic guideline *Bioavailability Studies in Man*. The new European guidelines are to a large extent harmonised with the current US Food and Drug Administration (FDA) guidelines. *Investigation of Bioavailability and Bioequivalence* covers oral immediate-release products with systemic effects. It contains detailed recommendations on design, data analysis and reporting. The requirements are summarised in Table 1.

Table 1. Summary of current EC requirements

Main variables	AUC and C_{max}. T_{max} only when there is a clinically relevant claim for rapid release
Logarithmic transformation	AUC and C_{max}
Statistics	<5% risk of erroneously accepting bioequivalence, i.e. a 90% confidence interval should be within the bioequivalence range
Acceptance ranges	AUC: 80–125% C_{max}: 80–125%, but a wider range may be accepted due to the larger variability T_{max}: clinically determined
Assumed distribution	AUC: parametric C_{max}: parametric T_{max} non-parametric

The three main variables discussed in the EC guideline are AUC, C_{max} and T_{max}. However, assessment of T_{max} is only required when there is a relevant claim for rapid release. Because of the multiplicative pharmacokinetic model behind AUC and C_{max}, it is recommended that these variables are log transformed to fit the additive ANOVA model. AUC and C_{max} are assumed to have a parametric distribution, while a non-parametric test is suggested for T_{max}.

The bioequivalence requirements are based on a maximal consumer (or regulatory) risk of less than 5% of erroneously concluding bioequivalence. Based on this, it has been shown that the limits of a 90% confidence interval should be fully contained within the accepted bioequivalence range.

The acceptance range for AUC is normally 80–125%. A tighter acceptance range may be required for some drugs with a narrow therapeutic range, while in other cases a larger acceptance range may be accepted. However, for the vast majority of all drugs the 80–125% range is applied.

The guideline recognises that C_{max} in many cases is more variable and a wider range than 80–125% may be accepted. The Swedish Medical Products Agency (MPA), however, believes strongly that one should be very careful when choosing an acceptance range for C_{max} (or any other variable) outside the 80–125% range. From a statistical point of view, it is not correct to discuss retrospectively the acceptance range based on the variability observed in the conducted study. One would then lose the control over the alpha-level and one may penalise companies that do everything to reduce variability in analytical methods, sampling times, etc. If the company would like to argue for a wider acceptance range this should be stated in the clinical trial protocol and preferably discussed with the regulatory agency before the study is performed.

If T_{max} is considered to be important, the 90% confidence interval should be within a clinically determined range. Needless to say, this requirement has caused many extensive discussions between regulatory agencies and drug companies, e.g. acceptance limits for drugs with the indication 'acute pain'.

The validity of the standardised bioequivalence design

Design, conduct and analysis of bioequivalence studies have been discussed extensively in the literature and at meetings during the last 15–20 years. Some of the specific issues, as shown in Table 2 (left-hand column), have been discussed thoroughly. Unfortunately some of these questions are perhaps less important when it comes to the validity of the bioequivalence trial to the clinical situation. Issues shown in the right-hand column of Table 2 are in this context as (or perhaps even more) important and these will be discussed below.

Population versus individual bioequivalence

The bioequivalence requirements today focus on changes in mean values in a population and we attempt to estimate the relationship between the true mean values of the test in relation to the reference. However, we should ask ourselves if this is always sufficient. Perhaps we should ask different questions depending on the situation and what we are trying to prove. It seems difficult to conclude that two products are bioequivalent if only their means are the same but the distribution in inter-individual variability is significantly different. In some cases we would perhaps also like to know that the intra-individual variability is approximately the same to conclude that two products are equivalent, i.e. that the individual patient receives the same amount of drug regardless of whether he takes formulation 1 or 2. Figure 1 attempts to illustrate this idea. Depending on the situation and what we would like to prove (e.g., if the mean value of

Table 2. Bioequivalence issues

Thoroughly discussed	Should be further discussed
Logarithmic transformation of pharmacokinetic variables	Individual v. population bioequivalence
90% v. 95% CI	Measurements of rate of absorption
CI v. two one-sided tests	Chirality issues
	Influence of food

Questions to address?   **Variability to consider**

CT formation?   Prescribability?   Changes in mean values?

New dosage form?   Switchability?   Changes in intra-individual variability?

Manufacturing process? Interchangeability?   Changes in inter-individual variability?

Generic product?   'Product-by-subject'

                       Interaction?

Figure 1.

two products is the same in two populations or if two products can be interchangeably used in one patient) we should perhaps set different requirements.

To set such requirements we would have to ask ourselves questions like 'Will the new formulation replace the older formulation or will the new formulation only be used in previously untreated patients?'

The introduction of generic substitution and so-called reference prices in many countries in order to control the reimbursement costs have added extra dimensions to this problem. The current bioequivalence criteria were never intended to guarantee that two products (e.g., a generic and an innovator product) can be used interchangeably in one patient.

If we would like to establish bioequivalence based on not only the mean values but also the inter- (and perhaps also intra-) individual variability, we must use other statistical methods and other study designs. A short summary of these methods is given in Figure 2.

Depending on the question asked, different methods should be used:

Mean values: 2-period crossover
                      CI or two-one sided test

Inter-individual   2-period crossover
variability: Morgan-Pitman, CI

Intra-individual   3- or 4-period crossover,
variability: F-test, CI

'Switchability'   2-period crossover, Hauck-Anderson
                      3- or 4-period crossover, e.g. Schall-Luus,
                      Ekbohm-Melander, Sheiner

Figure 2.

Measurement of rate of absorption

It is significantly more difficult to describe the rate of input of drug into the systemic circulation than to estimate the total input (AUC or A_e). The current EC guidelines suggest that T_{max} should be used when there are clinical indications that rate may be important. There are, however, several problems connected with this:

- This requirement is difficult to regulate and it often leads to discussions between the regulatory agency and the applicant. In the ibuprofen example given in Table 3, the MPA believed the confidence interval for T_{max} was too wide to be able to conclude that the two products would relieve pain just as quickly. However, the company disagreed and finally a court had to decide in favour of the MPA. Ibuprofen is a drug with the indication 'acute pain' and there are no reasons for accepting a new generic product with significantly slower absorption. In other cases, however, it is more difficult. What is an acceptable range in T_{max} for a pain reliever such as ibuprofen?
- T_{max} is a rather insensitive measurement of rate of absorption. Many other variables (e.g., 'feathered slope', 'feathered AUC' and 'partial AUC') and combination of variables (e.g., C_{max}/T_{max} and C_{max}/AUC) have been suggested. Unfortunately, there are currently a lack of conclusive data showing that these measurements are more sensitive than T_{max} to changes in rate of absorption.

In an attempt to answer these questions, Professor Tom Tozer is currently conducting an extensive simulation study on behalf of the US FDA. In his study, Tozer looks at the performance of many suggested alternative variables (including the ones mentioned above), under different conditions. Hopefully, the outcome of these simulations can tell us if we should continue to use T_{max} as a measurement of rate or not.

Racemic mixtures of chiral drugs

'Should pharmacokinetic variables used in bioequivalence studies be based on the active enantiomer alone or is it sufficient to measure the total con-

Table 3. Estimated mean values (SD)

	Test	Reference	90% CI
AUC (μg h/ml)	96 (15)	95 (16)	96–105%
T_{max} (h)	2.2 (1.6)	1.1 (0.8)	135–267%
C_{max} (μg/ml)	18 (4)	21 (4)	78–94%

centration of the two enantiomers?' This is a relatively new question triggered by the fact that various chiral separation methods have improved rapidly during the last few years. Intuitively, it may seem tempting to answer this question with 'It should be based on the active enantiomer' as we are assuming that similar concentration–time curves result in similar clinical efficacy and safety. This assumption may be difficult to defend if we measure something that is not responsible for the clinical effect.

On the other hand, because we only attempt in these studies to prove that two different formulations behave similarly *in vivo* and given the fact that chemical properties important for a molecule to be released from the dosage form, such as pK_a and solubility, are identical for the two enantiomers, one could argue that the total concentration of the two enantiomers sufficiently reflects the qualities of the dosage forms.

It is our impression that, today, we do not have enough data to give a final answer to this question. This is supported by the following statement in the new EC guidelines: 'In due time attention has to be given to the requirements of the recommendation/guideline on enantiomers and diastereomers (in preparation) as far as relevant for bioavailability and bioequivalence studies'. A majority of the scientists we have discussed this topic with would still question the need for enantioselective analytical methods in studies with immediate-release dosage forms. However, when it comes to slow-release dosage forms containing drugs with saturable enantioselective first-pass metabolism (i.e., rate of release from the dosage form is important) such as verapamil, I personally believe that selective analytical methods should be used.

The influence of food

The vast majority of the bioequivalence studies conducted today are performed in fasting healthy volunteers. This is done regardless of whether the drug is recommended to be taken with food or not. The reason for this is the hope of reducing the variability believed to be caused by concomitant intake of food. It is time to question this design in the light of our current knowledge of food effects. The following should be considered:

- The test situation, where subjects fast overnight and then do not eat anything before lunch, does not reflect the eating habits of most people.
- The rate of absorption of some drugs is slow. In these cases, it is not sufficient to recommend the drug to be taken before meals if one would like to avoid the effects of food. Several studies submitted to the MPA have demonstrated that the effect of food on some drugs was similar if the drug was taken with food or 2 h before the meal.
- Food influences stomach emptying and gastric blood flow for several hours.

- Food effects are common. Recently I did a small survey of 45 applications for new systemic drugs intended to be given orally. Thirty-three of these applications contained food effects studies. In 18 of these studies (55%), the extent of bioavailability was affected by food and in 19 (58%) the rate of absorption. The pharmacokinetics of only seven of the 33 drugs (21%) were unaffected by concomitant intake of food.
- Different food effects are not only observed between different drugs but also different dosage forms. Perhaps the most well-known example of this is the behaviour of various theophylline slow-release formulations. For some of these formulations, the extent of bioavailability is clinically significantly decreased when given with food, while the opposite is observed for other formulations. Such differences between formulations are not only observed for slow-release formulations but also for some immediate-release formulations such as doxycycline monohydrate versus doxycycline carrageenate (the latter being significantly less influenced by food—data submitted to the MPA).
- Food effects are difficult to predict.

For some drugs, it seems reasonable to question the validity of bioequivalence data obtained in fasting subjects to the clinical situation. Designs that reduce variability can only be accepted if they do not question the external validity of the result. In addition, based on our experience at the MPA, concomitant food intake does not always increase the inter-individual variability. There are many examples of the opposite.

Conclusions

There is a need for relatively simple *in vivo* techniques to demonstrate that extensive clinical efficacy and safety data obtained with one dosage form are transferable to another similar dosage form containing the same drug. As a result, the standardised design of bioequivalence studies and regulatory requirements for demonstrating bioequivalence are similar all over the world. This should not be interpreted as if these issues are simple and that scientists all over the world share a common view of the potential problems. The vast number of meetings discussing these issues demonstrate the opposite.

Unfortunately, mainly pharmacokineticists and statisticians have participated in these meetings and the discussions have therefore focused on some pharmacokinetic and statistical issues. Other questions which may be of equal or even more importance when it comes to the validity of the standardised test situation to the clinical situation have not been fully discussed.

13 THE 'CLINICAL TRIAL' OF THE CLINICAL TRIAL

Alvan R. Feinstein
Yale University School of Medicine, New Haven, and
Department of Veterans Affairs Medical Center, West Haven,
Connecticut, USA

Introduction

To evaluate the current status of randomised controlled trials (RCT), we need to consider how and why they were developed. The event commonly hailed as the introduction of modern randomised trials occurred in the UK about 45 years ago. The trial was done to decide whether a proposed new treatment—in this instance, streptomycin for advanced tuberculosis—was efficacious enough to warrant industrial production.

Initial progress of randomised controlled trials

Like all new advances in medicine, randomised trials went through a slow, grudging period of initial acceptance. Many physicians did not like the trials because of the abandonment of clinical judgement. Doctors were also unhappy about the ethics of possibly giving patients inferior treatment. A further medical objection was that the research protocols were too rigid and not clinically realistic. Although these complaints were eventually counterbalanced by the many advantages of randomised trials, the complaints can still be supported and are still offered today.

Role of thalidomide

The major stimulus to the rapid growth and acceptance of randomised trials occurred after the thalidomide disaster of the early 1960s, when regulatory agencies demanded that pharmaceutical companies use RCT to obtain evidence of 'safety and efficacy' for all new drugs. They were increasingly being discovered or developed during an 'explosion' in

Clinical Measurement in Drug Evaluation. Edited by W. S. Nimmo and G. T. Tucker
© 1995 John Wiley & Sons Ltd

pharmaceutical research; and the profits made the pharmaceutical companies become major industrial giants. As randomised trials became used for testing all of the new agents, the trials became a relatively commonplace event in medical thought and clinical practice.

Two interesting ironies about the established acceptance of the trials are, first, that current regulations would not prevent another thalidomide disaster. An agent can be developed, tested in animals whose fetuses are not susceptible to the teratogenic action of the drug, and shown to have unequivocal efficacy for symptoms such as nausea in people who are not pregnant. After regulatory approval, when the drug comes on the market and is then received for the first time by pregnant women, the thalidomide story could occur all over again.

A second interesting irony is that all of the demands for safety and efficacy were placed almost exclusively on pharmaceutical products. No similar demands were made for demonstrating the efficacy of surgical operations or of the many technological procedures that are not pharmaceutical products. The consequence of this narrow-focused vigilance has been the almost undisciplined growth of the many surgical and technological procedures today whose high costs are not accompanied by evidence of efficacy.

Current status of randomised controlled trials

In their current status, RCT have been accepted as the 'gold standard' for evaluating therapy despite the absence of any 'clinical trials' comparing randomised trials versus other forms of evaluation to prove that RCT are indeed the only gold standard. Because no other methods have been scientifically approved, we are left with two major problems. The first is that double-blind randomised trials cannot be feasible for many therapeutic evaluations such as surgery, non-pharmaceutical forms of psychotherapy, and many issues in pharmaceutical treatment itself. The second major problem is that randomised trials are not applicable for scientific questions in the long-term safety of therapy, for studies of risk factors in the aetiology of disease, or for the evaluation of informational technology, such as radiological imaging. How do we evaluate the many cogent questions that cannot be answered with randomised trials?

Misconceptions about randomised controlled trials

Many physicians, scientists and statisticians have the fundamental misconception that the results of randomised trials are intended for use in thoughtful clinical practice. They are not. Randomised trials are aimed at showing that treatment A is, on average, more efficacious than treatment B or placebo. The trials have been magnificent for demonstrating average efficacy in the special circumstances in which the trials are conducted. Nevertheless, the results of the selected outcomes in an average patient may not be pertinent for the total outcomes and other effects that must be noted in cogent clinical subgroups when physicians make therapeutic decisions for individual patients in ordinary clinical practice.

Development of statistical hegemony

The goal of showing average efficacy then led to the development of the statistical hegemony that dominates the current approach to designing and analysing results for randomised trials. To be approved, new therapeutic agents required unbiased, randomised trials. Consequently, statistical principles were used to establish a set of demands and requirements that would presumably provide the unbiased evidence. These demands included efficient criteria for admission, the use of standard dosage regimens, appropriate patterns of randomisation, a reliance on 'hard data', the use of double-blind observations, the development of intention-to-treat (ITT) analysis, and concepts of ample sample sizes for 'statistical significance'. The statistical principles have been excellent and successful for the goal of showing the average efficacy of treatment. On the other hand, each of these statistical principles have been accompanied by adverse clinical and scientific side-effects.

Adverse scientific side-effects

The efficient admission criteria have been excellent for the 'internal validity' of the therapeutic comparison conducted within a trial, but the results may then lack 'external validity' because of the restricted spectrum of clinical conditions in the group that was admitted to the trial.

The standard dosage regimens, which readily permit double-blind observations and statistical analyses of variance, are inappropriate for ailments where the dosage must be 'titrated' for each patient, and cannot be given according to a rigid single schedule. Furthermore, because the standard dosage regimens may not be maintained by individual patients, a careful analysis of results would have to consider changes, contaminations or other violations of the assigned regimen. All of these violations could be ignored, however, with an ITT analysis.

With randomisation we could believe that prognostic differences among patients were equally distributed at baseline. Hence, there would be no need to consider or to develop suitable taxonomies for prognostic staging systems. Consequently, such taxonomies have not been developed; and suitable data may not even be collected for their application either within or outside the analysis of randomised trials.

The reliance on hard data has given us information that can be regarded as trustworthy, but the hard data often do not correlate with, or reflect, crucial prognostic distinctions and outcomes that are expressed in soft data for such entities as patterns of symptoms, severity of illness, severity of co-morbidity, or functional capacity. Because all of this crucial human information is ignored, patients now regularly complain (quite appropriately) about the dehumanisation of the modern clinical approach to therapy.

Double-blind observations are good 'window dressing' to suggest that the observations are objective, but the masks are often perforated by various side-effects of treatment; or the double-blind observations may be inapplicable for evaluating things like surgery or other treatments that cannot be given in a double-blind manner. Furthermore, the use of the double-blind technique allows a persistent neglect of the need to develop better mechanisms for collecting, classifying and 'hardening' crucial 'soft data'. The policy seems to be that as long as we don't know which treatment the patients are getting, we don't have to notice how they respond and react.

The ITT analyses allegedly avoid the 'bias' introduced by post-randomisation events such as compliance or changes in treatment, although these events are crucial clinical issues in evaluating the total course of treatment. We assume that the changes in assigned regimen occur randomly in both of the compared groups. Very often, however, the changes are made not at random, but in response to good or bad things whose identity is left unstipulated and unrecorded. Perhaps the most obvious hazard of ITT analyses is that the results may lack clinical 'common sense'. It seems silly to analyse people as having had surgical treatment when they were assigned to it but never received it. Conversely, it also seems silly to analyse other people as not having received surgical treatment when they violated the protocol and had the operation shortly after beginning the assigned course of medical therapy.

The ample sample sizes used for 'statistical significance' have had at least three sets of adverse effects. One of them has been the almost exclusive focus on the probabilistic α and β levels for p-values and confidence intervals, while inadequate or no attention has been given to the δ and ζ levels needed for demarcating the large or tiny quantitative effects that denote 'clinical' significance or insignificance. A second problem is that the current doctrine of 'large, simple trials' is excellent for getting statistical significance in showing the average efficacy of treatment, but the results are generally useless for clinical application afterwards. Finally, the sample sizes used in clinical trials have been needlessly inflated, and trivial clinical distinctions have become statistically significant, with the huge, costly trials produced by the current Neyman–Pearson calculations aimed at getting 'doubly significant' results.

Problems in compliance

The famous Coronary Drug Project two decades ago offers an example of the problems produced by the hegemony and rigidity of statistical doctrines. In that trial, the success rates were found to be higher in compliant than in non-compliant patients for the active treatment, but also for the placebo group. Because the contrast of results for compliant versus non-compliant active treatment might have led to a misleading conclusion, the findings were therefore used as a major buttress to support the principle of ITT analysis.

The emphasis on the ITT principle—to the exclusion of everything else that was learned in that trial—has had many deleterious scientific consequences. First, compliance itself was the only significant effective factor in that trial, but was ignored thereafter. In customary forms of science, the investigators would try to determine the mechanism by which compliance produced its strikingly successful results. What was the mechanism? Did the compliant patients have psychic factors that affected both their compliance and their favourable outcomes? Did the compliant patients in the placebo group also maintain effective co-therapy and is their success due to that co-therapy? In customary forms of science, someone would try to find out what made compliance such an effective agent, if for no other reason than the possibility of isolating that factor and then marketing it. Obsessed with the statistical dogmas, however, the investigators made no attempt to do any further study of this important scientific finding.

A separate problem that occurs when an ITT analysis is done, with no acknowledgement of either compliance or of changes in therapy, is wrong conclusions about therapy. The average dosage in the trial will inevitably be regarded as higher than what was actually used. The conclusions will also be wrong about average efficacy and perhaps safety of the tested products, because we will not know which patients were or were not taking the products, and why the change was made in those who stopped.

Scientific challenges and opportunities

The current status quo offers many scientific challenges and opportunities for improvement. Within the format of randomised trials, improvements in soft data and development of an appropriate taxonomy for soft data can lead to more homogeneous clinical groups and more frequent outcome events for the research. Thus, relief of pain and better functional capacity may occur much more frequently than reinfarction or death. With these more-frequent endpoints, the trials could be done with smaller sample sizes, with more clinically applicable results for the data, and with more enthusiastic participants among both doctors and patients, who would be pleased to be involved in a trial that seems aimed at realistic clinical goals.

With other improvements, we can try to monitor compliance, determine the reasons why treatments were changed, and analyse the results appropriately. These post-randomisation phenomena will not have the sacred statistical imprimatur of randomisation, but the results can provide worthwhile scientific knowledge. The additional knowledge can increase the current relatively low productivity of expensive randomised trials that are aimed only at average efficacy, and that provide information only for that average goal.

Another important set of challenges and opportunities is to develop alternatives to randomised trials. One of the most magnificent contributions of randomised trials has been their demonstration of scientific principles that do not require randomisation. Among such principles are appropriate eligibility criteria, objective observations, and analyses that account for everyone in the cohort who began treatment. These principles can now be used to obtain valid or persuasive results from non-randomised observational data.

For example, by applying the same admission criteria, classification of treatment and outcome events, augmented with a suitable prognostic stratification, Ralph Horwitz *et al.*, using an observational clinical cohort at Yale–New Haven Hospital, obtained the same results as the well-known randomised BHAT or Beta Blocker Heart Attack Trial. In several other instances, observational groups—when followed with the same admission criteria and the same non-randomised principles used in a randomised trial—have yielded results similar to those of the trial.

Although necessary in developing alternatives to randomised trials, we need to improve the quality of soft data for such phenomena as symptoms, co-morbidity, severity of illness, functional capacity, 'health status' and 'quality of life'. These improvements will require developing 'measurements' that use clinimetric principles, based on patient care, rather than the current psychometric tactics, based on statistical strategies or non-clinical authoritative doctrines. The improved soft data could also be used, of course, to improve substantially the clinical and scientific quality of randomised clinical trials themselves.

Finally, we could make better use of populational and vital statistics data if we could convert them into trustworthy scientific information. That information, as currently obtained from death certificates and other untrustworthy sources of data, is a bizarre anti-scientific anomaly in the era of molecular biology and magnificent technology. Drastic improvements are needed to bring the scientific quality of populational and vital statistics data up to a standard that might have been satisfactory, if achieved, for the middle of the twentieth century. If the nineteenth and early twentieth centuries were the eras that established the use of vital statistics and populational data, the twenty-first century can be the era when the information begins to develop the bare elements of scientific quality. The improvements, if initiated even in small regions, could provide valuable supplemental data for what is found with randomised trials and non-randomised observational cohort studies.

14 PATIENT COMPLIANCE WITH PRESCRIBED DRUG REGIMENS: OVERVIEW OF THE PAST 30 YEARS OF RESEARCH*

John Urquhart
University of Limburg, Maastricht, The Netherlands, and APREX
Corporation, Fremont, California, USA

Introduction

Crucial to the study of any phenomenon, biomedical or otherwise, is the ability to make reliable measurements. In therapeutics, a major factor that has long been unmeasurable is outpatient compliance with prescribed drug regimens. Compliance is best defined as:

> the extent to which the actual time history of dosing corresponds to the prescribed time history of dosing.

Thus, the basis for measuring compliance is the reliable recording of dosing times, together with means for analysing and interpreting the clinical or pharmacological implications of discrepancies between actual and prescribed dose timing.

Measured and expressed in this manner, compliance quantifies the patient's exposure to drug, the importance of which is directly related to the drug's therapeutic power. Of the many ways to express therapeutic power, the most useful in the present context are the slopes of the relations between the drug's dose and its various biological actions, for these

* Reprinted, with permission, from the Cinquième Entretiens du Centre Jacques Cartier: Pharmacoépidémiologie Prescription et Utilisation des Médicaments, Épidémiologie Clinique, vol. IV, Édition Fondation Marcel Mérieux, Lyon, 1993.

Clinical Measurement in Drug Evaluation. Edited by W. S. Nimmo and G. T. Tucker
Published 1995 by John Wiley & Sons Ltd

dose–response relations predict the consequences of under- or over-dosing. Obviously compliance is irrelevant for an agent whose dose–response relations have zero slope, i.e. no discernible biological actions, and it has relatively little importance for drugs with low-slope or shallow dose–response relations. With pharmacologically active agents, however, under-compliance deprives patients of therapeutic benefit, over-compliance can create toxicity, and certain instances of erratic dosing may create rebound or other types of hazardous effects. The interpretation of erratic dosing does not fit the dose–response rubric, which is a steady-state construct. Erratic dosing has to be dealt with separately as an inherently time-dependent, dynamic phenomenon.

Overall, the clinical interpretation of compliance data is specific to drug, to disease, and to the severity of disease.

Besides its historical focus, this chapter is orientated around the three important aspects of patient compliance:

- Its reliable measurement.
- Its clinical pharmacological and therapeutic correlates.
- Its impact on the interpretation of drug trials.

Reflecting this orientation, Table 1 lists 13 key events in the field during the past three decades since the first description of means for measuring compliance. The chapter is organised to discuss these items. It does not address the behavioural aspects of compliance, about which much has been written, but is unfortunately still mostly based on unsatisfactory methods for measuring compliance.

First concept of a special-purpose device to record dosing times

The notion of using a special-purpose device to measure compliance began in the early 1960s with the writings of a tuberculosis researcher, Dr Thomas Moulding [1]. Moulding recognised the need to track the time history of dosing, but, as his work preceded the micro-electronic revolution, he relied on indirect means for estimating when dosing had occurred. His device was a cabinet that stored drug dosage forms in small individual trays, with photographic film exposed to a radioactive source until the drug was removed from the tray. Practical implementation of this approach was precluded by several factors, including phobias about radioactivity, but it nevertheless stands as a historical landmark in the field for being the first means for recording the time history of dosing by outpatients. Accordingly, Table 1 begins with Moulding's concept.

Table 1. Key events in the history of the compliance field

1. 1962: first device to measure outpatient dosing times [1]
2. 1962: demonstration that ignoring compliance in outpatient drug trials leads to underestimation of drug effects, both beneficial and toxic [2]
3. 1976: first electronic monitor of outpatient dosing [3]
4. 1980: compliance-stratified reanalysis of Coronary Drug Project results demonstrates the potential for bias in equating compliance with exposure to the test drug [4]
5. 1984: NIH-sponsored conference on use of low-dose chemical markers to measure compliance [5]
6. 1985: FDA relabels cholestyramine using compliance-stratified data from Lipid Research Clinics--Coronary Primary Prevention Trial [6,7]
7. 1986: electronic monitoring data demonstrate white-coat compliance and drug holidays [8,9]
8. 1987: digoxin and phenobarbitone identified and qualified as reliable, low-dose chemical markers [10,11]; first electronic monitors enter the scientific products marketplace [12]
9. 1988: hazards of drug holidays identified for drugs having rebound effects [13]
10. 1989: chemical marker studies show that pill counts 'grossly overestimate' compliance [14]
11. 1990: Efron–Feldman method (1990 JASA Applications Lecture) [15]
12. 1991: Hutt and Lasagna show that conventional statistical policies used to analyse pre-market drug trials result in misleading labelling [16]
13. 1992: use of electronic monitoring data to project the time history of the concentration of drug in plasma in outpatients [17]

Numbers in brackets are reference numbers.

Variable compliance as a natural experiment in dose ranging

Variable compliance is prevalent, both in medical practice and clinical trials. In fixed-dose, controlled trials, variable compliance creates a natural experiment in dose ranging. The person who seems first to have grasped this point as a potentially important heuristic tool was C. R. B. Joyce, whose work [2] is the second listing in Table 1. This theme recurs and is reinforced in items 6, 9, 11 and 13 in Table 1.

PHARMACOLOGICAL CORRELATES OF COMPLIANCE

The importance of dose timing follows from basic concepts of pharmacokinetics (PK) and pharmacodynamics (PD) that describe how and why drug action waxes and then wanes in the aftermath of a single dose, and how and why dosing must follow a certain time sequence if drug action is to be maintained. Thus, defining 'compliance' in terms of the time history of dosing opens the way to projecting (i.e., modelling), with the aid of pharmacokinetic and pharmacodynamic information on the drug in question, the time history of drug actions in the outpatient setting. This type of modelling is a powerful tool for understanding successes and failures of outpatient pharmacotherapy. Rubio *et al.* have recently made the first such projections [17], which is the last item in Table 1.

Thus, 'compliance' should not be thought of as a simple percentage of prescribed doses taken. There are now many examples of excessively long intervals between doses that allow drug action to fade, even when, in the long run, approximately the correct number of doses end up being taken. Urquhart [18] illustrates how poor timing with diuretic dosing during a few days can precipitate costly complications of fluid retention and pulmonary congestion in heart failure patients, even if, over the longer run, correct numbers of doses are taken.

COMPLIANCE DATA CAN HELP IDENTIFY SUBOPTIMAL REGIMENS

Many writings on compliance are based on an assumption that any deviation from the prescribed regimens is, *ipso facto*, bad. In fact, many recommended regimens are suboptimal, with recommended doses usually much higher than necessary [19]. The pre-market overestimation of dose requirements has multiple causes and is a whole topic in itself; one factor, certainly, is a strong desire to avoid non-response, much of which stems from unrecognised poor and partial compliance in trials [20]. One of the ways to avoid overestimating dosing requirements is to heed the natural experiment in dose ranging created by variable compliance.

Obviously, good compliance is undesirable with irrationally prescribed drugs [21].

Beginnings of electronic monitoring of compliance

In the mid-1970s, the electronic revolution intersected with growing recognition of the need for practical and reliable means for measuring compliance. The author, then directing research at ALZA Corporation, initiated an effort to develop objective means to measure compliance with antiglaucoma eye-drops. An ALZA engineer, Fred Glover, invented the first electronic compliance monitor which incorporated into the drug package circuitry for time keeping, event monitoring and data storage [3]. This device compiled a time history of outpatients' dosing with antiglaucoma eye-drops by recording times when two events coincided: removal of the cap from the eye-drop container, and inversion of the container. This device was the first embodiment of the principle later termed 'medication event monitoring'—recording the time and date of use of the drug package in a manner necessary to administer a dose. A medication event does not, of course, prove that dosing occurred, but non-occurrence of a medication event around the time of a scheduled dose is a virtually certain sign that dosing failed to occur as scheduled.

Several dozens of Glover's device were fabricated at ALZA, which sponsored a clinical trial of the devices by Dr Michael Kass at Washington University [22], the third item in Table 1.

Kass's study showed the predominance of delayed and omitted doses as the main form of non-compliance. Several years later, Norell in Sweden published similar data on compliance in glaucoma treatment based on data from an electronically monitored holder for a standard eye-drop dispenser [23]. Kass's definitive papers were not published until 1986–7 [8,9,24], because he sought to reduce the size of the Glover device, whose components pre-dated the advent of microcircuitry, and so was substantially larger than a conventional eye-drop dispenser. There were, however, no striking qualitative differences between his earlier findings with the larger device and his later findings with the smaller one.

Controversy about the interpretation of compliance data

In 1980, compliance research was dealt a severe setback by a myopically interpreted reanalysis of the Coronary Drug Project (CDP) trial of clofibrate [4]—item 4 in Table 1. The reanalysis was undertaken to ascertain if patient compliance data might help explain the negative results of a trial in which high hopes had been vested for a positive outcome with clofibrate, an early cholesterol-lowering agent. The results of that reanalysis are shown in Table 2: patients who had taken $\geqslant 80\%$ of prescribed doses of either clofibrate or placebo had an approximately 40% lower mortality

Table 2. Five-year mortality in Coronary Drug Project patients by treatment group, according to five-year averages of estimated compliance

Compliance (% of prescribed doses estimated to have been taken)	Treatment group			
	Clofibrate		Placebo	
	Patients (*n*)	Mortality (%)	Patients (*n*)	Mortality (%)
$\geqslant 80$	708	15.0	1813	15.1
< 80	357	24.6	882	28.2
All patients	1065	18.2	2695	19.4

Source: Coronary Drug Project Research Group [4].

than those who had taken <80% of either. The authors concluded as follows:

> Analyses of data from the Coronary Drug Project have demonstrated the great difficulty, if not impossibility, of drawing any valid conclusions from findings about mortality or morbidity in subgroups defined by patient responses—such as adherence or biochemical response—to a treatment. [4]

As Feinstein has pointed out, the strikingly lower mortality among good compliers with placebo is a far bigger beneficial 'effect' than any yet found in all the studies on cholesterol reduction in coronary heart disease. Why was this not a strong stimulus to compliance research? In fact, but for the innovative work on compliance in the already-begun Helsinki Heart Study, this report appears to have inhibited research in the field throughout most of the 1980s. A major change occurred when the work of Efron and Feldman [15] was chosen for the JASA Applications Lecture at the 1990 meeting of the American Statistical Association (item 11 in Table 1).

REANALYSING THE REANALYSIS

Both Hasford [25] and the author [7] have identified a number of substantial methodological problems in the design and methods of the CDP trial as they relate to the assessment and use of compliance data. Most important, however, is that this was a secondary prevention trial whose participants entered the trial with established coronary heart disease—all patients having had at least one myocardial infarction. At enrolment, about half the patients were taking diuretics, cardiac glycosides, nitrates or other powerful cardiovascular drugs; more began such treatment during the five-year duration of the trial. Correct versus incorrect dosing with these agents of proven therapeutic power can have—depending on disease severity—major impact on morbidity and mortality because of suboptimal treatment of cardiomyopathy, fluid retention, rhythm disturbances and the like. Correct versus incorrect dosing with these non-trial agents was reflected by the measure of placebo compliance during the trial, because compliance with concomitantly prescribed agents is usually similar [12,26]. The CDP reanalysts asserted that multivariate analysis was unable to find a basis for the correlation between mortality differences and placebo compliance. The burden of proof, however, rests with the reanalysts as to whether the data and methods were robust enough to demonstrate what is, in fact, such a clinically obvious basis for the association of compliance behaviour, morbidity and mortality.

Analogous considerations apply to the reanalysis of the Beta Blocker Heart Attack Trial [27], as discussed in Urquhart [7].

Development of useful chemical markers to estimate compliance

Nevertheless, efforts continued to find reliable measures of compliance. In 1984, the National Institutes of Health sponsored a conference on methods for assessing compliance (item 5 in Table 1). The consensus at this conference was that the ideal chemical marker was one that had a very short residence time in the body [5]. This was wrong, because it soon became clear from electronic monitoring data that compliance usually improves in the day or two prior to a scheduled visit [8,9,24,28]. As item 7 in Table 1 indicates, this phenomenon has come to be known as 'white-coat compliance'—a term coined by Alvan Feinstein [29]. A chemical marker with a short residence time is destined only to reflect compliance during the phase of 'white-coat compliance', and thus to overestimate usually prevailing compliance and miss clinically important underdosing. The prevalence of this pre-visit improvement in compliance is one of the main reasons that poor or partial compliance so often escapes clinical detection [9,13,16,18,28,29].

As item 8 in Table 1 indicates, the groups in Helsinki [10] and in Leeds [11] independently demonstrated the value of long residence time, low-dose markers—digoxin or phenobarbitone. The Helsinki group appear to have limited their work to the five-year trial of gemfibrozil [30], but the Leeds group, under Morgan Feely's direction, have performed studies in a variety of therapeutic settings showing the extent to which partial compliance is both unrecognised and a major source of problems in patient management—arthritis [31], anticoagulation [32] and thyroid disease [33]. Pullar and Feely [34] provide a good summary of the Leeds group's work.

From the perspective of drug trials, one of the most valuable contributions of the low-dose chemical marker methods has been to show how conventional tablet counting overestimates patient compliance—item 10 in Table 1. In a single instant, patients can and do discard tablets and create the illusion of full compliance. The Leeds group demonstrated this unequivocally [14], and Rudd and his colleagues at Stanford have shown that compliance estimated from returned tablet counts rises in proportion to the excess numbers of dosage forms dispensed to the patients [35]—also evidence that many patients simply discard all or most of the dosage forms before returning the containers to the investigative staff. Patients with chronic obstructive pulmonary disease have also been shown to discard unused inhalational drug just before a scheduled visit [36].

HOW GOOD IS COMPLIANCE IN CLINICAL TRIALS?

Many clinical researchers feel that compliance in drug trials is appreciably better than in medical practice, because patients have volunteered for the trial and understand its purposes. While these are considerations, one should note that over 35% of patients in the carefully executed Helsinki Heart Study (HHS) of gemfibrozil, a twice-daily lipid-lowering agent, materially underdosed, based on a three-method assessment of compliance [37]. This underdosing reflected itself in major dilution of the drug's effects on all cholesterol fractions and triglycerides [30].

Labelling implications

This dilutional effect of poor compliance also occurred in the Lipid Research Clinics–Coronary Primary Prevention Trial (LRC-CPPT) of cholestyramine [38]. The data, taken from the drug's US labelling, are shown in Table 3, and are the basis for item 6 in Table 1. Inclusion of this information in labelling [6] informs physicians, patients and payers about the effect of variable dosing on cholesterol reduction and coronary risk reduction. As Hutt and Lasagna have pointed out (item 12 in Table 1) [16], this compliance-stratified labelling is an important regulatory precedent, because it avoids the mislabelling created by conventional biostatistical analyses that link a recommended dosage with effects created by a much lower dosage—the average dose actually taken by trial participants. The resulting mislabelling is not only a biostatistical issue, but an economic and ethical issue as well.

ECONOMIC ISSUE

Subsequent pharmaco-economic interpretations of the LRC-CPPT have amply demonstrated that accurate cost-effectiveness assessments require understanding of dose-dependent effects, associated costs, and the range of compliance in representative patient populations [39–41].

Table 3. Relation of reduction in cholesterol to reduction in coronary heart disease (CHD) risk

No. of doses per day	No. of patients	Total cholesterol lowering (%)	Reduction in CHD risk (%)
0–2	439	4.4	10.9
2–5	496	11.5	26.1
5–6	965	19.0	39.3

Dose = 4g packet of cholestyramine.

All patient, compliance-blind averages:

cholesterol lowering	8.5%
reduction in CHD risk	19.0%

Sources: QUESTRAN [6]; LRC-CPPT [38].

ETHICAL ISSUE

The ethical issue arises when fully compliant patients are misled into rejecting treatment based on misinformation about the magnitude of drug benefits. A fully compliant patient can directly perceive the associated costs and common side-effects of dosing according to the label's instructions, but must rely on the label for information on the magnitude of long-term therapeutic benefits, because these are usually not perceivable by the individual patient, e.g. in hypertension or dyslipidaemias. If the long-term benefits are based on a compliance-blind, all-patient average, they will usually be substantially diluted, as Table 3 illustrates using the only example of a long-term medication whose therapeutic benefit is stratified by compliance in its labelling. In the usual case where labelling gives only the compliance-blind average benefit, the patient is confronted by full-dose costs and side-effects and a diluted estimate of benefits. Some fully compliant patients will reasonably conclude that the trade-off is unsatisfactory and thus be deprived of valuable therapy. In this and other ways, the minority of patients who substantially under-comply in drug trials are able to disenfranchise the compliant majority.

PLACEBO EFFECTS

In contrast to results in the CDP trial, there was no association between outcomes and placebo compliance in either the HHS or LRC-CPPT [30,38]. Efron and Feldman did find a weak association between placebo compliance and reductions in cholesterol levels in the Stanford subset of LRC-CPPT [15]—an effect perhaps mediated by better compliance with a low-cholesterol diet among the better compliers with placebo. The crucial point is that both LRC and Helsinki were primary prevention trials, carried out in healthy subjects enrolled only on the basis of their having elevated lipid concentrations, but without evidence of existing coronary heart disease. Thus, except for the few patients who developed coronary heart disease during these trials, interpretation is uncomplicated by use of concomitant, powerful non-trial medications capable of influencing the trial's outcome variables.

The LRC-CPPT was the first demonstration that intervening to normalise uncomplicated hypercholesterolaemia can reduce the risk of developing coronary heart disease. It led, in 1985, to the relabelling of cholestyramine, in turn triggering not only item 6, but also items 11 and 12 in Table 1.

Interpretation of drug 'holidays'

Electronic monitoring promptly demonstrated what has become a frequently observed pattern of partial compliance: the multi-day interruption in dosing [8,9,24,26,42,43]. As first noted in 1988 [13], these drug 'holidays' have potentially three different pharmacodynamic effects:

A. They represent a period of lapsed drug action.
B. They usually begin with an abrupt halt in dosing, which may trigger hazardous rebound effects.
C. They usually terminate with an abrupt resumption of full-strength dosing, which may transiently cause overdose effects in drugs that require initial dose titration.

With respect to item B, Psaty *et al.* have demonstrated the risk of incident coronary disease due to rebound effects occurring in partially compliant patients prescribed beta blockers for mild–moderate hypertension [44]. Lasagna has summarised it well [45]:

> In the past, I have often told students and physicians that a patient's condition would not improve if they failed to take a medication as prescribed, nor would they be harmed by the absence of the drug (except in the sense that no therapeutic benefit would result). It is now known, however, that with certain drugs, rebound phenomena occur when treatment is withdrawn, increasing the risk for exacerbation of the condition being treated or for some other untoward event.

Item C is yet to be demonstrated. A likely example is the reflex tachycardia occurring episodically in patients treated with nifedipine; eventually someone will study the extent of correlation between its occurrence and the resumption of dosing after nifedipine holidays. Another possible example of this phenomenon may be the disappointing results in the CAST trial, in which mortality with encainide [46] or flecainide [47] was higher than with placebo. Both agents are specifically labelled as requiring very careful, gradual escalation in dose when treatment is initiated [46,47]. But what happens to the already-titrated patient whose dosing lapses for several days, and then abruptly resumes full-strength dosing? Unfortunately, the CAST trial did not include electronic compliance monitoring, which could have indicated the incidence of multi-day drug holidays in this patient group, and whether there was any temporal association of serious episodes of arrhythmia with drug holidays. This may be another example where a minority of non-compliant patients has disenfranchised the compliant majority who could benefit from the drugs.

In overview

Initial recognition of the problems created by prevalent poor compliance was catalysed during the 1970s by Lasagna in the USA [48], by Sackett and Haynes in Canada [49,50], and by Weber in Germany [51,52]. By 1980, however, it was clear that the field was stalled for want of adequate methods, and all these workers turned their attention to other fields, though both Lasagna [20,45] and Weber [43] returned to contribute to the field when electronic monitoring became possible. Another early contributor to the field was Peck [53,54], who has recently integrated patient compliance into a general model of the sources of variance in drug responses [55]. Along with the work of Rubio [17], it anticipates future efforts to model the PK/PD consequences of variable dosing.

The Efron–Feldman paper [15] was published together with commentaries by four leading figures in biostatistics [56–58]. They capture the ambivalent sense of challenge created when statistical thinking confronts the magnitude of variance in drug response created by the patterns of dosing that actually prevail in randomised controlled trials. In his recent presidential address to the American Society of Clinical Pharmacology and Therapeutics, Sheiner has directly challenged the prevailing statistical policy of ignoring compliance [59].

Two recent reviews [60,61] give additional perspectives on non-compliance in drug trials.

Looking ahead

Items 11–13 in Table 1 suggest that we shall see increasing use of the principle initially demonstrated by Dick Joyce in 1962 (item 2, Table 1) of availing ourselves of the natural experiment in dose ranging imbedded in every outpatient drug trial. The Efron–Feldman method [15] is only a beginning of serious statistical attention being paid to improving the analyses of these natural experiments, as references [56–58] suggest. The big fear, raised to feverish levels by the reanalysis of the CDP trial of clofibrate [4], is a major, hidden bias that leads to a wrong conclusion. That reanalysis has itself now been reanalysed enough to close the book on this unsatisfactory episode, drawing from it two already obvious conclusions:

- Placebo controls help avoid mistaken conclusions, but, as Efron and Feldman note [15], they cannot completely exclude the hypothetical possibility that some factor linked to compliance behaviour may modulate drug action.
- Trials are difficult to interpret when they include patients who take powerful non-trial medications whose compliance-dependent actions can influence trial outcome.

It is in the nature of biostatisticians and epidemiologists to pose 'what if?' questions whenever experimental designs are insufficiently rigorous to rule them out. Sheiner has countered this approach by acknowledging the possibility but questioning the likelihood or incidence of such complications [59]. The work of Rubio *et al.* [17] (item 13, Table 1) opens the door to formal pharmacokinetic and pharmacodynamic analyses capable of creating mechanistic foundations to strengthen the interpretation of the natural experiment in dose ranging.

Little thought has yet been given to designing randomised controlled trials in ways specifically aimed at strengthening the interpretation of the imbedded natural experiment in dose ranging. That may be the next area of importance advance. The trial design of Johnson, Whelton and McMahon [62] illustrates one such approach.

As the accelerating pace of events listed in Table 1 indicates, compliance research has been reanimated since 1986 and has begun to make important progress. Its revival has been triggered by the advent of reasonably reliable, if still imperfect, methods. There will undoubtedly be refinements of the methods for measuring compliance, but it seems clear that the long-standing methodological blockade has been lifted. An important next step will be regulatory action to resolve the mislabelling problems created by ignoring widespread poor compliance in trials of new drugs [16]. There is an urgent need for better understanding of the adverse consequences of drug holidays, as the examples of beta blockers, encainide and flecainide suggest.

Meanwhile, a new type of natural experiment is gaining increasing attention: the assessment of outcomes of medical care [63]. A great deal of wishful thinking and political activity has already been invested in 'outcome research' in hopes that observational studies in this new dress will prove to be an economical short-cut in the assessment of the effectiveness and economics of medical interventions. It is an area where patient compliance is an obviously important determinant of good versus poor outcomes, with direct impact on costs. Focused attention on improving compliance promises to be an important tool in cost containment.

Patient compliance is only one of several variables for evaluating the proficiency of medical care. Besides patients' abilities and willingness to follow prescribed regimens of drug, diet or exercise, one must evaluate as well the diagnostic acumen and interventional skills of physicians and surgeons—not easy measurements to make. In addition to overcoming these methodological hurdles, 'outcome research' will require novel study designs if it is to avoid the rediscovery of lessons long-since learned about observational studies.

Acknowledgements

The author is indebted to the Fondation Marcel Mérieux for permission to reprint this paper, and thus give it circulation in the English-speaking world.

References

1. Moulding T. Proposal for a time recording pill dispenser as a method for studying and supervising the self-administration of drugs. Am Rev Respir Dis 1962; 85: 754–757.
2. Joyce CRB. Patient co-operation and the sensitivity of clinical trials. J Chronic Dis 1962; 15: 1025–1036.
3. Glover F. US Patent 4 034 757, 1976.
4. Coronary Drug Project Research Group. Influence of adherence to treatment and response of cholesterol on mortality in the coronary drug project. N Engl J Med 1980; 303: 1038–1041.
5. The papers from the NIH symposium are published in Controlled Clin Trials 1984; 5: 459–567.
6. QUESTRAN (cholestyramine). Physicians' Desk Reference. Oradell, NJ: Medical Economics Data, 1992; 710–711.
7. Urquhart J. Patient compliance as an explanatory variable in four selected cardiovascular studies. In: Cramer JA, Spilker B (eds), Compliance in Medical Practice and Clinical Trials. New York: Raven Press, 1991; 301–322.
8. Kass MA, Meltzer D, Gordon M, Cooper D, Goldberg J. Compliance with topical pilocarpine treatment. Am J Ophthalmol 1986; 101: 515–523.
9. Kass MA, Gordon M, Meltzer DW. Can ophthalmologists correctly identify patients defaulting from pilocarpine therapy? Am J Ophthalmol 1986; 101: 524–530.
10. Mäenpää H, Javela K, Pikkarainen J, Malkonen M, Heinonen OP, Manninen V. Minimal doses of digoxin: a new marker for compliance to medication. Eur Heart J 1987; 8 (Suppl I): 31–37.
11. Feely M, Cooke J, Price D et al. Low-dose phenobarbitone as an indicator of compliance with drug therapy. Br J Clin Pharmacol 1987; 24: 77–83.
12. Data on file, APREX Corporation, Fremont, CA.
13. Urquhart J, Chevalley C. Impact of unrecognized dosing errors on the cost and effectiveness of pharmaceuticals. Drug Inform J 1988; 22: 363–378.
14. Pullar T, Kumar S, Tindall H, Feely M. Time to stop counting the tablets? Clin Pharmacol Ther 1989; 46: 163–168.
15. Efron B, Feldman D. Compliance as an explanatory variable in clinical trials. J Am Statist Assoc 1991; 86 (413): 7–17. See also discussion following on pp 18–25.
16. Lasagna L, Hutt PB. Health care, research, and regulatory impact of noncompliance. In: Cramer JA, Spilker B (eds), Compliance in Medical Practice and Clinical Trials. New York: Raven Press, 1991; 393–403.
17. Rubio A, Cox C, Weintraub M. Prediction of diltiazem plasma concentration curves from limited measurements using compliance data. Clin Pharmacokinet 1992; 22: 238–246.
18. Urquhart J. Time to take our medicines, seriously. Inaugural professorial lecture, University of Limburg, Maastricht, April 3, 1992. Pharm Weekbl 1992; 127: 769–776.
19. Temple R. Dose–response and registration of new drugs. In: Lasagna L, Erill S, Naranjo CA (eds), Dose–Response Relationships in Clinical Pharmacology. Amsterdam: Elsevier, 1989; 145–167.
20. Lasagna L. Pharmacometry in man: the state of the art. In: Lasagna L, Erill S, Naranjo CA (eds), Dose–Response Relationships in Clinical Pharmacology. Esteve Foundation Symposia, vol 3. Amsterdam: Excerpta Medica, 1989; 1–7.
21. Weintraub M. Intelligent noncompliance and capricious compliance. In: Lasagna L (ed), Patient Compliance. Mount Kisco, NY: Futura, 1976; 39–47.

22. Kass MA, Zimmerman T, Yablonski M, Becker B. Compliance to pilocarpine therapy. Invest Ophthalmol (ARVO abstracts supplement) 1977; 108: abstract 2.
23. Norell SE, Granstrom PA, Wassen R. A medication monitor and fluorescein technique designed to study medication behaviour. Acta Ophthalmol 1980; 58: 459.
24. Kass MA, Gordon M, Morley RE, Meltzer DW, Goldberg JJ. Compliance with topical timolol treatment. Am J Ophthalmol 1987; 103: 188–193.
25. Hasford J. Biometric issues in measuring and analyzing partial compliance in clinical trials. In: Cramer JA, Spilker B (eds), Compliance in Medical Practice and Clinical Trials. New York: Raven Press, 1991; 265–281.
26. Cramer J, Ouelette VL, Mattson RH. How can non-compliance be measured? Epilepsia 1988; 29(5): 705.
27. Horwitz RI, Viscoli CM, Berkman L et al. Treatment adherence and risk of death after a myocardial infarction. Lancet 1990; 336: 542–545.
28. Cramer JA, Scheyer RD, Mattson RH. Compliance declines between clinic visits. Arch Intern Med 1990; 150: 1509–1510.
29. Feinstein AR. On white-coat effects and the electronic monitoring of compliance. Arch Intern Med 1990; 150: 1377–1378.
30. Manninen V, Elo MO, Frick H et al. Lipid alternations and decline in the incidence of coronary heart disease in the Helsinki Heart Study. JAMA 1988; 260: 641–651.
31. Pullar T, Peaker S, Martin MFR, Bird HA, Feely MP. The use of a pharmacological indicator to investigate compliance in patients with a poor response to antirheumatic therapy. Br J Rheumatol 1988; 27: 381–384.
32. Kumar S, Haigh JRM, Rhodes LE et al. Poor compliance is a major factor in unstable outpatient control of anticoagulant therapy. Thromb Haemost 1989; 62: 729–732.
33. Penn ND, Speaker S, Griffiths AP, Feely M, Tindall H. Use of a pharmacological indicator to monitor compliance with thyroxine. Eur J Clin Pharmacol 1988; 35: 327–329.
34. Pullar T, Feely M. Problems of compliance with drug treatment: new solutions? Pharm J 1990; 245: 213–215.
35. Rudd P, Byyny RL, Zachary V et al. The natural history of medication compliance in a drug trial: limitations of pill counts. Clin Pharmacol Ther 1989; 46: 169–176.
36. Tashkin DP, Rand C, Nides M et al. A nebulizer chronolog to monitor compliance with inhaler use. Am J Med 1991; 91 (Suppl 4A): 33S–36S.
37. Mäenpää H, Manninen V, Heinonen OP. Comparison of the digoxin marker with capsule counting and compliance questionnaire methods for measuring compliance to medication in a clinical trial. Eur Heart J 1987; 8 (Suppl I): 39–43.
38. Lipid Research Clinics Coronary Primary Prevention Trial results: (I) Reduction in incidence of coronary heart disease; (II) The relationship of reduction in incidence or coronary heart disease to cholesterol lowering. JAMA 1984; 251: 351–374.
39. Weinstein MC, Stason WB. Cost-effectiveness of interventions to prevent or treat coronary heart disease. Annu Rev Public Health 1985; 6: 41–63.
40. Oster G, Epstein AM. Cost-effectiveness of antihyperlipemic therapy in the prevention of coronary heart disease. JAMA 1987; 258: 2381–2387.
41. Himmelstein DU, Woolhandler S. Costs and effects: the lipid research trial and the Rand experiment. N Engl J Med 1985; 311: 1512–1513.
42. Cramer JA, Mattson RH, Prevey ML, Scheyer RD, Ouellette VL. How often is

medication taken as prescribed? A novel assessment technique. JAMA 1989; 261: 3273–3277.

43. Kruse W, Weber E. Dynamics of drug regimen compliance: its assessment by microprocessor-based monitoring. Eur J Clin Pharmacol 1990; 38: 561–556.

44. Psaty BM, Koepsell TD, Wagner EH, LoGerfo JP, Inui TS. The relative risk of incident coronary heart disease associated with recently stopping the use of beta blockers. JAMA 1990; 263: 1653–1657.

45. Lasagna L. Noncompliance data and clinical outcomes: impact on health care. Primary Cardiol 1992; 18 Suppl 1: 36–39.

46. ENKAID (encainide hydrochloride). Physicians' Desk Reference. Oradell, NJ: Medical Economics Data, 1992; 704–707.

47. TAMBOCOR (flecainide acetate). Physicians' Desk Reference. Oradell, NJ: Medical Economics Data, 1992; 1315–1317.

48. Lasagna L (ed). Patient Compliance. Mount Kisco, NY: Futura, 1976.

49. Sackett DL, Haynes RB (eds). Compliance with Therapeutic Regimens. Baltimore: Johns Hopkins University Press, 1976.

50. Haynes RB, Taylor DW, Sackett DL (eds). Compliance in Health Care. Baltimore: Johns Hopkins University Press, 1979.

51. Gundert-Remy U, Montmann U, Weber E. Studien zur Regelmassigkeit der Einnahme der verordneten Medikamente bei stationaren Patienten, I. Methodik und Basisdaten, II. Erlauternde Feststellungen zu sozialen und Krankeitsbedingten Faktorn sowie zur Selbsteinschatzung der Erkrankung durch den Patienten. Innere Medizin 1973; 27 and 73.

52. Weber E. Compliance als unterbewertetes Problem der Pharmakotherapie. In: Weber E, Gundert-Remy U, Schrey A (eds), Patienten Compliance. Workshop am 14 Mai 1977 uber Verbesserung der Arzt-Patienten-Beziehung in Frankfurt a.M. Baden-Baden: Verlag Gerhard Witzrock, 1977.

53. Peck CC. Qualitative aspects of therapeutic decision making. In: Melmon KL, Morrelli HF (eds), Clinical Pharmacology: Basic Principles in Therapeutics. New York: Macmillan, 1978; 1063–1083.

54. Peck CC. Should we improve patient compliance with therapeutic regimens, and, if so, how? In: Lasagna L (ed), Controversies in Therapeutics. Philadelphia: Saunders, 1980; 559–566.

55. Harter JG, Peck CC. Chronobiology: suggestions for integrating it into drug development. Ann NY Acad Sci 1991; 618: 563–571.

56. Zeger SL, Liang K-Y. Comment: dose–response estimands. J Am Statist Assoc 1991; 86 (413): 18–19.

57. Meier P. Discussion. J Am Statist Assoc 1991; 86 (413): 19–22.

58. Rubin D. Comment: dose–response estimands. J Am Statist Assoc 1991; 86 (413): 22–24.

59. Sheiner LB. The intellectual health of clinical drug evaluation. Clin Pharmacol Ther 1991; 50: 4–9.

60. Vander Stichele R. Measurement of patient compliance and the interpretation of randomized clinical trials. Eur J Clin Pharmacol 1991; 41: 27–35.

61. Kruse W. Patient compliance with drug treatment: new perspectives on an old problem. Clin Invest 1992; 70: 163–166.

62. Johnson BF, Whelton A. A study design for comparing the effects of missing daily doses of antihypertensive drugs. Am J Therapeutics (in press).

63. Ellwood P. Shattuck lecture: outcomes management. N Engl J Med. 1988; 318: 1549–1556.

PART IV
MEASUREMENT OF ADVERSE EVENTS

15 PREDICTION OF DRUG INTERACTIONS: IMPLICATIONS OF RECENT ADVANCES IN DRUG METABOLISM

G. T. Tucker
University of Sheffield, The Royal Hallamshire Hospital,
Sheffield, UK

Selection of studies

In drug development, the selection of drug interaction studies is usually based on two main criteria: the likelihood of co-prescription and the therapeutic index. Classically, studies are done using antipyrine as a model inhibitee and cimetidine as a ubiquitous inhibitor, while the list of low therapeutic index compounds that are of concern includes warfarin, oral contraceptives, phenytoin, theophylline and cyclosporin. The problem with this approach is 'how long is a ball of string?'—where does the list end? An alternative approach, for those interactions involving changes in drug metabolism, is to make intelligent use of the recent expansion of knowledge of the substrate selectivity of isoenzymes, particularly amongst the cytochrome P450 superfamily. This offers a more focused identification of interactions that might need to be assessed, but also helps to exclude those combinations that it may not be necessary, and may therefore be unethical, to study. Rather than carrying out extensive 'box-ticking' volunteer studies with 'classical' compounds such as antipyrine (where understanding of isoform selectivity is incomplete), prior identification of the enzymes involved in the metabolism of a new drug should direct volunteer studies to the interactions that might be relevant, and give confidence to assess the less likely ones by less stringent population kinetic studies in patients.

Clinical Measurement in Drug Evaluation. Edited by W. S. Nimmo and G. T. Tucker

In vitro screens

CYTOCHROMES P450

The cytochrome P450 monooxygenases comprise the most important class of enzymes with respect to drug metabolism. Therefore, the prediction of drug interactions involving this enzyme system will be emphasised. Cytochromes P450 are grouped according to their amino acid sequence into families and subfamilies which apply across different species; a greater than 40% homology defines a family and a greater than 55% homology defines a subfamily. The symbol CYP is used to denote both the human cytochrome P450 gene and enzyme. This is followed by an arabic numeral denoting the family, a capital letter designating the subfamily and then another arabic numeral representing the individual gene/enzyme [1]. For example, CYP2D6 refers to debrisoquine hydroxylase—a human form of cytochrome P450 which shows a marked genetic polymorphism. In humans, five CYP subfamilies appear to be principally involved in drug metabolism, namely CYPs 1A, 2C, 2D, 2E and 3A.

PROBE SUBSTRATES, INHIBITORS AND INDUCERS

The broad structural characteristics of substrates for each of the main CYP isoforms involved in human drug metabolism have been discussed by Smith and Jones [2] (Table 1). A list of some probe substrates and relatively potent and selective inhibitors is shown in Table 2. It should be

Table 1. Substrate structure–activity relationships of cytochrome P450 isoforms ([2]; Smith, personal communication)

CYP1A	Neutral, flat aromatic compounds, tricyclic or above
CYP2A	Neutral, bicyclic, planar compounds with a minimum of one aromatic ring
CYP2D6	Arylalkylamines with site of oxidation 5–7 Å from protonated nitrogen
CYP2E	Small, polar molecules. Lower rotational and tumbling energy for binding, at a non-specific site
CYP2C9	Neutral or acidic molecules with site of oxidation 5–8 Å from H-bond donor heteroatom
CYP3A	Neutral or basic molecules with site of oxidation determined by ease of electron or hydrogen atom abstraction

Table 2. Xenobiotic substrate probes, selective inhibitors and regulation of human cytochrome P450 isoforms

Isoform	Model substrate	Selective inhibitors	Regulation
CYP1A1	Benzo(a)pyrene		Induced in cigarette smokers
CYP1A2	Caffeine, phenacetin	Furafylline	Induced in cigarette smokers
CYP2A6	Coumarin		
CYP2C9/10	Tolbutamide, phenytoin, S-warfarin	Sulphaphenzole	Induced by rifampicin, phenobarbitone
CYP2C19	S-Mephenytoin, omeprazole, proguanil		Genetic polymorphism (3% PM in C; 20% in O)
CYP2D6	Debrisoquine, sparteine, metoprolol, dextromethorphan	Quinidine	Genetic polymorphism (8% PM in C)
CYP2E1	Chlorzoxazone, ethanol, N-nitroso-dimethylamine, 4-nitrophenol	Diethyldithiocarbamate	Induced by ethanol
CYP3A4/5	Cyclosporin, nifedipine, erythromycin, lignocaine, midazolam, caffeine, ethynyloestradiol	Ketoconazole (low conc.) gestodene	Induced by dexamethasone, rifampicin; 3A5 polymorphic (present in 30%)

PM, poor metaboliser phenotype; C, Caucasian; O, Oriental.
Source: Birkett *et al.* [48].

noted that the list includes many of the low therapeutic index drugs of concern with regard to drug interactions. Thus, in principle, it is increasingly possible to predict which kinds of compounds a new drug might inhibit or be inhibited by. The selectivity of enzyme inducers is rather less than that of inhibitors. CYP2D6 is not inducible, polycyclic hydrocarbons induce 1A, phenobarbitone and rifampicin induce 2C, ethanol induces 2E and rifampicin and dexamethasone induce 3A. CYPs 2D6 and 2C19 exhibit marked genetic polymorphism.

LABORATORY METHODS

A variety of laboratory methods, each with different advantages and disadvantages, may be used to identify the roles of specific CYP isoforms and to screen for likely interactions *in vitro*.

Animals

In spite of considerable amino acid sequence similarity in enzymes across species, even small differences can alter the catalytic activity dramatically. For example, the 6- and 8-hydroxylation of warfarin is catalysed by CYP1A1 in the rat but not in the mouse, despite 93% homology in the enzyme sequence [3]. *S*-mephenytoin is 4-hydroxylated by a member of the 2C subfamily in man but this reaction is carried out by CYP3A in the rat [4,5]. Thus, predictions of metabolically based drug interactions from animal data alone are generally inadequate.

Human liver microsomes

Access to human liver tissue is possible through non-profit making sources in the USA. Microsomes are easy to prepare and retain their activity with respect to cytochromes P450 when stored at $-80\ ^{\circ}\text{C}$. Limitations to the use of microsomes include a short incubation time, necessitating the development of sensitive assays for metabolites of low-extraction compounds, inability to study induction, and the difficulty of assessing the contribution of oxidative metabolism to net drug clearance without independent data on other pathways of drug elimination. It is also important to study a sufficiently wide range of samples from different livers to ensure that results are representative.

The availability of microsomes from livers of genotyped individuals facilitates recognition of the role of CYP2D6 in the metabolism of a compound. Thus, studies using 'poor metaboliser' and 'extensive metaboliser' microsomes, along with the use of quinidine and quinine as inhibitors, can be diagnostic [6].

Human liver hepatocytes/slices

A major advantage of these systems is the ability to study enzyme induction. However, a considerable disadvantage at the present time is that the preparations have to be used fresh, although developments in cryopreservation may ultimately remove this need. Improvements in the ability to maintain liver cells in culture are also anticipated.

Expression systems

Human cell lines, yeast and bacteria expressing single or multiple CYPs are becoming increasingly available. If validated adequately, their use can confirm the participation of a single enzyme in the metabolism of a compound. For example, yeast expressing human CYP2D6 [7] has been used to establish a role for this enzyme in the metabolism of 'Ecstasy' (methylenedioxymethamphetamine), with implications for genetic differences in susceptibility to its toxic effects [8]. Perhaps in the future an array of expressed human enzymes, present in relation to their quantitative importance, may be used as an 'artificial liver' for studying drug metabolism?

Antibodies

In principle, the availability of a specific antibody raised against a particular enzyme allows its role in the metabolism of a drug to be delineated. Two approaches can be used. The first uses non-inhibitory antibodies and involves correlating the patency of the metabolic pathway of interest with the immunoblot intensity for the enzyme across a series of livers. This can then be confirmed by using inhibitory antibodies to block the metabolic pathway. In practice, the applicability of these approaches depends upon the specificity of the antibodies used. While some, such as the anti-LKM$_1$ antibody to CYP2D6, are highly specific [9], others should be used with great care.

Molecular modelling

Models of the active sites of several of the cytochromes P450 are in the process of being refined. For example, in the case of CYP2D6 these range from templates based upon structure–metabolism relationships to representations based upon protein structure [10]. Ultimately, a combination of approaches, including systematic structure–activity studies, site-directed mutagenesis, use of single-enzyme expression systems and molecular modelling, should improve our ability to visualise the topography of active sites and, thereby, to predict interactions *in computro*.

APPLICATIONS

A number of studies illustrating the potential value of the *in vitro* screening approach to the identification of metabolism-based drug interactions in man have appeared in the recent literature. The following are some examples.

CYP2C9

The 7-hydroxylation of the more active S isomer of warfarin is the major metabolic pathway and is mediated almost entirely by CYP2C9. Thus, studies in microsomes or expression systems with S-warfarin, or other known substrates of this isoform (e.g., tolbutamide), have been proposed to predict likely inhibitors *in vivo* [11,12].

CYP2C19

The aliphatic hydroxylation of omeprazole is a major route of elimination, and systematic *in vitro* studies using human liver microsomes have shown it to be mediated primarily by CYP2C19, with a contribution from CYP3A4 [13]. This would have predicted earlier *in vivo* findings that omeprazole exhibits polymorphic metabolism co-segregating with the oxidation of S-mephenytoin, and that it inhibits the metabolism of diazepam, another 2C19 substrate [14,15].

CYP2D6

Interactions involving CYP2D6 have been predicted from *in vitro* studies of several new CNS-active drugs, including paroxetine [16], minaprine [17] and clozapine [18], although in the last case it appears that oxidation by the enzyme is not a major pathway. Based upon a simple template in which the site of oxidation is located 5–7 Å from a binding site between the basic nitrogen of the substrate and a carboxylic acid group within the enzyme, Koymans *et al.* [19] predicted that four out of 14 potential metabolic routes for four new drugs are CYP2D6 mediated. The drugs and routes predicted to be via 2D6 were: alfentanil (none), astemizole (O-demethylation), risperidone (7- and 9-alicyclic hydroxylation) and nebivolol (aromatic hydroxylation). All but the O-demethylation of astemizole were confirmed by *in vitro* and *in vivo* studies. Thus, in turn, potential interactions with other known CYP2D6 substrates could be anticipated.

CYP3A4

Using human liver microsomes and hepatocytes 59 drugs representative of 17 different therapeutic classes have been assigned as inhibitors or inducers of or non-interactors with CYP3A4-mediated metabolism of cyclosporin [20].

CYP1A2

Relationships between the structures of quinoline antibacterials, their effects on bacterial growth and their ability to inhibit caffeine 3-demethylation were defined by Fuhr *et al.* [21]. An optimal structure which maximises antibacterial effect while minimising the potential for CYP1A2 inhibition was suggested.

Cimetidine

When incubated with human liver microsomes cimetidine appears to inhibit CYP2D6 and a form of CYP3A more than CYPs 1A2 and 2C9 [22].

Phase II enzymes

In vitro studies with suitably fortified human liver microsomes may also be useful in predicting interactions involving phase II drug-metabolising enzymes. Thus, potential interactions between tertiary amine drugs (e.g., chlorpromazine, tricyclic antidepressants, lamotrigine), that undergo *N*-glucuronidation, and the glucuronidation of steroids have been screened in this way [23,24].

Substrate and/or inhibitor or inducer?

When using *in vitro* screens it is important to appreciate that compounds should be studied both as potential substrates and as inhibitors. Thus, there are many examples where inhibitors apparently are not themselves substrates for particular enzymes. These include: quinidine (inhibitor but not substrate of CYP2D6; substrate but less potent inhibitor of CYP3A4); many beta blockers (inhibitors of CYP2D6 in relation to their lipid solubility, but not all substrates of the enzyme [25,26]); mexiletine (substrate of CYP2D6 but inhibitor of theophylline, a substrate of CYP1A2 [27]).

The structures of both timolol and moclobemide contain a morpholino group. Since cleavage of this ring in timolol is known to be mediated by CYP2D6 [28], it might be anticipated that the same would be true for moclobemide. However, whereas the morpholino group of timolol aligns with the oxidative site of the simple 2D6 template, that of moclobemide probably anchors to the anion binding site, thereby blocking the oxidative site with the metabolically inert chloro group at the other end of the molecule. This might explain why moclobemide is a potent inhibitor of CYP2D6 *in vivo*, but does not appear to be a substrate for the enzyme [29].

Screening of the ability of a new compound to inhibit is relatively straightforward by judicious use of probe substrates. However, identification of enzymes involved in its metabolism may be more difficult if its metabolism is slow and sensitive assays for products are not available.

Inducers of particular forms of cytochrome P450 are also not necessarily substrates of those forms. For example, omeprazole is metabolised primarily by CYPs 2C19 and 3A4, yet it is a weak inducer of CYPs 1A1 and 1A2 [30,31].

In vitro–in vivo scaling

A number of factors must be considered when extrapolating the results of *in vitro* studies to expectations *in vivo*. Thus, the equation below shows that, assuming competitive inhibition, the decrease in clearance of an inhibitee, and hence its steady-state plasma concentration (C_{ss}), will depend critically on the fraction of the dose normally metabolised by the pathway that is inhibited (f_m), and the ratio of the concentration of the inhibitor at the enzyme site (I) to the inhibition constant (K_i) [32]:

$$\frac{C_{ss}(inhibited)}{C_{ss}(normal)} = \frac{1}{[f_m/(1+(I)/K_i)+(1-f_m)]}$$

The equation stresses the insensitivity of net drug clearance to inhibition when f_m is less than 0.5. However, the value of f_m may be difficult to evaluate *in vitro*, especially from experiments using microsomes (since they do not routinely measure both phase I and II metabolic products), and especially if only loss of parent drug is monitored (when the pattern of metabolism may vary with the dose added). In addition, if two or more cytochromes P450 have been identified as being involved in the metabolism of a compound, the amounts of those enzymes as a fraction of total P450 must be considered when weighting their importance. Furthermore, this proportion may vary considerably in different individuals especially if one or more of the enzymes are inducible. For example, although 2C19 was identified *in vitro* as a major enzyme metabolising omeprazole [13], the role of CYP3A4 may be dominant in some subjects since this is the most abundant P450 in human liver and it is inducible. The relative importance of renal and metabolic routes and of hepatic and extrahepatic metabolism also needs to be known in order to assess the value of f_m. The gut, for example, has considerable CYP3A4 activity [33]. Finally a low value of f_m will clearly be of more significance if the metabolite itself has potent pharmacological activity or toxicity.

Ideally, it could be argued that the $(I)/K_i$ ratio should be expressed in terms of free inhibitor and inhibitee concentrations at the enzyme site. Although free plasma concentration of inhibitor at steady state (Cu_{ss}) is likely to approximate to that at the enzyme site *in vivo*, there are difficulties in equating total concentrations of substrate and inhibitor added to an *in vitro* incubate with those at the enzyme site because of partitioning into the lipid environment of the enzyme and non-specific binding [34]. Thus, the K_i value obtained *in vitro* will reflect the partition characteristics of both inhibitor and inhibitee. Further complications arise if it is considered that concentrations 'seen' by the enzyme are not those in the aqueous phase—the enzyme binding site may be aqueous- or lipid-facing or, more likely, a mixture of both [34]. Also, the mechanism of inhibition by many compounds is not competitive, but mediated by a metabolite, an intermediate complex, or involves covalent binding. For this reason, when using some probe inhibitors *in vitro*, such as furafylline [35] and cimetidine [36], it is necessary to pre-incubate them to allow adequate formation of the inhibiting species. Thus, scaling of *in vitro* to *in vivo* $(I)/K_i$ ratios is not straightforward. Nevertheless, a knowledge of *in vitro* inhibitor concentrations relative to Cu_{ss} values can be of prognostic value provided that the difficulties are appreciated. Yet another point to consider is the fact that enzymes will be subjected to much higher drug concentrations during 'first pass' through the liver after oral drug administration. However, a reasonable estimate of drug concentration going to the liver via the hepatic portal vein may be obtained from the product of the dose and the absorption rate constant divided by assumed hepatic portal blood flow.

In summary, *in vitro* screens and 'enzyme profiling' offer a useful early-warning system for the rational selection of *in vivo* studies provided that there is careful thought and synthesis of all information available on the disposition and kinetics of the compound involved. Two examples will now be discussed where information from such screens might have pre-empted some dangerous drug interactions following the introduction of new drugs into clinical practice.

Case studies

SELECTIVE SEROTONIN REUPTAKE INHIBITORS AND TRICYCLIC ANTIDEPRESSANTS

The standard 'package' of metabolism and pharmacokinetic studies carried out during the development of paroxetine (a selective serotonin reuptake inhibitor, SSRI) indicated that its kinetics were complex, that it is not a general inducer or inhibitor of hepatic drug oxidation, and that it has little or no effect on the pharmacokinetics of other drugs examined [37]. Unfortunately, the latter compounds were classical *in vivo* probes such as antipyrine and warfarin. Subsequently, just prior to registration, it was shown both *in vitro* and *in vivo* that paroxetine is oxidised largely by CYP2D6 and that it is also a potent inhibitor of this enzyme [16,38–40]. Thus, an appropriate pro-active warning about interactions with other substrates of

CYP2D6 was formulated for the UK Data Sheet. In contrast, fluoxetine which, along with its major active nor-metabolite, also inhibits CYP2D6 [16,41], was introduced into clinical practice without the benefit of this knowledge. If this information had been available earlier perhaps a number of cases of severe cardiotoxicity resulting from co-administration of fluoxetine with tricyclic antidepressants might have been avoided [42]. Thus, many tricyclic antidepressants are metabolised to a significant extent by CYP2D6, explaining why the addition of fluoxetine to therapy increased their plasma concentrations by up to 300%, with subsequent toxicity.

TERFENADINE–KETOCONAZOLE

In 1989 astute clinical observation linked the occurrence of a rare, life-threatening ventricular arrhythmia (*torsades de pointe*) in an otherwise healthy woman with an interaction between her antihistamine (terfenadine) and antifungal (ketoconazole) medication [43]. Additional cases were identified through the US Food and Drug Administration's (FDA's) spontaneous reporting system, leading to the circulation of 'Dear Doctor' letters in August 1990 in the USA and in July 1992 in the UK.

There would be little reason to suspect an interaction between terfenadine and ketoconazole on the basis of their respective pharmacological actions. However, in retrospect, it is clear that an important interaction should have been predictable from a knowledge of drug metabolism and an appropriate appreciation of the cardiovascular effects of terfenadine. Terfenadine is a pro-drug, which undergoes extensive biotransformation on first pass through the liver. Thus, plasma concentrations of parent drug are virtually undetectable under normal conditions, and the combination of antihistaminic activity and minimal sedation is due to a zwitterionic C-oxidation product which does not pass the blood–brain barrier. Using human liver microsomes it has been shown that both C-oxidation and N-dealkylation of terfenadine are mediated by CYP3A4 [44]. *In vitro* studies have also shown that, at concentrations below about 10 μM, ketoconazole is a potent and selective inhibitor of this enzyme [45]. Therefore, when ketoconazole is co-administered with terfenadine its systemic availability becomes appreciable, resulting in arrhythmia mediated by the parent compound [46].

Unlike ketoconazole, fluconazole is a much less potent inhibitor of CYP3A4. Inhibition constants with respect to the oxidation of cyclosporin by human liver microsomes are 0.3 and 63 μM, respectively [45]. Therefore, it comes as no surprise to learn that during co-administration of terfenadine with the recommended 200 mg daily dose of fluconazole, plasma concentrations of unchanged terfenadine remain undetectable and there are no significant changes in cardiac repolarisation [47].

Conclusion

A case can be made for early *in vitro* studies using human liver tissues and enzymes to flag out potential drug interactions involving changes in drug metabolism. Although interpretation of such data is not without its problems, this information does promise to minimise the 'box-ticking' approach to selection of drug interaction studies in healthy volunteers. By helping to focus on relevant *in vivo* studies, *in vitro* screens could have significant economic and ethical advantages for drug development.

References

1. Nelson DR, Kamataki T, Waxman DJ et al. The P450 superfamily: update on new sequences, gene mapping, accession numbers, early trivial names of enzymes, and nomenclature. DNA Cell Biol 1993; 12: 1–51.
2. Smith DA, Jones BC. Speculations on the substrate structure–activity relationship (SSAR) of cytochrome P450 enzymes. Biochem Pharmacol 1992; 44: 2089–2098.
3. Kaminsky LS, Dannan GA, Guengerich FP. Composition of cytochrome P-450 isozymes from hepatic microsomes of C57BL/6 and DBA/2 mice assessed by warfarin metabolism, immunoinhibition and immunoelectrophoresis with anti-(rat cytochrome P450). Eur J Biochem 1984; 141: 141–148.
4. Shimada T, Misono KS, Guengerich FP. Human liver microsomal cytochrome P-450 mephenytoin 4-hydroxylase, a prototype of genetic polymorphism in oxidative drug metabolism: purification and characterization of two similar forms involved in the reaction. J Biol Chem 1986; 261: 909–921.
5. Shimada T, Guengerich FP. Participation of a rat liver cytochrome P-450 induced by pregnenolone 16alpha-carbonitrile and other compounds in the 4-hydroxylation of mephenytoin. Mol Pharmacol 1985; 28: 215–219.
6. Otton SV, Crewe HK, Lennard MS, Tucker GT, Woods HF. Use of quinidine inhibition to define the role of sparteine/debrisoquine cytochrome P450 in metoprolol oxidation by human liver microsomes. J Pharmacol Exp Ther 1988; 247: 242–247.
7. Ellis SW, Ching MS, Watson P, Lennard MS, Tucker GT, Woods HF. Catalytic activity of human debrisoquine 4-hydroxylase (CYP2D6) heterologously expressed in *Saccharomyces cerevisiae*. Biochem Pharmacol 1992; 44: 617–620.
8. Tucker GT, Lennard MS, Ellis SW et al. The demethylenation of methylenedioxymethamphetamine ('Ecstasy') by deprisoquine hydroxylase (CYP2D6). Biochem Pharmacol 1994; 47: 1151–1156.
9. Zanger WM, Hauri HP, Loeper J, Homberg JC, Meyer UA. Antibodies against human cytochrome P450db1 in autoimmune hepatitis type II. Proc Natl Acad Sci USA 1988; 27: 8256–8260.
10. Koymans L, den Kelder GMDO, te Kopelle JM, Vermeulen NPE. Cytochromes P450: their active-site structure and mechanism of oxidation. Drug Metab Rev 1993; 25: 325–387.
11. Rettie AE, Korzekwa KR, Kunze KL et al. Hydroxylation of warfarin by human cDNA-expressed cytochrome P-450: a role for P-4502C9 in the etiology of (S)-warfarin–drug interactions. Chem Res Toxicol 1992; 5: 54–59.
12. Heimark LD, Wienkers L, Kunze K et al. The mechanism of the interaction between amiodarone and warfarin in humans. Clin Pharmacol Ther 1992; 51: 398–407.

13. Andersson T, Miners JO, Veronese ME, Tassaneeyakul W, Meyer UA, Birkett DJ. Identification of human liver cytochrome P450 isoforms mediating omeprazole metabolism. Br J Clin Pharmacol 1993. Br J Pharmacol 1993; 36: 521–530.
14. Andersson T, Regardh C-G, Dahl-Puustinen ML, Bertilsson L. Slow omeprazole metabolizers are also poor *S*-mephenytoin hydroxylators. Ther Drug Monit 1990; 12: 415–416.
15. Andersson T, Cederberg C, Edvarsson G, Heggelund A, Lundborg P. Effect of omeprazole treatment on diazepam plasma levels in slow versus normal rapid metabolizers of omeprazole. Clin Pharmacol Ther 1990; 47: 79–85.
16. Crewe HK, Lennard MS, Tucker GT, Woods FR, Haddock RE. The effect of selective serotonin reuptake inhibitors on cytochrome P4502D6 (CYP2D6) activity in human liver microsomes. Br J Clin Pharmacol 1992; 34: 262–265.
17. Marre F, Fabre G, Lacarelle B et al. Involvement of the cytochrome P-450IID subfamily in minaprine 4-hydroxylation by human hepatic microsomes. Drug Metab Dispos 1992; 20: 316–321.
18. Fischer V, Vogels B, Maurer G, Tynes RE. The antipsychotic clozapine is metabolized by the polymorphic human microsomal and recombinant cytochrome P450 2D6. J Pharmacol Exp Ther 1992; 260: 1355–1360.
19. Koymans L, Vermeulen NPE, van Acker SABE et al. A predictive model of substrates of cytochrome P450–debrisoquine (2D6). Chem Res Toxicol 1992; 5: 211–219.
20. Pichard L, Fabre I, Fabre G et al. Cyclosporin A drug interactions: screening for inducers and inhibitors of cytochrome P-450 (cyclosporin A oxidase) in primary cultures of human hepatocytes and in liver microsomes. Drug Metab Dispos 1990; 18: 595–606.
21. Fuhr U, Strobl G, Manaut F et al. Quinolone antibacterial agents: relationship between structure and in vitro inhibition of the human cytochrome P450 isoform CYP1A2. Mol Pharmacol 1993; 43: 191–199.
22. Knodell RG, Browne DG, Gworzdz GP, Brian WR, Guengerich FP. Differential inhibition of individual human liver cytochromes P-450 by cimetidine. Gastroenterology 1991; 101: 1680–1691.
23. Sharp S, Mak LY, Smith DJ, Coughtrie MWH. Inhibition of human and rabbit liver steroid and xenobiotic UDP-glucuronosyltransferases by tertiary amine drugs: implications for adverse drug reactions. Xenobiotica 1992; 22: 13–25.
24. Magdalou J, Herber R, Bidault R, Siest G. In vitro *N*-glucuronidation of a novel antiepileptic drug lamotrigine, by human liver microsomes. J Pharmacol Exp Ther 1992; 260: 1166–1173.
25. Al-Asady SAH, Black GL, Lennard MS, Tucker GT, Woods HF. Inhibition of lignocaine metabolism by beta-adrenoceptor antagonists in rat and human liver microsomes. Xenobiotica 1989; 19: 929–944.
26. Ferrari S, Lemman T, Dayer P. The role of lipophilicity in the inhibition of polymorphic cytochrome P450IID6 oxidation by beta-blocking agents in vitro. Life Sci 1991; 48: 2259–2265.
27. Hurwitz A, Vacek JL, Botteron GW, Sztern MI, Hughes EM, Jayaraj A. Mexiletine effects on theophylline disposition. Clin Pharmacol Ther 1991; 50: 299–307.
28. Lennard MS, Lewis RV, Brawn LA et al. Timolol metabolism and debrisoquine oxidation polymorphism: a population study. Br J Clin Pharmacol 1989; 27: 429–434.
29. Gram LF, Brøsen K and the Danish University Antidepressant Group. Moclobemide treatment causes a substantial rise in the sparteine metabolic ratio. Br J Clin Pharmacol 1993; 35: 649–652.

30. Diaz D, Fabre I, Daujat M et al. Omeprazole is an aryl hydrocarbon-like inducer of human hepatic cytochrome P450. Gastroenterology 1990; 99: 737–747.
31. McDonnell WM, Scheiman JM, Traber PG. Induction of cytochrome P4501A genes (CYP1A) by omeprazole in the human alimentary tract. *Gastroenterology* 1992; 103: 1509–1516.
32. Rowland M, Matin SB. Kinetics of drug–drug interactions. J Pharmacokin Biopharm 1973; 1: 553–567.
33. Kolars JC, Awni WM, Merion RM, Watkins PB. First-pass metabolism of cyclosporin by the gut. Lancet 1991; 338: 1488–1490.
34. Parry G, Palmer DN, Williams DJ. Ligand partitioning into membranes: its significance in determining K_M and K_S values for cytochrome P-450 and other membrane bound receptors and enzymes. FEBS Lett 1976; 67: 123–129.
35. Sesardic D, Boobis AR, Murray BP et al. Furafylline is a potent and selective inhibitor of cytochrome P4501A2 in man. Br J Clin Pharmacol 1990; 29: 651–663.
36. Jensen JC, Gugler R. Cimetidine interaction with liver microsomes in vitro and in vivo: involvement of an activated complex with cytochrome P-450. Biochem Pharmacol 1985; 34: 2141–2146.
37. Kaye CM, Haddock RE, Langley PF et al. A review of the metabolism and pharmacokinetics of paroxetine in man. Acta Psychiatr Scand 1989; 80 (Suppl 350): 60–75.
38. Skjelbo E, Brøsen K. Inhibitors of imipramine metabolism by human liver microsomes. Br J Clin Pharmacol 1992; 34: 256–261.
39. Bloomer JC, Woods FR, Haddock RE, Lennard MS, Tucker GT. The role of cytochrome P4502D6 in the metabolism of paroxetine by human liver microsomes. Br J Clin Pharmacol 1992; 33: 521–523.
40. Sindrup SH, Brøsen K, Gram LF. Pharmacokinetics of the selective serotonin reuptake inhibitor paroxetine: nonlinearity and relation to the sparteine oxidation polymorphism. Clin Pharmacol Ther 1982; 51: 288–295.
41. Otton SV, Wu D, Joffe RT, Cheung SW, Sellers EM. Inhibition by fluoxetine of cytochrome P450 2D6 activity. Clin Pharmacol Ther 1993; 53: 401–409.
42. Westermeyer J. Fluoxetine-induced tricyclic toxicity: extent and duration. J Clin Pharmacol 1991; 31: 388–392.
43. Peck CC, Temple R, Collins JM. Understanding consequences of concurrent therapies. JAMA 1993; 269: 1550–1552.
44. Yun C-H, Okerholm RA, Guengerich FP. Oxidation of the antihistaminic drug terfenadine in human liver microsomes: role of cytochrome P-450 3A(4) in *N*-dealkylation and *C*-hydroxylation. Drug Metab Dispos 1993; 21: 403–409.
45. Maurice M, Pichard L, Duajat M et al. Effects of imidazole derivatives on cytochromes P450 from human hepatocytes in primary culture. FASEB J 1992; 6: 752–758.
46. Honig PK, Wortham DC, Zamani K, Conner DP, Mullin JC, Cantilena LR. Terfenadine–ketoconazole interaction: pharmacokinetic electrocardiographic consequences. JAMA 1993; 269: 1513–1518.
47. Honig PK, Wortham DC, Zamani K, Mullin JC, Conner DP, Cantilena LR. The effect of fluconazole on the steady-state pharmacokinetics and electrocardiographic pharmacodynamics of terfenadine in humans. Clin Pharmacol Ther 1993; 53: 630–636.
48. Birkett DJ, Mackenzie PI, Veronese ME, Miners JO. In vitro approaches can predict human drug metabolism. Trends Pharmacol Sci 1993; 14: 292–294.

16 WHAT NUMBER OF PATIENTS IS NECESSARY TO ESTABLISH DRUG SAFETY?

Peter R. Jackson, Erica J. Wallis, Wilfred W. Yeo and Lawrence E. Ramsay

Royal Hallamshire Hospital, Sheffield, UK

Introduction

It is a truism that no drug can be proven safe. The best we can hope for is a degree of certainty that the benefits of using a drug exceed any risk [1]. At the time of registration, information on efficacy is generally better than that on safety. A new drug will have been used by less than 1500 patients on average [2] and for a relatively short duration. Furthermore the patients included in pre-registration trials and the investigators who treated them tend to be highly selected. It is no surprise therefore that important adverse drug reactions continue to emerge after registration when the drug is used more widely and less selectively. Because of this, various methods of monitoring the safety of drugs in general use have evolved, for example voluntary reporting systems, post-marketing surveillance studies, automated record linkage, hospital-based schemes and disease registries. Despite this our methods for ensuring drug safety remain imperfect. Absolute safety is unattainable and the nearer to absolute safety are the demands of the public or governments, the more expensive will be the necessary studies [3]. Part of the problem is the need to treat very large numbers of patients before rare but nevertheless serious adverse reactions can be excluded with reasonable certainty. Added to this is the considerable difficulty in recognising and verifying adverse drug reactions. Discussion of the numbers of patients needed requires some understanding of the various methods employed to establish drug safety or detect drug hazards. These can be considered in three

Clinical Measurement in Drug Evaluation. Edited by W. S. Nimmo and G. T. Tucker
© 1995 John Wiley & Sons Ltd

steps: detecting signals of possible risk, establishing a causal relation, and determining the frequency or magnitude of the risk. Further detail of these methods and examples of systems which have been implemented can be found in Stephens' textbook [3].

Recognising adverse drug reactions: risk signalling

Detecting signals of possible hazard remains the most difficult aspect of pharmacovigilance. Predicting or detecting risk at an early stage is generally less of a problem with type A reactions, which are related to the pharmacological properties of a drug and may therefore be anticipated. Some estimate of the incidence and importance of such reactions is often possible before registration. However, type B reactions, which are, by definition, unrelated to the known pharmacological activity of the drug and therefore unpredictable, still have a remarkable capacity to surprise despite the great increase in awareness in recent years. It seems remarkable in retrospect that unique or near-unique syndromes such as phocomelia with thalidomide, the oculomucocutaneous reaction to practolol, or subacute myelo-optic neuropathy with clioquinol escaped detection for so long. Systems of pharmacovigilance have improved immeasurably since these episodes, and because of them, but we should not imagine that similar problems will not occur in the future. For an example of the continuing frailty of pharmacovigilance systems, consider the persistent dry cough which commonly complicates angiotensin converting enzyme (ACE) inhibitor treatment. This adverse reaction escaped detection through the entire pre-registration programme (considered capable of detecting reactions occurring at a frequency of one in 100 [3]) and even after marketing—yet it occurs in no less than 15% of all patients, and 20% of all women treated [4,5]. Evidently we can still be embarrassed by an adverse reaction with a clinical presentation never previously associated with drug therapy. ACE inhibitor cough might be considered a 'clinical nuisance' rather than a 'clinical catastrophe' in Feinstein's terminology [6], but it illustrates the important point that an adverse reaction may be harmless in itself but not in its consequences. Many patients were subjected to repeated courses of antibiotics, repeated chest X-rays, and even invasive procedures such as bronchoscopy before persistent dry cough was recognised as an adverse drug reaction. As discussed later, 'clinical nuisances' may also herald 'clinical catastrophe' adverse drug reactions. Bearing in mind that ACE inhibitors were evaluated in the 'modern' era of pharmacovigilance it is plain that signalling of adverse reactions continues to rely heavily upon the clinical acumen and alertness of individual doctors, and on their willingness to report or publish their observations.

VOLUNTARY REPORTING SYSTEMS

The detection of rare adverse events still depends heavily upon voluntary reporting schemes or registries such as the yellow card system run by the Medicines Control Agency in the UK. Prescribers report possible drug-related events by entering on a card details of the drug involved, the nature of the adverse event and some demographic data before sending it to a central registry. Details of similar national systems are given by Stephens [3]. Important requirements for such schemes are clear objectives, an adequate rate of reporting, the technology to handle and review reports efficiently, reliable methods of assessment to generate risk signals and the ability to initiate, or have initiated, other methods of study to validate or refute any signals which emerge. The objectives are easy to define—to detect and quantify adverse effects of drugs that may be fatal or cause serious disability, especially if this is irreversible [7], or to detect 'clinical catastrophes' [6]. Ideally the system should not be overwhelmed by trivial adverse reactions—clinical nuisances [6]—but unfortunately apparently trivial adverse reactions may have serious implications. For example, dry eyes are a common clinical nuisance, but detection and signalling of dry eyes in patients on practolol might well have provided a vital early clue to the oculomucocutaneous syndrome [7]. The UK yellow card system strikes a sensible balance by encouraging reports for new drugs of *all* possible adverse reactions, no matter how trivial, for two years after marketing. For established drugs, only reports of serious or previously unknown adverse reactions are requested. One major drawback of these systems is the low rate of voluntary reporting, even for new drugs or serious adverse reactions. Reporting rates may be improved by making reporting compulsory as in Sweden [3], by payment for reports [8], and perhaps by accepting reports from paramedical groups such as pharmacists or nurses. Short of these measures, features likely to enhance reporting rates include having a system which is widely known to prescribers, convenient and simple to use, and perceived as competent and useful. Advances in computer methods may have improved the handling and review of voluntary reports and have enabled also the sharing of data between national registries [3]. Assessment of the data for signals of potential hazard remains the most taxing step in these systems. The data are inherently biased because reporting doctors have already attributed causality, and further bias may arise following published reports or regulatory warnings of specific adverse reactions. The numerator (number of reports) is imprecise because of incomplete reporting, and the denominator (exposure to the drug in question) is also unknown, although it can be estimated approximately from prescription or sales figures. These systems therefore generate rather crude signals, and rarely provide proof of causality or a reliable estimate of the frequency or magnitude of any risk. They generally have to be backed by additional methods for establishing causality, such as case–control studies, cohort studies or analyses based on data collected by automated record linkage.

Methods of generating signals from voluntary reporting systems do not appear to be uniform. Some depend largely upon intuitive assessment by people with knowledge and experience of adverse reactions. Others [9] employ formal methods such as algorithms (see below) to assess the likelihood of causality. Predictably the likelihood of a causal relation is rated higher by reporting doctors than by assessors [9] (predictably because the reporting doctors would not have reported otherwise). Surprisingly, mathematical or statistical methods of generating or verifying signals do not appear to have been developed or used to a great extent. Tubert and colleagues have proposed a test based upon the Poisson distribution [10]. Given an approximate estimate of the background incidence of an adverse event in a population not receiving the drug, and an approximate estimate of the exposure of subjects to the drug, the number of events observed can be compared with the number predicted. Should these differ significantly, confirmatory studies can be mounted to verify the adverse reaction. The sensitivity and specificity of the method can be varied by adjusting the probability at which one would accept the occurrence of a difference by chance. Interestingly, the small dispersion of the Poisson distribution means that this does not alter markedly the size of the difference needed to flag a possible drug-related adverse event. Advantages of such methods include the fact that the event need not be linked to drug use by individual doctors, and demonstrable freedom from bias on the part of assessors. We doubt whether such methods will be universally applicable or will replace intuitive assessment, but they could prove a useful adjunct to informal expert assessment of spontaneous reports.

Those charged with interpreting possible signals from voluntary reporting systems have to tread a remarkably fine line, and the stakes are high. On the one hand, failure to act on a signal will leave patients exposed to a drug which has an adverse risk–benefit balance, resulting in harm to patients and to public confidence in drug safety. On the other hand, regulatory action on a 'false alarm' will cause anxiety to patients and doctors, can lead to unnecessary withdrawal of a valuable drug, and carries enormous financial penalties for companies which have developed drugs to the stage of marketing. Increasingly these decisions excite the attention of the media and pressure groups. Intuitive assessment of such signals is inevitably prone to error and bias, even when performed by those with skill and experience in interpreting adverse reactions. There is a strong case for developing and using statistical methods to support and complement intuitive assessment.

PUBLISHED CASE REPORTS

Reports of single cases or small series of putative adverse reactions have proved remarkably successful in providing early warnings of major drug hazards. Concerns have been expressed that such reports may be flawed scientifically, biased, and may damage unfairly the reputation of drugs. Reporting may also be delayed because investigators wish to 'collect' a larger series [3] or by a lengthy editorial process. However, the value of case reports has been defended [11], correctly, because they have an excellent track record in signalling important adverse drug reactions. Notable successes of anecdotal reporting include phocomelia with thalidomide, aplastic anaemia with chloramphenicol and phenylbutazone, pseudomembranous colitis with antibiotics, halothane jaundice, subacute myelo-optic neuropathy with clioquinol, thromboembolism with oral contraceptives and the oculomucocutaneous syndrome with practolol [12]. Occasional red herrings may be a price well worth paying for the safer use of drugs. Published cases are also incorporated into many voluntary reporting schemes by systematic scanning of the literature.

UNCONTROLLED POST-MARKETING SURVEILLANCE STUDIES

Post-marketing surveillance studies lie somewhere between adverse reaction registries and randomised controlled trials. Most have been uncontrolled cohort studies designed without a specific hypothesis and without predetermined statistical power. They are therefore generally descriptive and capable only of generating hypotheses or signals, and not of testing hypotheses or proving causality. Potential problems with post-marketing surveillance studies were foreshadowed as long as two decades ago by Feinstein [6], who indicated that 'the job will not be easy'. Shortly afterwards an editorial concluded that such studies had not proved successful, were expensive, and had not detected major new adverse reactions [13], while Castle *et al.* [14] detailed many potential problems. Unfortunately these gloomy predictions have proved largely correct. Many post-marketing studies have been unsatisfactory [2] because they had no comparator group, prescribing was open to selection bias, recruitment was slow and often incomplete, and reporting of the results was unsatisfactory [2]. Additional concerns are that new drugs may be prescribed specifically because of such studies, prescribers may have a financial incentive to participate, some studies may have an element of 'concealed marketing' [15] and few studies seem to incorporate any verification of the data collected. Waller *et al.* [2] concluded that such studies have made only a limited contribution to the assessment of drug safety. We are concerned about the ethics of studies which may prompt the prescribing of newly marketed drugs to patients who have not given informed consent.

HOSPITAL-BASED SCHEMES AND DISEASE REGISTRIES

Other methods which have aimed to provide signals of drug hazard have included intensive surveillance of hospital admissions and inpatients [16,17]. These have provided much useful information on the incidence, prevalence and importance of adverse drug reactions in the patient populations studied, but they are not particularly well suited to early signalling of adverse reactions to new drugs. Disease registries based on pertinent specialities such as haematology, nephrology or neurology, to which serious adverse drug reactions present commonly, are better suited to providing signals for new drugs. Examples are given by Stephen [3]. In our view speciality-based registries have not been developed and exploited to the full, particularly in the UK.

SUMMARY

These methods of generating hazard signals all have strengths and weaknesses, but all have a role to play. Spontaneous reporting to journals and adverse reaction registries are likely to remain the mainstays of pharmacovigilance in the foreseeable future. In a detailed analysis of the history of selected major adverse drug reactions, Venning [12,18] concluded that anecdotal reports, often of single cases, were the commonest initial signals for such reactions. The remainder were signalled from cohort studies or from series of cases. He concluded that voluntary reporting systems such as the yellow card system had made a negligible contribution. This is correct for the reactions analysed, but there seems little logic in concluding that published case reports are invaluable while reporting systems, which rely on similar reports, are not. In the last three years, the UK yellow card system has given prescribers early warning of several important adverse reactions through its regular bulletin *Current Problems in Pharmacovigilance*. These include hepatotoxicity with terbinafine, withdrawal symptoms and involuntary movements with paroxetine, myocarditis with clozapine, aplastic anaemia with remoxipride and ileocaecal strictures with high-potency pancreatins. Venning also emphasised that case-orientated approaches had proved superior to drug-orientated methods for signalling and verifying adverse drug reactions, supported the development of speciality-based disease registries and stressed the importance of recording 'events' rather than 'adverse reactions'.

Verifying adverse drug reactions

ASSESSING INDIVIDUAL EPISODES

In Venning's analysis of selected important adverse reactions, causality was proved by study of individual cases in almost half of the instances studied [18]. In most, the syndrome was unique or nearly unique, and, in a few, causality was clinched by rechallenge or by experimental findings in individual patients. Despite these notable successes, the assessment of individual putative adverse reactions is subjective and imprecise [19]. In Feinstein's words [6], 'after we work our way through all the majesty of the computer print-out and the glory of the statistics we find that the decision-making mechanism for identifying adverse reactions depends on the vagaries of clinical judgement of an array of unstandardised physicians'. He stressed the importance of developing reproducible methods for diagnosing adverse drug reactions, and several groups responded by devising formal methods or algorithms for assessing putative adverse reactions [20–23]. These methods reduce variability within and between observers [21] and, at least in some cases, show good agreement between methods [24]. However, in the absence of a gold standard—the absolute truth—they may conceivably reduce the variability around the wrong conclusion. Algorithms prompt systematic rather than haphazard consideration of the facts, and are now used routinely in some adverse drug reaction registries [9], but none can compensate for the incomplete information [25] which is often available to registries. The criteria used may also be inappropriate, misleading or biased in some situations. These criteria are generally the previous experience with a drug, alternative causes for the event, temporal relationship, dose or concentration effect, dechallenge and rechallenge. There are important systematic biases in diagnosing adverse drug reactions [25]. It is easy to 'nail' drugs which provide clear objective evidence of toxicity in the form of a plasma concentration (e.g., digoxin or phenytoin) or pharmacological effect (e.g., prothrombin time, hypoglycaemia), and those reactions which are distinctive (e.g., serum sickness, drug-induced lupus). However, for the pharmacovigilance of new drugs, the inclusion of prior knowledge of adverse reactions with a drug is a particular drawback. In Bayesian parlance the prior probability puts older drugs and those causing type A reactions at a 'disadvantage' because more is known about their adverse effects. Algorithms are much less useful for diagnosing reactions to new chemical entities or new type B reactions, which by definition are previously unknown.

Furthermore, these methods are incapable of dissecting out non-specific adverse reactions, i.e. those which closely simulate naturally occurring disease or actually cause an increased incidence of such disease [3]. Such reactions can be detected only by an increase in the incidence of events in a group of patients receiving the target drug when compared with a population which is identical apart from the use of the drug. The methods for verifying adverse reactions described below all depend to some extent on this form of statistical verification. The selection of matching populations is a major problem. Unless subjects give consent to be randomised to active drug or placebo in controlled trials it is difficult to exclude selection bias and potential confounding variables. Nevertheless comparison with a control population remains a mainstay of adverse event confirmation.

AUTOMATED RECORD LINKAGE

These methods make use of large and comprehensive record linkage systems which include details of drugs prescribed and outcome measures such as hospital admission, operations or death. They require large computer databases and have been used extensively in the USA, where health maintenance organisations hold computerised records for their patients and the procedures which they undergo [3]. In spite of their sophistication, these systems are not generally useful for generating hypotheses or signals. The testing of all possible linkages between all possible data sets stratified for all confounding factors poses too great a computing burden for any system yet envisaged. To detect a drug-associated risk of one in 10 000 or less for a drug used quite widely requires data on a base population of 3–5 million, and a great deal of money [26]. Data linkage systems therefore still require the human element to pose specific questions, i.e. their main use is in testing hypotheses or signals of possible risk generated by case reports, adverse reaction registries, or clinical trials. They provide immediate and inexpensive access to data already collected for other purposes. As the database contains demographic and clinical information not available in most voluntary reporting systems, preliminary stratification for important explanatory variables is often possible. Thus cases and controls can be assembled rapidly to conduct a case–control study. However, few hypotheses are amenable to testing using *only* the information available on computer file, and it is necessary generally to obtain access to the medical records and often to patients themselves to verify drug exposure and to validate the outcomes [27]. These systems are suited best to detecting adverse reactions which trigger events that can be monitored easily such as prescription of other drugs, hospital admission or death.

According to Shapiro [27] the important weaknesses of automated record linkage are that exposure to the drug, and the outcomes, tend to be ill defined, control for confounding factors may be inadequate and the statistical power may be low because the number of patients exposed to a target drug may be relatively small even in very large databases. These criticisms are justified only when automated record linkage data are employed inappropriately. When used properly, automated record linkage offers probably the best prospects for improving pharmacovigilance [26]. In the UK, databases suitable for record linkage are smaller than those in the USA because of differences in the health care systems. However, studies have been published from MEMO in Tayside [28], and VAMP [29], which operates through computers in general practices.

CONTROLLED POST-MARKETING SURVEILLANCE STUDIES

Some post-marketing studies have utilised non-random control or reference populations, and are therefore capable potentially of proving causality or providing accurate estimates of rate of risk. Prescription event-monitoring schemes such as that of Inman's Drug Safety Research Unit [30] have some advantages over the uncontrolled post-marketing surveillance studies discussed earlier. There is often access to a control population or cohort of patients who have been exposed to a drug similar to the target drug. The method is designed to detect 'events' rather than adverse reactions, i.e. the participating doctors do not have to impute causality to any events which arise. Because patients are identified through a routine prescription, the studies are observational and treatment is not altered deliberately for the sake of the study. The patients included are therefore more likely to be representative of patients in general, and there are few concerns about ethical, financial or commercial aspects. Among the problems of prescription event monitoring are the relative weakness of the control data [26], falling response rates (perhaps because of competition from uncontrolled post-marketing schemes) [30] and the fact that those who prescribe new drugs and thus contribute to such studies are not typical of all prescribing doctors [30]. In the UK, heavy prescribers of new drugs tended to be older, male, and to have qualified outside the UK [30]. Typical prescription event-monitoring studies are capable of detecting events only if they have a frequency of greater than one in 3000 [30] and they cannot therefore replace voluntary reporting systems or journal reports.

CASE–CONTROL STUDIES

Case–control studies have, as their starting point, the putative adverse reaction and therefore they require a signal of possible risk, for example from voluntary reporting schemes. Patients (cases) with the supposed adverse reaction are compared with matched patients (controls) without the reaction, and the two groups are compared as regards their exposure to the suspect drug. The method is well suited to the study of rare adverse events and those which occur very late during drug use—events which cannot be examined by prospective studies because of the number of patients or duration of treatment needed. Case–control studies are retrospective and their validity is entirely dependent upon careful choice of control subjects and rigorous avoidance of bias and potential confounding factors. These sources of error can never be excluded with absolute certainty and the results of case–control studies must always be viewed with caution. Confidence in the findings is increased when case–control studies in different settings reach the same conclusion. The outcome of case–control studies is expressed as relative risk, and they do not give a direct measure of absolute frequency. Measures of relative risk can themselves be valuable for ranking different agents within a single class of drugs. For example, it was possible to rank non-steroidal anti-inflammatory drugs as regards their propensity to cause upper gastrointestinal bleeding or perforation in a series of case–control studies [31]. They were in broad agreement in showing that ibuprofen had a smaller risk and azapropazone and piroxicam higher risks when compared with other non-steroidal drugs studied. Absolute risk can be measured if all the cases in a defined population have been identified, as may be the case when a case–control study is 'nested' within a cohort study. The absolute risk can also be approximated by calculating the attributable risk—the proportion of all cases which may be attributed to the drug—and applying this to the frequency of the condition in the whole population if this is known.

RANDOMISED CONTROLLED TRIALS

Randomisation eliminates various sources of bias and is required to prove or disprove safety in the true sense. For example, only randomised controlled trials could show the adverse risk–benefit outcomes for clofibrate [32] and class I antiarrhythmic drugs [33]. Similarly such trials were needed to confirm the favourable risk–benefit outcome for antihypertensive drug treatment and for ACE inhibitors in heart failure. The disadvantages for establishing drug safety are that randomised trials are generally small and often include highly selected patients, so that the findings may not be generalisable to all patients who will use the drug in ordinary practice. Furthermore the emphasis in random controlled trials is generally on drug efficacy, and methods of recording, analysing and reporting adverse drugs events are often unsatisfactory. A major development recently has been the mounting of very large pragmatic (no frills) randomised trials, for example the ISIS trials examining interventions in acute myocardial infarction. These trials rely on randomisation of large numbers of patients, minimal exclusions, simple data collection and 'hard' endpoints such as death or recurrent myocardial infarction. They have provided valuable information on the true balance of benefit and risk for the interventions studied. Another recent trend has been the increasing use of methods of meta-analysis to draw together and analyse statistically the results of trials of single drugs which were themselves often too small to provide conclusive answers. These analyses now have considerable influence but disturbing evidence of their fallibility is emerging. For example, the purported efficacy of magnesium or nitrates in acute myocardial infarction, shown in meta-analyses at a high level of significance, was not confirmed and was in fact refuted by the results of a single very large trial. An example of controlled trials failing to resolve important questions about the risk and benefit of therapy is the continuing controversy about the safety of lipid-lowering drugs. In reviewing the same data some take the view that these drugs increase non-coronary mortality substantially and significantly, and should therefore be used only in patients at very high risk of coronary death [34], whereas others dismiss this risk and favour much wider use of lipid-lowering drugs [35].

Quantifying the risk

Following a signal of possible risk and validation of causality, there is a need to quantify the risk. This cannot be considered in isolation and must be balanced against the benefit of a drug. Quantifying risk involves assessment of the frequency, severity and importance of adverse reactions. Measurement of frequency is not easy, and methods for measuring and weighting the severity and importance of adverse reactions are even less well developed.

COUNTING ADVERSE DRUG REACTIONS

Spontaneous reporting schemes do not provide accurate estimates of frequency of adverse reactions, as the true number of cases is underestimated because of under-reporting and the denominator is not known. It has been suggested that there may be some relation between the number of spontaneous reports and the true frequency of an adverse reaction [26] but this seems unlikely intuitively because the threshold for reporting is likely to vary with other factors such as the severity of the reaction or the degree of certainty about causality. As a rule, voluntary reporting rates will not even provide reliable estimates for the relative safety of drugs in the same class. Controlled post-marketing surveillance studies are capable of estimating the frequency of adverse drug reactions but the accuracy of such estimates will depend on the adequacy of the control group or population, the response rate of participating doctors, whether 'events' or 'adverse reactions' are recorded and the severity of the adverse reaction in question. Post-marketing surveillance studies are likely to underestimate substantially the true frequency of 'clinical nuisance' reactions such as ACE inhibitor cough [5,26]. They are suited better to determining the frequency of serious events or adverse reactions but, because such reactions are usually rare, the number of patients included is usually too small. These studies fall between two stools—they are insufficiently detailed for the study of nuisance reactions and too small for the study of clinical catastrophes. Uncontrolled cohort studies provide useful estimates of frequency only if the adverse reaction is unique or reliably identifiable.

Failing this, formal methods such as algorithms for assessing causality may have some role but they are far from perfect. Case–control studies estimate relative risk, but can provide indirect estimates of absolute frequency in the circumstances discussed earlier.

When expressing the frequency of adverse reactions, confusion may arise because estimates will differ in cross-sectional surveys and prospective cohort studies. The best methods of analysis are life table methods, which take account of the changing denominator resulting from loss of cases for various reasons. Failure to use life table methods tends to underestimate the true frequency of adverse reactions [5,36]. While it can be difficult to determine accurately the frequency of adverse reactions, particularly for uncommon or rare events, there has often been a failure to perform even the simple studies needed to quantify the risk of well-established side-effects. For example, it was assumed widely that hydralazine caused rarely a lupus-like reaction when the drug was used at a maximum daily dose of 200 mg. It did not require a large, elaborate or expensive study to show that this was clearly untrue [36].

WEIGHTING ADVERSE DRUG REACTIONS

Safety is a relative concept, and knowledge of the frequency of adverse events is of little value in isolation. The beneficial effects of the drug also have to be considered. Occasional cases of marrow aplasia may be accepted with an anti-cancer drug which is valuable in advanced malignancy but would be totally unacceptable with a 'me-too' antibiotic. Several different adverse events may contribute to the overall burden of a drug and less frequently there may be more than one benefit. Some integral measure or weighting system for risk and benefit is required. For deaths caused or prevented, the all-cause mortality meets this need. However, the effect of a drug on total mortality will often be small and a trial in many thousands of patients will be required to answer the question conclusively. With smaller numbers, trial outcomes are often equivocal, with failure to show benefit possibly a result of small numbers or an approximate balance between adverse and beneficial effects of drug treatment on mortality. This is illustrated well by trials of the drug treatment of hyperlipidaemia. The 'small' numbers in such trials mean that they have shown no significant reduction in overall mortality. Does the failure to reduce mortality simply reflect the inadequate size of studies or does it indicate an adverse effect of treatment on non-coronary mortality [34,35]?

For non-fatal adverse effects, scoring methods for quality of life have been developed as summative measures but no single method has been accepted universally as an adequate measure of overall health. Quality-of-life scores need to be calibrated against life events that can be understood generally. Some quality-of-life scores appear insensitive to adverse events which can be measured by direct questioning, and there has been a tendency to choose scores which are 'focused' on the adverse events anticipated. This actually negates the advantage of 'general' quality-of-life scores, as their main purpose is to provide a patient-derived weighting of overall well-being regardless of the presence or absence of specific adverse effects. In other words, focused quality-of-life scales may increase the sensitivity of a trial for specific adverse events but only by sacrificing their ability to estimate the impact of these side-effects on perceived health. More complex issues arise when the benefit of the drug is purely on morbidity but at some cost in terms of mortality. Dead patients provide no score for quality of life, but they can be allocated an arbitrary score so that their data are retained in the analysis. The magnitude of the arbitrary score for death may influence unduly the outcome of the risk–benefit equation. Doctors or epidemiologists have set these arbitrary scores but it is known that doctors and patients have markedly different views on risk taking [37]. Future quality-of-life instruments should ask patients perhaps what risks they are prepared to take to gain any benefit. For example, are patients willing to accept a tiny risk of *torsades de pointes* with terfenadine to avoid the drowsiness caused by chlorpheniramine?

The number of patients for trials examining quality of life will depend on the difference to be detected and the standard deviation of this score and can be estimated by standard power calculations. Trials aiming to detect small differences require very large numbers of patients. In the absence of large trials, risk and benefit may need to be assessed separately and then included in a risk–benefit equation using patient-derived weighting. This is especially important when the risk includes a small chance of serious adverse events such as death. In this circumstance the variance of the quality-of-life scores may differ between the drug and placebo populations, and power calculations based on pilot studies excluding data from patients who died may prove invalid.

We have to confess to some scepticism about the value of many of the quality-of-life 'instruments' and studies which seem to have proliferated in recent years. These studies are enormously time consuming for patients, tedious for investigators, and a nightmare for statisticians—yet the end-product appears to be an arbitrary summation and weighting of measurements derived from a collection of arbitrary scales purported to measure different aspects of life and health satisfaction. We doubt whether we are alone in having some difficulty in understanding exactly what the final numbers mean. It would be interesting to see some of the more complex instruments pitted head-to-head against simple five-point scores or 10 cm visual analogue scales which enquire whether patients are happy with their life and their health.

How many patients are required?

INTERPRETATION OF OBSERVATIONS OF ZERO ADVERSE EVENTS

In many prospective studies, no serious untoward events will occur. What comfort can be drawn from such zero observations? What do they tell us about the safety of the drug concerned? As experience with the drug increases in further trials, or when the drug is released for general use, a somewhat different picture may emerge. Clinicians tend to be too readily impressed by trials in which no adverse event occurs, and it is not uncommon to read that drugs proved 'safe' in reports of trials with sample sizes measured in tens rather than hundreds. An observation of no adverse events provides much less reassurance for larger populations than is generally thought. What statistical rules tell us how big a risk has been excluded? Suppose that no serious adverse reactions are observed in a trial of a new drug in 100 patients. Can we conclude that the drug is relatively safe? The outcome is in fact compatible with a frequency of serious adverse events of 3% when the drug is used by a large number of patients. The predictive value of the result observed for the more general case is described by the confidence interval—the range which will embrace the majority of outcomes observed if the trial was performed repeatedly. This also predicts the likely outcome when the drug is released for general use in a similar population. The confidence interval can be selected to include any percentage of all outcomes desired but is calculated commonly to embrace 95% of all values—the 95% confidence interval. Except in extremely small trials, the upper 95% confidence limit for an observation of no events is approximated by the expression $(300/n)\%$, where n is the number of subjects who received the drug [38] (Table 1). This formula is invaluable for tyro investigators as the calculation does not even need the back of an envelope—yet few feats inspire quite as much awe (during scientific meetings for example) as the instantaneous calculation of confidence intervals.

The 95% confidence interval calculated in this situation differs from that usually estimated. In most circumstances the range selected is symmetrical about the average, with 2.5% of possible values excluded at each tail of the distribution. In the present case, the lower end of the distribution is con-

Table 1. Confidence interval above zero events

Trial size	10	15	50	100	500	1000	10000
Risk excluded	1:4	1:6	1:17	1:34	1:167	1:333	1:3333

Risk excluded in trials of given size when no events occur.

strained by zero, as it is impossible to observe a negative number of adverse effects. The 5% of values which fall outside the 95% confidence interval are all therefore at the upper end of the distribution. For simplicity we will use asymmetric confidence intervals for all calculations in this chapter, because when considering drug safety we are not usually interested in the possibility of having fewer serious adverse reactions than placebo.

The confidence intervals for a zero observation shown in Table 1 give food for thought. Phase I and II trials are unlikely to uncover any but the most common events. At the time of licensing, an average of 1500 patients will have been treated with a new drug [2]. A clean sheet at that stage is quite compatible with a true frequency of clinical catastrophes as high as one in 500. If the sheet is still clean after a post-marketing surveillance study of 10 000 patients, the true incidence of disasters may still be uncomfortably high at one in 3333. Add to that the distinct possibility that serious adverse reactions may not be readily recognisable and may be overlooked, and one starts to grasp the enormousness of the task of proving a new drug 'safe'.

SAMPLE SIZE TO EXCLUDE RARE EVENTS

The numbers in Table 1 cannot be used to calculate the size of a prospective trial needed to exclude an adverse event at a given frequency. Because of the play of chance, adverse events will be observed in some studies even when the true risk of an adverse event is below the frequency that the investigator wishes to exclude. Allowance therefore has to be made in the sample size calculation for the possibility of observing the adverse event in the treated group. In other words, the trial has to be large enough to cope with the chance of an adverse event occurring, which in a smaller trial would give an inflated impression of the risk of the drug. The numbers in the trial must therefore be set to provide a reasonable chance that a one-sided test will show the rate to be below a predetermined acceptable rate. This is akin to the calculation of trial size for randomised trials. There is no certainty that this can be attained, but the sample size can be calculated to provide a given power—e.g. a 90% probability of attaining the desired outcome. Stephens [3] suggests that three questions should be answered before estimating a size for such trials. First, a frequency threshold must be set above which the occurrence of adverse events would be unacceptable. This threshold will obviously vary according to the severity of the adverse event sought. Then the statistical questions relating to power must be considered. What level of significance is desired in the one-tailed test if the observed frequency is below the threshold? Also how capable should the trial be of giving such a result if the true frequency lies below the threshold? The answers to these questions may be

Table 2.

Incidence to be excluded	No of patients in treated group
1 in 10	99
1 in 100	999
1 in 1000	9999
1 in 10000	99999

The number of patients required in the treatment group to give a 90% chance of excluding the given incidence at the 95% level, assuming a drug-specific adverse event.

Table 3. Trial size to produce a given number of adverse events

Expected incidence	Required no adverse events				
	1	2	3	4	5
1:10	30	48	63	78	92
1:100	300	475	630	776	916
1:1000	2996	4744	6296	7754	9154
1:10000	29958	47439	62958	77537	91536

The number of patients required is calculated from the Poisson distribution as that number which has a 95% chance of producing the desired number of events *or greater*.

used to determine the number of subjects to be studied (Table 2). Table 2 gives the numbers of patients required for a study to have a 90% chance of showing an upper 95% confidence interval to exclude an adverse event more frequent than a chosen threshold. Stephens [3] also includes a further point relating to the number of adverse events required to convince investigators that they are drug specific. This might be of academic interest but is not in fact needed to exclude a frequency of adverse events above the threshold. Furthermore, comparison of Tables 2 and 3 shows that trials of size sufficient to exclude a frequency above a threshold will also provide enough adverse events to determine whether or not they are drug related unless the true frequency of the adverse event is well below threshold.

SAMPLE SIZE TO DETECT AN INCREASE IN THE BACKGROUND FREQUENCY OF EVENTS

Adverse reactions are commonly non-specific; i.e. they may mimic closely naturally occurring events or increase the incidence of naturally occurring events. At the 'clinical nuisance' level, drugs may cause symptoms such as headache, dizziness or tiredness, all of which are remarkably common in untreated subjects and therefore in placebo-treated comparator groups. At the more serious end of the spectrum, sudden death caused by class I anti-arrhythmic drugs [33] does not differ from sudden death which occurs in patients with coronary heart disease—who may be taking such a drug. To detect and quantify such effects, the frequency observed in a group receiving the test drug has to be compared either with the frequency of the event in the population, or with the frequency in a control group of patients. If the population incidence of an adverse event is known accurately, for example from previous large surveys, the number of patients required will be smaller because only one group is needed. However, it is uncommon for the background frequency of adverse events to be known with sufficient accuracy. More often the new drug has to be compared with a comparator group, ideally in a random placebo-controlled study. When a randomised control group is not available, for example in post-marketing surveillance studies, selection of a suitable comparator group is difficult. In general they should have the disease for which the drug is being prescribed, as the disease may itself cause or be associated with relevant events. Even then the group prescribed a new drug may differ subtly from patients with the same condition because of biases influencing prescribers or patients.

Again the questions posed by Stephens might be helpful but in addition to those considered for drug-specific adverse events some estimate is required for the background frequency of the event in the population. If this is known with accuracy then approximately double the number of subjects are required than for the detection of drug-specific adverse events even if the drug causes a 100% increase in frequency (Table 4). When the background frequency is less well defined even more subjects will be required in both test and control group (Table 4). To limit the number of subjects exposed to the drug the design may be weighted to have multiple control subjects for each one receiving the test drug. However, the maximum effect such a design can have is limited to halving the size of the test group (Table 4).

It should be noted that these sample sizes are strictly applicable only when the analysis is restricted to a single endpoint. When numerous endpoints or events are tested some 'significant' associations between the drug and 'adverse events' are likely to occur by chance. Testing multiple hypotheses is not good statistical practice and will throw up spurious associations. Most post-marketing surveillance studies are not set up to examine a specific endpoint or event, and they must generally be regarded as generating signals or hypotheses. Additional studies will usually be needed to confirm or refute possible associations which emerge using, for example, case–control methods.

SAMPLE SIZE FOR CASE–CONTROL STUDIES

Surprisingly little has been written about the calculation of sample size for case–control studies. The number of patients studied often appears

Table 4. Size of each group when adverse event occurs in untreated population

	Added risk from drug		
Control incidence known precisely			
Background risk	1:100	1:1000	1:10 000
1:10	10 300	954 000	94 700 000
1:100	1 950	114 000	10 500 000
1:1000	1 020	19 800	1 150 000
Control incidence unknown			
Background risk	1:100	1:1000	1:10 000
1:10	20 000	1 910 000	190 000 000
1:100	3 300	221 000	21 000 000
1:1000	1 450	33 500	2 230 000
Control incidence unknown 5 controls per case			
Background risk	1:100	1:1000	1:10 000
1:10	11 900	1 150 000	114 000 000
1:100	1 880	132 000	12 600 000
1:1000	720	19 000	1 330 000

The number of patients required in the treatment group to give a 90% chance of excluding the given incidence at the 95% level.

remarkably similar to the number available to the investigator. The outcome of case–control studies is expressed as relative risk. However, it is possible to estimate the sample size needed to exclude a given absolute risk related to a drug. The assumptions required are the proportion of patients in the population using the drug and the background frequency of the putative adverse event in the population. Negative case–control studies cannot be interpreted without some estimate of their power. Methods are available for calculating confidence intervals for the estimate of absolute risk, given the outcome of the study and the background incidence of the adverse event in the whole population [39]. Although case–control studies usually have greater power than prospective cohort studies, the number of patients needed may still present difficulty. When the proportion of the population receiving the drug is small, and the increased risk associated with the drug use is not high, the fraction and hence number of patients exposed to the drug in both case and control groups will be low. Case–control studies will also have low statistical power when the index drug is used by almost all of a population. For example, a case–control study in hypertensive patients would be most unlikely to show an adverse effect associated with beta blocker treatment if 90% of all patients

Table 5. Number of events to be studied in case–control study

	Added risk from drug			
Drug use 1:10				
Background risk	1:10	1:100	1:1000	1:10 000
1:10	312	20 200	1 910 000	190 000 000
1:100	24	393	24 500	2 310 000
1:1000	8	25	402	25 000
1:10 000	6	8	25	402
Drug use 1:100				
Background risk	1:10	1:100	1:1000	1:10 000
1:10	2 690	182 000	17 300 000	1 730 000 000
1:100	151	3 340	221 000	21 000 000
1:1000	18	155	3 410	225 000
1:10 000	6	18	155	3 500
Drug use 1:1000				
Background risk	1:10	1:100	1:1000	1:10 000
1:10	26 500	1 800 000	172 000 000	>3 200 000 000
1:100	1 440	32 900	2 190 000	208 000 000
1:1000	132	1 470	33 600	2 230 000
1:10 000	18	133	1 470	33 600

The number of patients required in the treatment group to give a 90% chance of excluding the given incidence at the 95% level.

were taking a beta blocker. The statistical power of case–control studies may be increased somewhat and the number of subjects needed may be reduced by individual matching of case and control subjects. In practice the advantage of matching is often lost because of non-response or missing data, and the results have to be analysed on an unmatched basis. The statistical power can also be enhanced by using multiple control subjects for each case. Table 5 shows that fewer subjects are required when drug use is high, risk from the drug is high and background risk is low. Impossibly high numbers of events would still be required if drug use is low and the extra risk from receiving the drug is small.

Conclusions

The search for rare but serious adverse drug reactions cannot be compared with looking for a needle in a haystack—it is much more difficult than that. There is no certainty that there is a needle to find, or there may in fact be several needles. Some needles will be recognisable instantly as such; others look entirely unlike any needle previously seen, and yet others are indistinguishable in appearance from the hay which conceals them. Some very dangerous needles are not detected, and needles are sometimes spotted when they do not actually exist. The haystack keeps growing while the search goes on. Pharmacovigilance is not a suitable discipline for those who are uncomfortable with uncertainty. Living with uncertainty does seem to take its toll as the literature contains much bickering and even warfare between proponents of different systems of pharmacovigilance. Given all the difficulties, every method of signalling possible hazards has a role, they all need to be developed further and signals from any quarter should be welcomed. We also need all the tools at our disposal to follow up these signals, verify causality and quantify the risk. The number of patients necessary to establish drug safety is, in fact, infinite.

References

1. Langman MJS. This volume, Ch 18.
2. Waller PC, Wood SM, Langman MJS, Breckenridge AM, Rawlins MD. Review of company postmarketing surveillance studies. Br Med J 1992; 304: 1470–1472.
3. Stephens MDB. Post-marketing surveillance (PMS). In: The Detection of New Adverse Drug Reactions (2nd edn). New York: Mcmillan Press Ltd, 1988; 143–200.
4. Yeo WW, Foster G, Ramsay LE. Prevalence of persistent cough during long-term enalapril treatment: controlled study versus nifedipine. Q J Med 1991; 293: 763–770.
5. Yeo WW, Ramsay LE. Persistent dry cough with enalapril: incidence depends on method used. J Hum Hypertens 1990; 4: 517–520.
6. Feinstein AR. Clinical biostatistics XXVIII. The biostatistical problems of pharmaceutical surveillance. Clin Pharmacol Ther 1974; 16: 110–123.
7. Dollery CT. Detecting adverse reactions to drugs. Br Med J 1977; 2: 1592–1593.
8. Feeley J, Moriarty S, O'Connor P. Stimulating reporting of adverse drug reactions by using a fee. Br Med J 1990; 300: 22–23.
9. Miremont G, Harramburu F, Begaud B, Pere JC, Dangoumau J. Adverse drug reactions: physicians' opinions versus a causality assessment method. Eur J Clin Pharmacol 1994; 46: 285–289.
10. Tubert P, Begaud B, Harramburu F, Pere JC. Spontaneous reporting: how many cases are required to trigger a warning? Br J Clin Pharmacol 1991; 32: 407–408.
11. Anonymous. Communicating adverse drug reactions. Lancet 1978; i: 133.
12. Venning GR. Identification of adverse reactions to new drugs. III: Alerting processes and early warning systems. Br Med J 1983; 286: 458–460.
13. Anonymous. After practolol. Br Med J 1983; 2: 1561–1562.
14. Castle WM, Nicholls JT, Downey CC. Problems of post-marketing surveillance. Br J Clin Pharmacol 1983; 16: 581–585.
15. Anonymous. Postmarketing surveillance: how should doctors get involved? Drug Ther Bull 1988; 26: 89–91.
16. Hurwitz N, Wade OL. Intensive hospital monitoring of adverse reactions to drugs. Br Med J 1969; 1: 531–540.
17. Miller RR. Hospital admissions due to adverse drug reactions: a report from the Boston Collaborative Drug Surveillance Program. Arch Intern Med 1974; 134: 219–223.
18. Venning GR. Identification of adverse reactions to new drugs. IV: Verification of suspected adverse reactions. Br Med J 1983; 286: 544–547.
19. Karch FE, Smith CL, Kerzner B, Mazzullo JM, Weintraub M, Lasagna L.

Adverse drug reactions: a matter of opinion. Clin Pharmacol Ther 1976; 19: 489–492.

20. Kramer MS, Leventhal JS, Hutchinson TA, Feinstein AR. An algorithm for the operational assessment of adverse drug reactions. I. Background, description, and instructions for use. JAMA 1979; 242: 623–632.

21. Hutchinson TA, Leventhal JS, Kramer MS, Karch FE, Lipman AG, Feinstein AR. An algorithm for the operational assessment of adverse drug reactions. II. Demonstration of reproducibility and validity. JAMA 1979; 242: 633–638.

22. Naranjo CA, Busto U, Sellars EM et al. A method for estimating the probability of adverse drug reactions. Clin Pharmacol Ther 1981; 30: 239–245.

23. Karch FE, Lasagna L. Toward the operational identification of adverse drug reactions. Clin Pharmacol Ther 1977; 21: 247–254.

24. Busto U, Naranjo CA, Sellars EM. Comparison of two recently published algorithms for assessing the probability of adverse drug reactions. Br J Clin Pharmacol 1982; 13: 223–227.

25. Ramsay LE, Freestone S, Silas JH. Drug-related acute medical admissions. Hum Toxicol 1982; 1: 379–386.

26. Waller PC. Measuring the frequency of adverse drug reactions. Br J Clin Pharmacol 1992; 33: 249–252.

27. Shapiro S. The role of automated record linkage in the postmarketing surveillance of drug safety: a critique. Clin Pharmacol Ther 1989; 46: 371–386.

28. Beardon PHG, Brown SD, McDevitt DG. Post-marketing surveillance: a follow-up study of morbidity associated with cimetidine using record linkage. Pharm Med 1988; 3: 185–193.

29. Jick H, Jick SS, Derby LE. Validation of information recorded on general practitioner based computerised data resource in the United Kingdom. Br Med J 1991; 302: 766–768.

30. Inman W, Pearce G. Prescriber profile and post-marketing surveillance. Lancet 1993; 342: 658–661.

31. Bateman DN. NSAIDs: time to re-evaluate gut toxicity. Lancet 1994; 343: 1051–1052.

32. Committee of Principal Investigators. A cooperative trial in the primary prevention of ischaemic heart disease using clofibrate. Br Heart J 1978; 40: 1069–1118.

33. The Cardiac Arrhythmia Suppression Trial II Investigators. Effect of the anti-arrythmic agent moricizine on survival after myocardial infarction. N Engl J Med 1992; 327: 227–233.

34. Davey Smith G, Egger M. Commentary on the cholesterol papers: statistical problems. Br Med J 1994; 308: 1025–1027.

35. Law MR, Wald NJ. Commentary on the cholesterol papers: disagreements are not substantial. Br Med J 1994; 308: 1027–1029.

36. Cameron HA, Ramsay LE. The lupus syndrome induced by hydralazine: a common complication with low dose treatment. Br Med J 1984; 289: 410–412.

37. Ferner RE. Hazards, risks and reality. Br J Clin Pharmacol 1992; 33: 125–128.

38. Hanley JA, Lippman-Hand A. If nothing goes wrong, is everything all right? Interpreting zero numerators. JAMA 1983; 249: 1743–1745.

39. Fleiss JL. Determining sample sizes needed to detect a difference between two proportions. In: Statistical Methods for Rates and Proportions (2nd edn). New York: Wiley, 1981; 33–49.

17 ACCURACY OF ADVERSE DATA FROM POST-MARKETING STUDIES AND THE INFLUENCE ON EXTENSION OF LICENSED INDICATIONS

D. H. Lawson
Glasgow Royal Infirmary, Glasgow, UK

Introduction

The literature on 'adverse drug reactions' and 'post-marketing surveillance' studies is often confused by a lack of clarity in defining the terms used. For the purposes of this presentation, I shall define various terms carefully and can only hope that these definitions are acceptable widely (see Appendix).

The term post-marketing surveillance studies strictly refers to all studies undertaken on marketed drugs. However, it has often been used to refer to a subset of this wide spectrum, namely that which involves observational studies of a cohort of recipients of a drug, usually undertaken in the early to medium period after marketing. I feel uncomfortable with this restriction and would prefer that investigators replaced the term with more specific details of the type of study under discussion.

If we adopt a wide view of the nature of any study included in the term 'post-marketing studies', we see that they range in spectrum from the classic double-blind randomised controlled clinical trial (RCCT), through the controlled clinical trial (CCT) without blinding, via the observational cohort studies involving collection of 'event' information or 'suspected adverse reaction' information to the classic spontaneous reporting scheme for suspected adverse reaction (e.g., Yellow Card scheme in the UK). It is clear that just as the costs per patient fall dramatically as one progresses from the RCCT to the Yellow Card scheme, so the accuracy of the resulting information also falls. This does not, however, mean that the information is lacking in value because it is less than totally accurate, merely that the interpretation of the output of any such information system must be assessed appropriately in the light of its acknowledged limitations.

Adverse reactions

Adverse reactions information is very broad in its scope. Reactions may be classified as pharmacological or idiosyncratic in nature. Broadly, pharmacological reactions are predictable, dose related, reasonably frequent, relatively easy to quantify and can usually be defined fairly accurately [1]. They are often recognised pre-marketing and can be quantified accurately in post-marketing studies. The pre-marketing studies usually define their frequency in the 'idealised' patients entering into RCCT whereas the post-marketing studies define their frequency both amongst the routine patient-in-the-street and in unusual subjects such as those experiencing renal or hepatic impairment, those at the extremes of age and those of different ethnic background to the subjects entering into the original trial.

Conversely, the idiosyncratic type of reaction is much more elusive, being broader in scope, unpredictable in type and in whom it occurs, not clearly dose related and relatively infrequent in its manifestation. Rarely are idiosyncratic reactions uncovered in pre-marketing studies. This is the type of complex and unpredictable reaction, so difficult to evaluate, which must be addressed by our observational studies. Yet it is only easily approachable via the very study which itself is least accurate, least reproducible, and most open to a variety of interpretations of any association between an 'event' (which could be an idiosyncratic adverse drug reaction) and a drug.

Generally speaking, the more accurate the description of the 'event' the greater the likelihood of correct attribution of its cause will be. Similarly, the shorter the time-scale from exposure to a putative causal agent and onset of a suspect event, the greater the chance of correctly assessing the true nature of the association between drug and event. Conversely, the longer the time-scale, the lower the chance of establishing a link. A good example of this latter problem is the demonstration of delayed-onset rashes in patients receiving ampicillin [2,3]. Clearly, if a rash occurs a week or more after cessation of therapy, the likelihood of this being correctly established and attributed to the medication is diminished. A more recent example is the delay in recognising the possibility that flucloxacillin could be associated with a delayed-onset hepatitis [4]. Here again, the reaction was both a difficult one to recognise and evaluate as an entity and the relationship with the medication was difficult to prove given the delay of anything up to 1½–3 months after stopping treatment [5].

Thus, for our existing systems to evaluate a possible adverse reaction efficiently, the reaction should be easy to recognise or distinctive in nature and the duration between exposure and outcome should either be short or, if prolonged, the lesion should at least occur while the patient is taking the medication.

Types of post-marketing studies

With this background in mind, it is helpful to divide post-marketing studies into hypothesis-testing and hypothesis-generating studies. The former are by far the simplest to undertake. A defined problem is suspected to be caused by a drug. One has the option of assembling a large cohort of drug recipients and following them to determine whether any develop the problem of interest (the 'event'), i.e. undertake a cohort study—or one can assemble a number of patients who have developed the problem of interest and assess their history to determine whether any received exposure to the drug of interest, i.e. a case study.

In either instance, it is always preferable to have a comparator group to facilitate interpretation of the resulting information. Thus generally one would undertake a controlled cohort study or a case–control study. However, it is important to think clearly about the need for and nature of such comparator subjects. Several factors must be considered. *First, the cost*: if it costs little or nothing to collect information on comparative subjects, then clearly they should be included. However, if the costs are prohibitive, careful thought must be addressed towards the need to include such a group. *Second, the nature of the comparator group*: an ideal comparison subject is one who is as likely to be identical to the subject under study as possible in all respects save only for the problem under review. *Third, the need*: this is the aspect of comparators which causes me most concern. The purpose of the comparator is to provide evidence of background risk. If one knows from other sources that the background risk of an event or an exposure is very low, then there may be occasions when the cost of reconfirming this is out of all proportion to the benefit achieved. It is therefore my strongly held view that the tendency to dismiss uncontrolled studies on *a priori* grounds purely *because* they are uncontrolled is inappropriate. Each study should be evaluated carefully in the light of the problems it sets out to address. Perhaps examples of this will help our thinking.

At one point immediately after release of cimetidine, the first H2-receptor blocking drug, there was concern about possible bone marrow toxicity arising from the fact that the development of the first H2 blocking drug (metiamide) was discontinued because of bone marrow toxicity. A cohort of cimetidine recipients was assembled and there was much debate about the need for a comparator cohort. RCCT of several hundred exposed subjects had uncovered no bone marrow toxicity. There was no known relationship between the condition for which cimetidine would be prescribed and bone marrow problems. The background risk of bone marrow problems in the community under study was known to be approximately $1:50–100\,000$ subjects. Thus in a cohort of $10\,000$ cimetidine recipients the likelihood was that there would be no bone marrow problems whatsoever (or at most only one patient affected). Since the study could not be done in a record linkage scheme, there was a major cost in including a comparator—one comparator enrolled in the study cost the same as one new cimetidine recipient. Thus for the same cost, the manufacturer could double the size of the exposed cohort of cimetidine recipients or include a comparator group [6]: the benefit to be gained by including a comparator series was therefore doubtful.

In the late 1960s, a number of young women were noted to have developed vaginal adenocarcinoma in their teens and early twenties [7]. An extensive case series of these individuals uncovered an extremely high probability of maternal exposure to high-dose stilboestrol during pregnancy. While a control group of subjects would confirm that the background risk of this exposure was zero in a random group of some 70 subjects, this fact was known from first principles. Thus, again, rather than undertaking a full-blown case–control study, a case series fully and carefully evaluated, sufficed for the purpose and greatly reduced the time, effort and overall cost of the study.

To summarise, generally observational studies are more powerful if they include appropriate comparison subjects. However, there are many occasions where such subjects may not be required and studies should not be over-criticised for omitting comparators when they are unnecessary.

Associations between exposures and events

Observational controlled studies need careful and critical analysis. Associations between exposures and events can arise in many different ways. Foremost amongst the factors which must be taken into account are chance, confounding, selection bias and observational bias.

Chance can be assessed on a simple statistical basis and does not usually give rise to a problem. Errors in data collection will tend to reduce the chances of detecting a true difference and will not generate associations where none pre-exist. *Confounding* is a complex subject, which is addressed in standard epidemiological handbooks. Suffice it to say here that confounding can be very difficult to rule out even in carefully organised studies. Confounding occurs when a variable is linked independently to exposure and outcome. An example should clarify this. In the long-term controlled cohort study of cimetidine use previously referred to, we would expect to see a statistically valid association between cimetidine and lung cancer. This will not arise because cimeti-dine 'causes' lung cancer, but because cimetidine is used to treat peptic ulcer. Patients with peptic ulcer have an increased prevalence of smoking. Smokers have an increased incidence of lung cancer and there-fore cimetidine recipients are likely to be associated with lung cancer. Any association between the H2 blocker and lung cancer is likely to be due to confounding. Theoretically, one could, with vast cohorts, confirm the absence of an association between cimetidine and lung cancer in non-smokers and show that the frequency of lung cancer in cimetidine-taking smokers was no different from that in smokers who had never taken an H2 blocker; however, the cost of such a study would be prohibitive and the need for it at present seems absent.

Bias is a major problem in all studies. It is important to appreciate this and to emphasise that it affects *all* studies, whether randomised or not. The classic double-blind RCCT contains substantial bias; however, the effect of the double-blindness and the randomisation is to distribute this bias evenly across the trial between exposed and non-exposed. Thus the bias is evenly balanced and hence its effect is minimised. Books have been written about bias. Here, suffice it to emphasise that *before embarking* on an observational study, one should address carefully all facets of bias, paying particular regard to selection bias—am I including a truly random sample of exposed or have I some systematic distortion of selection *which could influence the outcome measures* I am reviewing? The next important bias to consider is *observation* or *observer bias*—do my investigators know the hypothesis I am testing? If so, could they (unconsciously) distort the result by looking more intensely for an outcome of interest amongst the exposed as compared to the non-exposed?

A third key bias is *outcome bias*. Are my patients with outcome X equally likely to enter into my study whether or not they are exposed to a drug of interest? For example, if I am concerned about an infection, e.g. pneu-monia—are all patients with this diagnosis equally likely to be hospita-lised or do those who are taking immunosuppressives, such as steroids, always gain admission whereas those with 'simple' pneumonia often stay at home and hence do not enter into my study? If so, we have a systematic bias that needs to be addressed in interpreting our data.

I have perhaps spent a long time emphasising matters which may seem to many of you to be self-evident. If so, please spread the message to your colleagues, particularly those in industry. In my discussions about adverse drug reactions, I still find a substantial confusion in industry about the topic. Some feel intuitively suspicious about handling data of less than perfect quality. Others are unhappy about addressing issues such as con-founding and selection bias, not realising that they are regularly dealing with this (albeit unconsciously) in their double-blind randomised con-trolled trials! Yet others hanker after the 'certainties' of their RCCT and wish for the ideal time when all adverse reaction data will be assessed by their 'strict' criteria. These individuals seem deeply troubled when I make two points to them. First, such a time will never come and adverse reaction data will always be subject to debate and uncertainty. Second, their ideal model—RCCT—is ideal only under extremely artificial conditions. Not only do they have randomisation of treatments to a small subsection of the population with definitively diagnosed conditions in the absence of specific co-morbidities, but they perform well only when looking at relatively short-term outcomes. Where a target outcome is separated from the randomisation by a period of more than six months or a year, the possibilities increase for the development of additional variables which could affect outcome within the confines of the study, i.e. the study becomes increasingly heterogeneous despite the initial randomisation. Thus interpretation of the final results of RCCT where the conclusions are years away from randomisation forces us to think of all the caveats present in standard observational studies before accepting a causal explanation for any statistically valid outcome.

Post-marketing surveillance studies

REVIEW

In the mid-1980s the Committee on Safety of Medicines (CSM) reviewed the area of post-marketing surveillance and came to certain conclusions [8]. The place of the spontaneously reported adverse reaction scheme was secure. This system was deemed to be invaluable and relatively cheap to run. The Committee, however, acknowledged that there was a need for newer approaches, particularly where long-term drug therapy was being considered for relatively benign or asymptomatic conditions. Perhaps the best example of this type of treatment is the long-term use of oral contraceptives and, more recently, hormone replacement therapy. Also included is long-term treatment of elevated lipids, asymptomatic hypertension and so forth. Here the Committee agreed with industry representatives and the Association of the British Pharmaceutical Industry that there was a need for a voluntary initiative to undertake post-marketing surveillance studies. These studies have two objectives: first, to test any hypothesis that has arisen during pre-marketing studies or trials; and, second, to reassure the users, manufacturers and regulators that the drug performs as well in practice as it did in the pre-marketing trial stage. This latter hypothesis-generating phase has been the cause of substantial concern. Partly this concern arises from lack of suitably trained expertise within industry—or indeed within academia—because the skills of pharmacoepidemiology are difficult to acquire, depending as they do upon a rare combination of substantial clinical and epidemiological expertise. Partly also it relates to concern that hypotheses could be generated in one data set and cannot be tested in other sources, thus placing a drug at a competitive disadvantage with other drugs in the class.

If one acknowledges these concerns and couples them to the undoubtedly expensive nature of most ad hoc studies of a post-marketing observational nature, it is clear that in late 1993 the development of a suitable framework for post-marketing surveillance studies is less far advanced than had been hoped. Individual studies have contributed significantly to our knowledge in this area and are worthwhile mentioning *en passant*. However, we have yet to establish and utilise in the UK a sufficiently powerful group of resources to provide the required framework for routine future studies.

What is required for success in this area? In my view, we need a series of methods ranging from the formal ad hoc study run by the company via a short-term high-density study such as can be undertaken by Professor Inman's group in Southampton—Prescription Event Monitoring [9]—or International Medical Statistics in London [10], to a formal record linkage scheme of the type conducted by the VAMP group [11]. In the future, it is my view that the most cost-effective schemes will be those involving record linkage. It is therefore to be hoped that the pharmaceutical industry will begin to appreciate the potential benefits of initiating and funding two or more such schemes in the UK. Prior to this happening, the current situation is less than perfect, but has significant potential. Clearly in the view of the Medicines Control Agency (MCA) the position is depressing. In a review of some 31 studies voluntarily reported to the MCA over a four-year period from 1987 to 1991, the authors concluded that 'company postmarketing surveillance studies have made only a limited contribution to the assessment of drug safety, principally because of weak study designs and difficulties in patient recruitment' [12]. They suggest that a diversity of methods for undertaking post-marketing surveillance studies are needed: few will argue with this. They also suggest that the logistic problems of recruitment should be overcome and again few will argue with this, although life can be difficult for a firm attempting to avoid accusations of using post-marketing surveillance studies as concealed marketing of a product yet bound to recruit a substantial number of recipients into an observational study! They also recommend that the studies are more focused on to potential issues, i.e. that they are more along the lines of hypothesis-testing studies and less along the lines of hypothesis generation. Speaking personally, I am not convinced that this course of action is wise at present because it seems to me that sooner or later we will have to undertake hypothesis-generating studies on most drugs given to relatively healthy people for long periods of time.

EXAMPLES

Let us turn to some examples of post-marketing surveillance observational cohort studies to assess the benefits and pitfalls. I will confine myself to reviewing some published information.

The first study to report a major cohort concluded that the post-marketing surveillance study added nothing to the knowledge of the drug in question [13]. This was reassuring as the drug was a single-dose analgesic preparation—buprenophine—whose evaluation should have been adequately completed at the time of licensing. The study demonstrated that one could identify and follow such patients to a suitable conclusion and it confirmed the view that post-marketing surveillance studies would be most valuable in patients taking long-term therapy.

Another study, the Cimetidine Postmarketing Surveillance Study, conducted by Colin-Jones and his colleagues [6,14] was an early attempt at a long-term observational cohort study. It provided reassuring information about the freedom from major toxicity of this new H2-receptor antagonist despite several logistic problems, the greatest of which was the relative paucity of information about continued exposure in the target recipients. The study provided strong reassurance to the licensing authorities as they moved to broaden the indication of this drug and subsequently to move it from a prescription-only medicine to a pharmacy sales product.

The initial paper from this group addressed the vexed issue of an association between cimetidine and gastric cancer. Following anecdotal case reports in the literature, the data in the cohort study were reviewed and demonstrated a strong association between cimetidine and gastric cancer. However, the investigators concluded that the drug had not caused the cancer, rather cancer had caused the drug! Specifically the symptoms of an as yet undiagnosed gastric cancer had led to prescription of cimetidine (presumably under the impression that the diagnosis was peptic ulcer). Careful review of the information on gastric tumours over many subsequent years confirm the likelihood that a causal interpretation of the initial association was unjustified [15]. In the absence of an ongoing, independently evaluated observational study, it is quite possible that the history of H2 blockade could have been substantially altered by these initial anecdotal reports of the association with gastric cancer.

In another observational cohort study, Chalmers and his colleagues [16,17] reported on an ad hoc study of captopril, a new angiotensin converting enzyme inhibitor, licensed for the treatment of moderate to severe hypertension. This cohort was assembled by collecting data from patients commencing on treatment by their general practitioners. Some 10% of patients so started had mild hypertension and the resulting information played a significant role in reassessing the licensing authority's approach to the safety of this product and permitted an extension of its licence from severe hypertension to that of mild to moderate hypertension.

Examples of an anecdotal case-reporting system providing data leading to changes in drug indications can also be found. The change in status of ibuprofen from a prescription-only medicine to pharmacy status was assisted by the low frequency of reports about serious suspected adverse reactions to the CSM whereas data from similar sources contributed to licence withdrawal in a number of other non-steroidal anti-inflammatory agents [18].

Spontaneous reporting schemes have been of great assistance to licensing authorities in monitoring drugs safety [19,20]; however, there are severe limitations in their use. One area where the newer systems can be of great assistance is in providing reassurance that a drug does not appear to be causing a problem with measurable frequency. In my view, this is a facet of post-marketing surveillance which is poorly appreciated. In using closed record linkage schemes for reviewing drug utilisation and linking this information with hospitalisation data, a potentially powerful tool becomes available not only for generating hypotheses, but also for testing hypotheses generated from other data systems. If the subsequent analysis proves to be negative, then either the drug is not causing the problem or the system is insufficiently sensitive to pick up the association. The latter can easily be tested by reference to other drugs and events, i.e. the record system can be validated for accuracy of dealing with the problem of concern. The former hypothesis, i.e. that the drug is not causing the problem with a measurable frequency, which depends upon the numbers exposed to the drug in question, can then be established.

Use of large automated record linkage systems for this purpose is infrequent to date, but I believe will increase. An example would be the controversy surrounding cataract and allopurinol, which used the Puget Sound Health Maintenance Organisation data to assess the problem [21].

Other USA databases, e.g. Medicaid (Tennessee) system, have been used to show a strong negative correlation between long-term thiazide use and reduction in osteoporosis [22].

Several key features of successful record linkage systems need to be understood. These are, first, the successful establishment of linkage of demographic and hospitalisation or death data to an average of 95% of participants is required. Second, clear separation of individuals in the same family with the same name is necessary. Likewise, an ability to record and link maternal exposure to neonatal outcomes is highly desirable. Longitudinal records over time are important even after employment ceases. Finally, perhaps the most important feature of all—the ability to examine original case record data. This latter is at the heart of all post-marketing surveillance data collection. We are agreed that no observational study can be completely accurate. We are also agreed that inaccuracies tend to dilute important findings rather than create spurious ones. Any research involving large linked databases which does not include sample screening of primary records to evaluate the accuracy of the computerised analyses, in my view, is flawed. Thus regular evaluation of primary records is a paramount feature of all successful record linkage schemes.

Conclusion

To conclude, post-marketing surveillance has developed dramatically over the last 30 years since recognition of the thalidomide disaster. Drug surveillance systems looking at medical inpatients have given us reasonably secure information on short-term toxicity patterns of inpatient drug use [23]. Spontaneous reporting schemes have mushroomed in the developed world and are used extensively by many licensing authorities. Their value as hypothesis-generating systems would be enhanced greatly by the development of newer systems to evaluate these hypotheses.

Current systems of conducting cohort and case–control studies are relatively expensive and for a variety of administrative reasons less effective than intended by the pharmaceutical industry or as envisaged by regulatory authorities. The most efficient way forward would seem to be to concentrate some resources on developing the infrastructure for viable long-term record linkage schemes. Such a facility covering a relatively stable population of some 5 million or more would have the potential for a substantial reduction in the overall costs of conducting ad hoc post-marketing surveillance studies while at the same time increasing the value of the resulting data. If we could see at least two such schemes in operation in the near future, we could have a most powerful set of information which could be used both in the hypothesis-testing and hypothesis-generating modes. Data from one set could be evaluated in the other and firms would no longer be at the mercy of the results of a single study, but rather would have two resources to question. At least one such system— that run by VAMP [11]—is already in functioning order in the UK and a system with a somewhat different slant is functioning in Tayside: Medicines Evaluation Monitoring Organisation (MEMO) [24].

The results of such systems are likely to prove generally reassuring to patients, regulators and industry alike, as was the case with the original hospital monitoring studies [23].

If we as members of the pharmaceutical science professions do not proceed along such lines voluntarily, our consumers are going to push for such an approach using powerful pressures and possibly legislation. I much prefer the flexibility inherent in a voluntary approach, i.e. the route we traversed when setting up the Spontaneous Reporting Scheme for adverse reactions. Moreover, a 'Freedom-of-Information' Act could cause great potential for misinterpreting anecdotal information if left in unskilled hands. Now is the time for industry to take the initiative and begin to adequately fund the infrastructure for record linkage. If seen as an insurance policy, this will be worth the cost when one appreciates that the resulting data will also be most useful in assessing the efficacy of drugs marketed on the basis of altering appropriate markers of disease and possibly indicating alternative uses of medication.

Appendix

'EVENT' DATA

In an observational study any new occurrence is an 'event' and should be recorded as such whether or not it is thought to be drug related. An example could be fractured femur consequent upon a road traffic accident in which the injured was involved as a passenger in a vehicle.

ADVERSE DRUG REACTION DATA

Any 'event' which is due to a drug is said to be an adverse drug reaction. An example would be haematuria in a patient taking warfarin therapy.

SUSPECTED ADVERSE DRUG REACTION

An 'event' which is thought by a practitioner to be due to a drug. An example would be an upper gastrointestinal bleed in an NSAID (non-steroidal anti-inflammatory drug) recipient or a fracture sustained during a fall in a patient taking hypotensive therapy.

'AD HOC' STUDIES

Ad hoc studies are observational studies set up to address a single issue or problem, e.g. a cohort study of an angiotensin converting enzyme inhibitor to determine its effectiveness as a hypotensive agent and its toxicity in everyday use or a case–control study of gastrointestinal bleeding in elderly subjects.

RECORD LINKAGE STUDIES

These are studies where investigators link two or more existing data resources to provide a powerful tool to generate or test hypotheses about possible adverse drug events. These usually involved linking a data set of exposures (e.g., prescriptions with a given time frame) and a data set of outcomes (e.g., death certificate data, hospital discharge diagnoses, general practice consultation records).

STUDY VALIDATION

This term is often very poorly used because it lacks definition. Some use it to imply that the data have been checked for accuracy of transfer from one data set (e.g., paper) to another (e.g., computer). Others use it to infer that independent sources have been used to verify the accuracy of certain items of 'raw data', e.g. diagnoses, operations. Until a generally accepted definition becomes available, it is better to avoid this term and be explicit in defining the nature of the 'validation' undertaken.

References

1. Rawlins MD. Adverse reactions to drugs. Br Med J 1981; 282: 974.
2. Shapiro SS, Slone D, Siskind V, Lewis GP. Drug rash with ampicillin and other penicillins. Lancet 1969; November: 969.
3. Arndt KA, Jick H. Rates of cutaneous reactions to drugs: a report from the Boston Collaborative Drug Surveillance Program. JAMA 1976; 235: 918.
4. Victorino RMM, Maria VA, Correia AP, de Moura MC. Flucloxacillin-induced cholestatic hepatitis with evidence of lymphocyte sensitization. Arch Intern Med 1987; 147: 987.
5. Committee on Safety of Medicines. Flucloxacillin-induced cholestatic jaundice. Curr Probl 1992; 35: 2.
6. Colin-Jones D, Langman MJS, Lawson DH, Vessey MP. Postmarketing surveillance of the safety of cimetidine: twelve month morbidity report. Q J Med 1985; 215: 253.
7. Herbst AL, Ulfelder H, Poskanzer DC. Association of maternal stilboestrol therapy with tumour appearance in young women. N Engl J Med 1971; 284: 878.
8. Grahame-Smith DG. Report of the Adverse Reactions Working Party to the Committee on Safety of Medicine, London. London: Department of Health, 1986.
9. Inman WHW. Postmarketing surveillance of adverse drug reactions in general practice. Br Med J 1982; 3: 85.
10. Hill PC, Bridgman KM. A postmarketing surveillance study to evaluate the safety of bisoprolol. Br J Clin Res 1992; 3: 85.
11. Jick H, Derby LE, Rodriguez LAG, Jick SS, Dean AD. Liver disease associated with diclofenac, naproxen and piroxicam. Pharmacotherapy 1992; 12 (3): 207.
12. Waller PC, Wood SH, Langman MJS, Breckenridge AM, Rawlins MD. Review of company postmarketing surveillance studies. Br Med J 1992; 304: 1470.
13. Harcus AW, Ward AE, Smith DW. Methodology of monitored release of a new preparation: buprenorphine. Br Med J 1979; 2: 163.
14. Colin-Jones D, Langman MJS, Lawson DH, Logan RFA, Paterson KR, Vessey MP. Postmarketing surveillance of the safety of cimetidine: ten year mortality report. Gut 1992; 33 (90): 1280.
15. Colin-Jones D, Langman MJS, Lawson DH, Vessey MP. Cimetidine use and gastric cancer: a preliminary report from a postmarketing surveillance study. Br Med J 1982; 285: 1311.
16. Chalmers D, Dombey SL, Lawson DH. Postmarketing surveillance of captopril (for hypertension): a preliminary report. Br J Clin Pharmacol 1987; 24: 343.
17. Chalmers D, Whitehead A, Lawson DH. Postmarketing surveillance of captopril for hypertension. Br J Clin Pharmacol 1992; 34: 215.
18. Committee on Safety of Medicines Update. Non-steroidal anti-inflammatory drugs and serious gastrointestinal adverse reactions: 2. Br Med J 1986; 292: 1190.
19. Rawlins MD. Spontaneous reporting of adverse drug reactions. II: Uses. Br J Clin Pharmacol 1988; 26: 7.

20. Rawlins MD. Spontaneous reporting of adverse drug reactions. I: The data. Br J Clin Pharmacol 1988; 26: 1.
21. Jick H, Brandt HE. Allopurimol and cataracts. Am J Ophth 1984; 98: 355.
22. Ray WA, Griffin MR, Downey W, Melton LJ III. Long-term use of thiazide diuretics and risk of hip fracture. Lancet 1989; April: 687.
23. Jick H. Drugs: remarkably non-toxic. N Engl J Med 1974; 291: 824.
24. Beardon PHG, Brown SV, McDevitt DG. Gastrointestinal events in patients prescribed non-steroidal anti-inflammatory drugs: a controlled study using record linkage in Tayside. Q J Med 1989; 71 (266): 497.

18 CONTROLLED CLINICAL TRIALS: CONTRIBUTION TO DRUG SAFETY

M. J. S. Langman
Queen Elizabeth Hospital, Birmingham, UK

Introduction

An initial judgement would suggest that controlled clinical trials present an inappropriate format for assessing drug safety. The archetypal clinical trial includes carefully selected patients where the drive is towards judging clinical efficiency. Those included, though having the disease to be studied, may nevertheless be selected using such vigorous criteria that they cannot be considered generally representative of drug recipients in practice. Thus they may not include the very elderly, or those receiving other treatments, whether for the same or other diseases, simultaneously.

These features make the classical explanatory trial a generally unsuitable format, but the pragmatic trial bears a greater relationship to practice, with the emphasis not upon 'can treatment be shown to work?' but upon 'does treatment ordinarily work?'

A second feature of a clinical trial which limits value in safety assessment is that studies are often too small to be likely to detect unexpected hazards. Anticipated pharmacological actions on systems outside those to be modulated may well be assessable, however.

Controlled clinical trials can nevertheless contribute to drug safety in at least four ways. First, standard clinical trials may make useful contributions in particular by confirming that dosages required to produce pharmacological effects are well judged. Larger trials with wide entry criteria may have particular value in judging safety in practice. Third, it may sometimes be possible by combining data by meta-analysis to demonstrate

This chapter was first published in Z. Bankowski and J. F. Dunne (eds), *Drug Surveillance, International Cooperation – Past, Present and Future, Proceedings of the XXVIIth CIOMS Conference (1993).*

Clinical Measurement in Drug Evaluation. Edited by W. S. Nimmo and G. T. Tucker
Published 1995 by John Wiley & Sons Ltd. © 1994 Council for International Organizations of Medical Sciences

safety issues which are not discernible in individual small studies. Fourth, the deliberate design of randomised trials of large size specifically to assess safety may make a valuable contribution.

Standard clinical trials

Provided they are conducted in sufficient detail they may, for instance, have special value in establishing firmly the lowest doses required—typically of hypotensive drugs. Thus, with hindsight, there may have been insufficient attention paid to the lowest possible doses of angiotensin converting enzyme inhibitors in treating hypertension and cardiac failure. The result was that when released for general use there was an undesirable level of adverse effects typically associated with overdosage, such as hypotension and renal failure.

One could speculate that such events could arise through anxiety to ensure an effective dose rather than to establish that which was least effective, and thus most commensurate with drug safety.

LARGE TRIALS

Balance between advantage and disadvantage: hypertension

The balance between advantage and disadvantage is sometimes clearly assessable. Thus, the MRC trial for mild hypertension randomly assigned treatment in general practice by beta blockade, propranolol or placebo, and examined benefits as well as drawbacks.

Table 1 displays patterns of adverse effects in the male entrants. Treatment was clearly not without its drawbacks. At the same time the rates of

Table 1. MRC trial in mild hypertension, using bendrofluazide, propanolol or placebo [1]

	Percentage (males)		
	Bendrofluazide	Propanolol	Placebo
Impaired g.t.t.	7.7	3.4	3.3
Gout	12.8	6.3	1.3
Raynauds	0	5.1	0.2
Lethargy	3.6	5.3	0.5
Patient number	2236	2385	4525

g.t.t., glucose tolerance test.
Stroke rates
Active treatment   1.4
Placebo   2.6
(per 1000 patient years).

stroke occurrence were reduced by nearly 50%. This apparently satisfactory result has to be placed in context of requiring nearly 1000 patient years of treatment to stop one such event.

It then has to be asked whether the treatment regime is one that should be accepted as a standard rather than as one which demonstrates achievable benefit, but probably better obtained by another route, using less unpleasant remedies.

Results obtained by the MRC trial can be compared with those in the Systolic Hypertension in the Elderly Programme (SHEP). This also used a diuretic (chlorthalidone rather than bendrofluazide), and a beta blocking agent (atenolol rather than propranolol). Treatment was demonstrably effective with a 36% reduction in stroke rates by active treatment. Adverse effects (Table 2) were not prominent, despite the fact that the stepped programme allowed combination of the active agents.

The contrast between the outcomes of the two studies in terms of adverse effects is quite striking, and difficult to explain. Nevertheless, one possibility derives from the rigorous entry criteria of the SHEP study [2]. This randomised 4927 individuals, but they were drawn from an initial possible entry group of 448 921. It could be asked whether the entry and conduct criteria, apparently reasonable in themselves, resulted in the inclusion of a group of highly motivated, stoical and atypical individuals in acceptance of drug problems. The criteria included four blood pressure measurements on two separate visits, physical examination, 12-lead electrocardiogram, behavioural assessment and measurement of blood levels of cholesterol, uric acid and others, as well as repeated measurements.

The application of quality-of-life analysis is often, and very reasonably, advocated. It is not always immediately obvious what the outcome means.

Table 2. Systolic hypertension in the elderly programme: 447 921 individuals identified [2]. Copyright 1991 American Medical Association

Met criteria	11.6%	Baseline visit 1	2.7%
Eligible base visit 2	1.7%	Eligible randomise	1.2%
	Randomised	1.1%	

	Adverse effects (%) in SHEP	
	Active	Placebo
Postural faintness	12.8	10.6
Tiredness	25.8	23.8
Cold hands	13.6	9.8
Any intolerable effect	28.1	20.8
Patients	2365	2371
Stroke rate per 100 per 5 years	5.2	8.2

Thus a recent study compared the effects of captopril and enalapril on quality of life [3] and established differences which, in the author's opinion, were 'substantial' and 'clinically meaningful'. Examination of the paper showed that the basis included a comprehensive self-administered questionnaire which included (*inter alia*) psychological well-being and general perceived health. In addition, the degree of distress due to side-effects and other effects was assessed. 'The conceptualisation of quality of life and the rationale for choosing these scales were based on previous studies.'

Difficulty inevitably arises for the ordinary clinician in deciding just what changes in responsiveness index units mean (Table 3). This does not necessarily imply criticism of the authors. Rating scales are accepted tools in psychological assessment. It is more that their transposition to the field of blood pressure measurement is novel, and weighting is problematic. Thus a rise of 18.1 for low-dose captopril looks impressive, and may be— with confidence intervals which do not overlap zero. However, a rise of 18.1 from a base of 427 is a change of less than 5%.

Expected untoward effects: thrombolytics and aspirin

Aspirin has clearly demonstrable effects in the prophylaxis of transient ischaemic episodes. Aspirin is also well known to exacerbate peptic ulceration. The UK TIA trial included 2436 patients who received placebo, aspirin 300 mg or 1200 mg daily for a mean period of four years, with overall beneficial effects [4]. Later examination of the data showed clear differences in the frequency of upper gastrointestinal bleeding, with evidence that aspirin 300 mg is above the no-effect level [5] (Table 4). Episodes were markedly more common in the first three months of treatment than later. However, difficulty arises in deciding whether this represents weeding out of a population of susceptibles, gastric adaptation, or perhaps

Table 3. Quality of life analysis [3]: use of angiotensin converting enzyme inhibitors in mild to moderately severe hypertension

Dose	Captopril	Enalapril
Low	+18.1	+5.9
Medium	−6.8	−4.3
High	−0.5	−10.7
Patient number	184	178

Scores represent overall quality-of-life changes from baseline in responsiveness units.

Table 4. Upper gastrointestinal bleeding in UK TIA study [5]

Bleeding from:	Placebo	Aspirin 300 mg	Aspirin 1200 mg
Gastric ulcer	Nil	1	8
Duodenal ulcer	Nil	6	9
Unknown site	2	8	11
Odds ratio		7.7	14.4
(all causes)		1.7–33.8	3.4–60

Table 5. Streptokinase for myocardial infarction (ISIS-2) [6].
© The Lancet Ltd 1988

	Treated	Controls
Stroke, haemorrhagic	7	0
Major bleed	46	18
Vascular death	791	1029
Total	8592	8595

reduced dosage with continued use. The trial itself showed an 18% reduction in vascular events with a 7% (non-significant) reduction in disabling stroke, or death.

Thrombolytics are now well established as treatments for acute myocardial infarction. Amongst potential adverse responses are haemorrhagic stroke and reperfusion arrhythmias.

The ISIS study [6] was conducted to a very simple protocol, and so likely to give generalisable results. Table 5 shows the overall outcome and clearly illustrates that the chances of haemorrhagic stroke or major bleeding were outweighed by the reduced changes of vascular death.

If treatment is effective then there is logic in administering it as early as possible. The ISIS-2 study was conducted in hospital, and it is noteworthy that a range of side-effects including arrhythmias, hypotension and bradycardia as well as allergic and gastrointestinal reactions were more common in drug than placebo recipients. Pre-hospital thrombolytic therapy could arguably therefore be less safe.

A recent randomised study in 5469 patients compared feasibility and safety of therapy by 'well equipped, well trained mobile emergency medical staff' with that given in hospital [7]. Table 6 shows the results. The pattern of arrhythmia occurrence differed but overall was, if anything, more frequent in late (in-hospital) recipients than in those treated before admission. Whether this would imply safety in less skilled hands before admission and in less vigorously selected patients is unclear.

Table 6. Thrombolysis for myocardial infarction: occurrence of ventricular fibrillation [7]

	Treatment	
Event occurrence	Pre-hospital	In hospital
A. Pre-admission	69	44*
B. Admission to injection 2	34	43
C. Rest of hospital stay	100	145**
Total treated	2750	2719

*$p < 0.02$; **$p < 0.002$.

Unexpected adverse effects: azothioprin

Occasionally clinical trials yield unexpected information, although generalisation can be difficult. The national Crohn's cooperative trial, in comparing azathioprin, prednisone and placebo in treating Crohn's disease, had six patients in a total of 113 who developed acute pancreatitis within a month of azathioprin prescription; none of the other treatment groups had similar problems [8]. Generalisation is difficult; inflammatory bowel disease may constitute a special risk since mesalazine—and also olsalazine and sulphasalazine treatment—occasionally have been associated with pancreatitis. On the other hand, post-transplant pancreatitis during immunosuppression is also well recorded [9].

META-ANALYSES

The importance of including all data sets: steroids and ulcer

Three studies of ulcer occurrence in steroid recipients have been conducted in which data were aggregated, and they illustrate the differences in conclusions which can be reached when data sets are included, or excluded [10–12]. Conn and Blitzer [10] initially examined 50 controlled trials and found no significant association. Messer and colleagues used 71 studies and, by contrast, detected an association (Table 7). Conn and Poynard in a further analysis claimed that 28 of the studies in Messer *et al.*'s analysis were inappropriately included, and that in 12 other factors could have explained ulcer occurrence, while a further group of seven studies were inappropriately omitted. In the circumstances ultimate truth is difficult to define. However, overall ulcer rates were quite low in all data sets. One could ask whether rigorous exclusion/inclusion criteria made it possible to underestimate the true burden of disease.

Conclusions which appear to differ from clinical experience

Divergence from expectation is brought out by a meta-analysis of 123 trials of non-steroidal anti-inflammatory drug (NSAID) therapy [13] (Table 7). Compared with the results of case–control analyses the risks seem strikingly underestimated. It is difficult to tell whether such underestimation could arise because trials were generally of short duration, so that side-effects did not occur, or because of vigorous selection criteria, or because the severity of arthropathy diverted attention this from possible gastro-intestinal effects.

Unexpected conclusions about the general value of treatment

Examination of data obtained in cholesterol-lowering treatment trials has generally shown disappointing overall results. The statistical overview presented by Ravnskov is one of the largest and Table 8 summarises the data. Taken overall there was no evidence of a reduction in death rates, although fatal coronary heart disease and non-fatal coronary events were marginally reduced. These trends were associated with a markedly raised frequency of non-medical deaths and cancer deaths, reported in subsets of

Table 7. Meta-analysis, non-aspirin NSAIDS: 123 trials

	Treated	Controls
Proven ulcer	2	0
Gross bleeding	24	8
Abdominal pain	175	118
Indigestion	116	64
Total	6460	6355

Table 8. Overview of cholesterol-lowering trials [14]

Measurement	No. of trials	Odds ratio	95% CI
All deaths	24	1.02	0.97–1.07
Fatal coronary heart disease	27	0.94	0.88–1.00
Non-fatal coronary heart disease	24	0.90	0.84–0.96
Non-medical deaths	12	1.55	1.11–2.16
All deaths [a]	12	1.05	0.95–1.17
Cancer deaths	14	1.15	0.91–1.45

[a]In the same trials where non-medical deaths were recorded separately.

Table 9. Outcome in Serevent National Surveillance Study [15]

No. included:	Salmeterol 16 787 %	Salbutamol 8383 %	r.r.
All deaths	0.32	0.24	1.35
All admissions	1.89	1.97	0.95
Other serious	2.09	2.09	1.00
Asthma related			
Deaths	0.07	0.02	3.00
Admissions	1.15	1.22	0.95
Other serious	1.18	1.19	0.99
Withdrawals	2.91	3.79	0.77**
Mild events	3.50	4.60	
Moderate events	4.40	5.00	
Severe events	9.90	11.60	
Total no.	879	520	

**p < 0.001.

studies. The bases of these findings are unclear but they cast doubt upon the wisdom of general attempts to lower serum cholesterol levels by the methods used.

TRIALS DESIGNED TO EXAMINE SAFETY ISSUES

Data obtained in comparisons of salmeterol and salbutamol present a good example, in which 25 070 asthmatic individuals were randomised 2 : 1 to these respective drugs [14]. Table 9 summarises the outcome during the 16-week period of surveillance. Such information could not have been gathered during routine surveillance, where potential biases would include a likely inclusion preferentially of severe cases in the new drug group. The slight (non-significant) excess of deaths in those given salmeterol contrasts with somewhat lower proportions of asthma-related events in the same group. Taken overall the picture is reassuring.

Conclusions

Randomised controlled trials can make valuable contributions to drug safety but their defects must be recognised. They include degrees of selection which can make generalisation difficult, failure to include high-risk groups or concurrent other drug users and failure to mirror marketplace practices.

References

1. Medical Research Council Working Party. MRC trial of treatment of mild hypertension: principal results. Br Med J 1985; 291: 97–104.
2. SHEP Cooperative Research Group. Prevention of stroke by hypertensive drug treatment in older persons with isolated systolic hypertension. JAMA 1991; 265: 3255–3264.
3. Testa MA, Anderson RB, Nackley JG, Hollenberg NK and the Quality-of-life Hypertension study group. N Engl J Med 1993; 328: 907–913.
4. Peto R, Gray R, UK-TIA Study Group. United Kingdom transient ischaemic attack (UK-TIA, aspirin trial: interim results). Br Med J 1988; 296: 315–320.
5. Shorrock CJ, Langman MJS, Warlow CP and UK-TIA Study Group. Risks of upper GI bleeding during TIA prophylaxis with aspirin. Gastroenterology 1992; 102: A165.
6. ISIS-2 Second International Study of Infarct Survival Collaborative Group. Randomised trial of intravenous streptokinase, oral aspirin, both or neither during 17 187 cases of suspected acute myocardial infarction. Lancet 1988; ii: 349–360.
7. European Myocardial Infarction Project Group. Pre-hospital thrombolytic therapy in patients with suspected acute myocardial infarction. N Engl J Med 1993; 328: 383–389.
8. Sturdevant RAL, Singleton JW, Deren JJ, Law DH, McCleery JL. Azathrioprin related pancreatitis in patients with Crohn's disease. Gastroenterology 1979; 77: 838–886.
9. Corrodi P, Knoblauch M, Binswanger U, Scholzel E, Largiader F. Pancreatitis after renal transplantation. Gut 1975; 16: 285–289.
10. Conn HO, Blitzer BL. Non-association of adrenocorticosteroid therapy and peptic ulcer. N Engl J Med 1976; 294: 473–479.
11. Messer J, Reitman D, Sacks HS, Smith H Jr, Chalmers TC. Association of adrenocorticosteroid therapy and peptic ulcer disease. N Engl J Med 1983; 309: 21–24.
12. Conn HO, Poynard T. Adrenocorticosteroid administration and peptic ulcer: a critical analysis. J Chronic Dis 1985; 38: 457–468.
13. Chalmers TC, Berrier J, Hewitt P et al. Meta-analysis of randomised controlled trials as a method of estimating rare complications of non-steroidal anti-inflammatory drug therapy. Aliment Pharmacol Ther 1988; 2S: 9–26.
13. Ravnskov U. Cholesterol-lowering trials in coronary heart disease: frequency of citation and outcome. Br Med J 1992; 305: 15–19.
15. Castle W, Fuller R, Hall J, Palmer J. Serevent nationwide surveillance study: comparison of salmeterol with salbutamol in asthmatic patients who require regular bronchodilator treatment. Br Med J 1993; 306: 1034–1037.

19 PREDICTING ADVERSE DRUG REACTIONS

Charles F. George
University of Southampton, Southampton, UK

Introduction

Medicine taking is a common occurrence. Surveys by us [1,2] indicate that at any one time between 44% and 48% of the adult population have been prescribed a medicine within the preceding month. In the UK men visit their general practitioners on average 3.5 times per annum and for women the figure is five [3]. About two-thirds of consultations end with the issuing of a prescription.

Given this massive consumption of medicines, it is not surprising that adverse drug reactions (a noxious change in the patient's condition which may necessitate reduction in dosage, withdrawal of the medicine, and/or the need for additional treatment) can arise. In this chapter I shall indicate some of the ways in which adverse drug reactions can be predicted and, therefore, avoided.

Pre-clinical toxicology testing

A major development in the 1930s was the introduction of sulphonamide drugs. Prior to their introduction mortality from lobar pneumonia was at least 27% and clinical trials of M&B693 by Evans and Gaisford [4] confirmed its efficacy with a reduction in mortality to 8%. Resolution of the illness was also much more rapid in the treated group. There was, thereafter, a rapid proliferation of sulphonamide drugs on both sides of the Atlantic. Many of these compounds were introduced without pre-clinical toxicology testing being performed. As a consequence, in the USA a major disaster occurred following the introduction of an elixir of sulphanilamide. At least 76 people are known to have died in the months of September and October, 1937. Detailed pathological evaluations by Geiling and Cannon [5] revealed that the causative agent was the 72% content of

Clinical Measurement in Drug Evaluation. Edited by W. S. Nimmo and G. T. Tucker
© 1995 John Wiley & Sons Ltd

diethylene glycol which precipitated acute renal failure. These authors set out the needs for the careful examination of acute and chronic toxicity in varying dosage levels in different species.

There can be no doubt that careful pre-clinical toxicity testing can enable the identification of substances which are too toxic to be given to man, as well as those organs which are at particular risk [6]. However, it is important that the studies are carried out in appropriate species, otherwise potential adverse effects will be missed. Thus, chloroquine retinopathy can be detected in pigmented species, but will not be found in the albino rat. Similarly, the failure to test thalidomide for possible teratogenic effects in the rabbit (or primate) resulted in a major disaster [7].

Despite the obvious attractions of pre-clinical toxicity testing, there is little doubt that, on occasions, problems are missed. Many of these reactions have an immunological basis. Good examples include the Coombs' positive red cells identified in patients on long-term methyldopa therapy [8]. Although this reaction is for the most part merely a nuisance when it comes to the cross-matching of blood, on occasions haemolysis can occur.

Central nervous system effects are sometimes missed during pre-clinical toxicity testing. For that reason it is most important that human volunteer/phase I testing in man is carried out by well-trained investigators. An example which I myself experienced was during the development of an inotropic agent known as AR-L57 [9]. In doses of 150 mg given intravenously over 6 min there was a positive inotropic action as evidenced by a shortening of the pre-ejection period. However, in doses which were without obvious inotropic effect (as well as those which had that action) the drug produced hemeralopia and xanthopsia which lasted from 3 to 12 min after the cessation of the intravenous infusion. It is my belief that no amount of animal testing would have allowed one to identify this problem since 'you can't talk to a rat'. Risks exist also when our knowledge of pharmacology is incomplete. In that context a good example is that of clonidine [10]. This stimulant of α-adrenoceptors was developed as a nasal decongestant. However, it had a powerful action on pre-synaptic α-adrenoceptors (which was not recognised at the time it was first given to man) and this had an unexpected action to lower blood pressure acutely.

Dose–response studies

As a past member of a section 4 committee (the Committee on Review of Medicines) and journal editor, I have been disappointed by the relative lack of attention paid by some pharmaceutical companies to exploration of the dose–response relationship of their new compounds. This, in my view, is one of the areas which needs to be addressed in future studies. Indeed, draft guidance has been prepared by the EC on this topic. Good dose–response data should allow one to identify the most suitable dosage regimen for formal clinical trials, for patient subgroups and in particular for defining an appropriate dosing interval. It is particularly helpful if an adequate assay method exists for the parent molecule and any active metabolites so that concentration–effect relationships can also be studied. Ideally, we would like to know the shape of the dose–response curve, the minimal effective dose/concentration of the drug (or its active metabolite) so as to predict the likely duration of effect. Examples of problems that can arise when these measures are not followed have been published recently [11].

Special groups

Brodie and Feely [12] have identified a number of patient groups who are at particular risk from drug therapy. In this chapter I shall focus on four of these: the elderly, patients with renal disease, those with liver damage and patients receiving multiple drug therapy.

THE ELDERLY

Old people receive a disproportionate number of medicines on prescription and, in addition, are more likely to develop adverse effects due to a combination of circumstances. Drugs with an action on the cardiovascular system, the central nervous system and musculoskeletal systems are particularly likely to be used in old people and for that reason it is essential that these are studied in this age group. Space does not permit a full review of the likely changes in pharmacokinetics and dynamics which can exist in an elderly population. There are, however, numerous reviews on this topic to which readers are referred [13–15].

Ideally pharmacokinetic studies should include both clearance and concentration–time data after intravenous and oral doses (provided that an intravenous formulation is available and a suitable method exists for measurement of the drug in body fluids). Those agents with significant pre-systemic metabolism are likely to show reduced systemic clearance after an intravenous dose (due to diminished liver blood flow and hepatic volume) and increased bioavailability after oral dosing: nifedipine and laevodopa represent good examples [16,17]. However, in addition to studying the pharmacokinetics of such agents it is important to examine their dynamic actions. In the case of nifedipine, intravenous administration to young people provoked a marked tachycardia but no change in blood pressure [16]. By contrast, in the elderly there was no increase in heart rate but a pronounced fall in blood pressure and hypotension occurred in some individuals. These changes are thought to reflect a combination of impaired baroreflex function, as well as problems with diminished adrenoceptor sensitivity [15].

RENAL DISEASE

Renal disease can have a profound effect on the elimination of polar substances, which include cardiac glycosides, amiloride, aminoglycoside antimicrobials and water-soluble β-adrenoceptor antagonists [15]. Thus, the introduction of atenolol in fixed (100 mg) doses led to the occurrence of excessive pharmacological effects in people with diminished renal reserve. Many of these people were elderly and the end result was bradycardia with syncope which led, on occasion, to hospitalisation following falls. Subsequently, smaller (50 mg and 25 mg) doses became available.

Unfortunately, many doctors still do not understand the principles of dosage adjustment in renal failure, especially the relationship between age, gender, weight and serum creatinine. These simple measurements can, however, allow fairly accurate predictions of creatinine clearance which can aid the adjustment of dosage in elderly people and others with diminished renal function.

HEPATIC DISEASE

Knowledge of whether or not a drug is bound to albumin and subject to metabolism by the liver is important in deciding if a problem is likely to occur in patients with hepatic disease. Assuming either of these to be the case, studies will need to be undertaken to define the effects in greater detail. It is, however, important to recognise that patients with hepatic disease represent a heterogeneous group. Changes in drug disposition/metabolism are most likely to be seen with agents which are subject to pre-systemic metabolism and/or are highly bound to serum albumin. The biggest alterations in disposition and metabolism tend to be seen in those patients who have evidence of decomposition, i.e. serum albumin concentrations below 30 g/l, raised serum bilirubin and either ascites or encephalopathy. Finally, portosystemic anastomoses will increase the bioavailability due to shunting of blood around the liver [18].

MULTIPLE DRUG THERAPY

Hitherto, studies of potential drug interactions have tended to be of a blunderbuss nature. But it is clear from Professor Tucker's chapter [19] that greater precision can be achieved from a knowledge of whether or not a new compound is metabolised and, if so, by which cytochrome P450. Suffice it to say that cytochrome P4503A is the enzyme most commonly involved in the metabolism of xenobiotics. It is responsible for the metabolic breakdown of many endogenous compounds, including steroid molecules. It is known that the oral contraceptive pill can be rendered useless by anticonvulsant drugs, including phenytoin and carbamazepine. This knowledge should have led to a systematic investigation of other substrates for this enzyme. Amongst these are the dihydropyridine calcium channel blocking drugs. There is good evidence that the metabolism of felodipine [20] and nifedipine is markedly increased, rendering these drugs almost useless in conventional doses.

The demonstration using an *in vitro* system of dependence upon this enzyme system should also lead to systematic investigation of the effects of various enzyme inhibitors. The latter include citrus juices containing flavanoids [21], antifungal agents including ketoconazole as well as the macrolide antibiotic, erythromycin. The knowledge that the new antihistamine, terfenadine [23], was subject to metabolism by the same enzyme system could have identified the need for systematic evaluation of interactions with these and other inhibitors. Had they been performed the occurrence of toxicity, which includes *torsades de pointes* [23], might have been anticipated.

In vitro studies might also be appropriate for preliminary work on potential interactions with warfarin and other agents with narrow therapeutic indices.

Post-marketing surveillance

From the foregoing it should, I hope, be apparent that the majority of adverse effects of drug treatment relate to the type A category, i.e. excessive pharmacological reactions. By contrast, type B reactions [24] are often bizarre and not generally to be expected from the known actions of the drug when given in usual therapeutic doses. Furthermore, they tend to be uncommon/rare but are serious, with a significant mortality.

The occurrence of the oculomucocutaneous syndrome with practolol [25] therapy provides an excellent example of a type B reaction which was neither predicted in advance of marketing of the medicine, nor was it reproduced in subsequent, more detailed toxicological testing. Even with existing tests for drug safety the total experience with a new chemical entity tends to amount to no more than 1000 patient years by the time of marketing. It therefore follows that rare events occurring at a frequency of less than one per 5000 people are unlikely to be detected during pre-marketing studies. Nevertheless, Skegg and colleagues [26] identified that an alternative system, namely event monitoring, should allow the detection of adverse events which mimic naturally occurring problems such as dry eyes. Clearly, the green card system introduced by Inman [27] allowed the demonstration of photosensitive reactions and onycholysis to benoxaprofen.

Conclusions

It is inevitable that if patients are to derive benefit from medicines some risk is attached. Nevertheless, highly toxic agents can be screened out during the development process, while the potential toxicity of others can be anticipated. Early clinical testing must be done by experts working in an appropriate environment. Careful attention needs to be paid to dose–response relationships and the minimum effective concentration of drugs or their active metabolites defined.

Since almost all new chemical entities will be used in old people, attention needs to be given to their study in this age group. Major routes of drug elimination need to be defined by a combination of *in vitro* drug metabolism studies and renal elimination *in vivo*. Given this information, it is possible to target appropriate interaction studies. By so doing it should be possible to minimise the risk of type A reactions occurring and at least identify the situations which predispose to their occurrence. Post-marketing surveillance is, however, necessary to identify type B reactions. Some system of event monitoring is desirable in order to reduce the risks of doctors overlooking problems which mimic naturally occurring disease.

References

1. Ridout S, Waters WE, George CF. Knowledge of and attitudes to medicines in the Southampton community. Br J Clin Pharmacol 1986; 21: 701–712.
2. Sullivan M, George CF. Medicine taking in the Southampton community: a second look. In preparation.
3. Office of Population Censuses and Surveys. General Household Survey 1982. London: HMSO, 1984.
4. Evans GM, Gaisford WF. Treatment of pneumonia with 2-(*p*-aminobenzene sulphonamido)pyridine. Lancet 1938; ii: 14–19.
5. Geiling EMK, Cannon PR. Pathologic effects of elixir of sulphanilamide (diethylene glycol) poisoning. JAMA 1938; 111: 919–926.
6. Zbinden G. Risk predicted from animal studies. In: Walker SR, Asscher AW (eds), Medicines and Risk/Benefit Decisions. Lancaster: MTP Press, 1987; 49–56.
7. Mellin GW, Katzenstein M. The saga of thalidomide. N Engl J Med 1962; 267: 1184–1192, 1238–1244.
8. Carstairs KC, Breckenridge A, Dollery CT, Worledge SM. Incidence of a positive-direct Coombs' test in patients on α-methyldopa. Lancet 1966; ii: 133–135.
9. George CF. The importance of clinical pharmacology in drug development. Clin Sci 1981; 60: 247–250.
10. Ehringer H. Die Wirkung von 2-(2,6-Dichlorophenylamino)-2-imidazolinhydrochlorid auf die Extremitätendurchblutung, den Blutdruck und die Venenkapazität bei Normotonikern. Arzneimittelforsch 1966; 16: 1165–1169.
11. George CF. The contribution of academic clinical pharmacology to medicines research. In: Stonier P (ed), Discovering New Medicines: Careers in Pharmaceutical Research and Development. Chichester: John Wiley & Sons Ltd, 1994; 48–57.

12. Brodie MJ, Feely J. Adverse drug reactions. Br Med J 1988; 296: 845–849.
13. Woodhouse KW, James OFW. Hepatic drug metabolism with ageing. Br Med Bull 1990; 46: 22–35.
14. Montamat SC, Cusack BJ, Vestal RE. Management of drug therapy in the elderly. N Engl J Med 1989; 321: 303–309.
15. George CF, Waller DG. Drug treatment. In: Martin A, Camm AJ (eds), Geriatric Cardiology: Principles and Practice. Chichester: John Wiley & Sons Ltd, 1994; 593–622.
16. Robertson DRC, Waller DG, Renwick AG, George CF. Age related changes in the pharmacokinetics and pharmacodynamics of nifedipine. Br J Clin Pharmacol 1988; 25: 297–305.
17. Robertson DRC, Wood ND, Everest H et al. The effect of age on the pharmacokinetics of levodopa administered alone and in the presence of carbidopa. Br J Clin Pharmacol 1989; 28: 61–69.
18. George CF, George RH, Howden CW. The liver and response to drugs. In: Millward-Sadler GH, Wright R, Arthur M (eds), Wright's Liver and Biliary Disease (3rd edn). London: Saunders, 1992; Ch 17, 423–458.
19. Tucker GT. Ch 15, this book.
20. Capewell S, Freestone S, Critchley JAJH, Pottage A, Prescott LF. Reduced felodipine bioavailability in patients taking anticonvulsants. Lancet 1988; ii: 480–482.
21. Bailey DG, Spence JD, Munro C, Arnold JMO. Interactions of citrus juices with felodipine and nifedipine. Lancet 1991; 337: 268–269.
22. Honig PK, Woosley RL, Zamoni K, Conner DP, Cantilena LR. Changes in the pharmacokinetics and electrocardiographic pharmacodynamics of terfenadine with concomitant administration of erythromycin. Clin Pharmacol Ther 1992; 52: 231–238.
23. MacConnell TJ, Stanners AJ. Torsades de pointes complicating treatment with terfenadine. Br Med J 1991; 302: 1469.
24. Rawlins MD, Thompson JW. Mechanisms of adverse drug reactions. In: Davies DM (ed), Textbook of Adverse Drug Reactions (4th edn). New York: Oxford University Press, 1991; 18–45.
25. Nicholls JT. Publication No. 7, Medico-Pharmaceutical Forum. London, 1978; 4–11.
26. Skegg DCG, Doll R. The case for recording events in clinical trials. Br Med J 1977; ii: 1523–1524.
27. Inman WHW. Prescription–event monitoring: a preliminary study of benoxaprofen and fenbufen. Acta Med Scand 1984; Suppl 683: 119–126.

PART V
THE EDINBURGH DRUG ABSORPTION FOUNDATION LECTURE

20 INTERACTIONS IN FIRST-PASS METABOLISM AND VARIABILITY IN DRUG RESPONSE

Pertti J. Neuvonen
University of Helsinki, Finland

Introduction

Incomplete oral bioavailability of drugs may occur as a result of poor absorption from the gastrointestinal tract or because of pre-systemic metabolism [1–4].

Pre-systemic extraction itself includes two components. The first is *intestinal* first-pass metabolism, either in the mucosa or by gastrointestinal tract flora [5,6]. Cyclosporin is an example of an important drug which undergoes extensive first-pass metabolism in the gastrointestinal mucosa [7].

The second component of pre-systemic extraction is *hepatic* first-pass metabolism. Many commonly prescribed drugs are subject to significant hepatic first-pass metabolism, e.g. propranolol, metoprolol, verapamil, felodipine, nisoldipine and morphine. These drugs have a high extraction ratio in the liver and high hepatic clearance.

The relative contributions of intestinal and hepatic metabolism to the pre-systemic extraction of most drugs in man is unclear. In either case, concomitant drug therapy causing inhibition or induction of metabolism can greatly alter first-pass metabolism.

The clinical consequences of these interactions depend on the extent and role of the pre-systemic metabolism; the metabolites may be totally inactive, they may have different selectivity from that of the parent drug, or they can be the active form of a drug. Ultimately, therapeutic index will determine the clinical importance of an interaction. Some examples of pre-systemic interactions causing significant or even serious variability in drug response will be presented.

Clinical Measurement in Drug Evaluation. Edited by W. S. Nimmo and G. T. Tucker
© 1995 John Wiley & Sons Ltd

Terfenadine

Terfenadine is the prototype of a new group of non-sedating anti-histamines. It is available without prescription in several countries. During its first pass, terfenadine is metabolised extensively to at least one active metabolite, terfenadine carboxylate, which has potent antihistaminic properties. A cytochrome P450 enzyme, CYP3A4, converts terfenadine to terfenadine carboxylate. As a result of this biotransformation, it is unusual to find parent terfenadine in the plasma of patients who are taking therapeutic doses of terfenadine. However, in cases of intentional overdose, terfenadine concentrations in plasma often are detectable in association with Q–T interval prolongation on the electrocardiogram (ECG), syncope or cardiac arrest.

A few years ago, the occurrence of a life-threatening ventricular arrhythmia in a healthy young woman led clinicians in the USA to consider the possibility that this was triggered by a drug–drug interaction arising from treatment with both terfenadine and ketoconazole [8]. Analysis of blood samples revealed that the patient had high concentrations of unmetabolised terfenadine. Following this initial report, several cases of terfenadine–ketoconazole interaction, with prolonged Q–T intervals, cardiac arrhythmias and even fatal cardiac arrest, have been observed [9,10].

Recently, we saw a prolonged Q–T interval and *torsades de pointes* ventricular tachycardia in a healthy 26-year-old woman who was treated with regular doses of terfenadine and itraconazole [11]. She had been taking terfenadine 60 mg twice daily for eight days. She then began taking itraconazole 100 mg twice daily for vaginitis. On the third evening of the concomitant medication she started to have syncopal episodes. On admission to hospital, a clearly prolonged Q–T interval was seen on the ECG, and several bursts of *torsades de pointes* ventricular tachycardia were documented (Figure 1), two of them associated with syncope. Terfenadine and itraconazole were discontinued, but concentrations of parent terfenadine were clearly detectable and elevated for 60 h after the last dose of terfenadine. The Q–T interval returned to the normal range within three days, at the same time as unmetabolised terfenadine was no longer observed in the plasma. When a provocation test using a single dose of 120 mg of terfenadine was performed seven weeks later, without itraconazole, no unmetabolised terfenadine was detectable in plasma at any time. Concentrations of its metabolite were high and declined normally. The ECG did not show significant prolongation of the Q–T interval.

Honig *et al.* [9] examined the effects of ketoconazole on the pharmacokinetics and pharmacodynamics of terfenadine in healthy volunteers. After achieving a steady state while taking terfenadine (60 mg every 12 h) for seven days, daily concomitant ketoconazole (200 mg every 12 h) was given. Only one of the six volunteers had detectable plasma concentrations

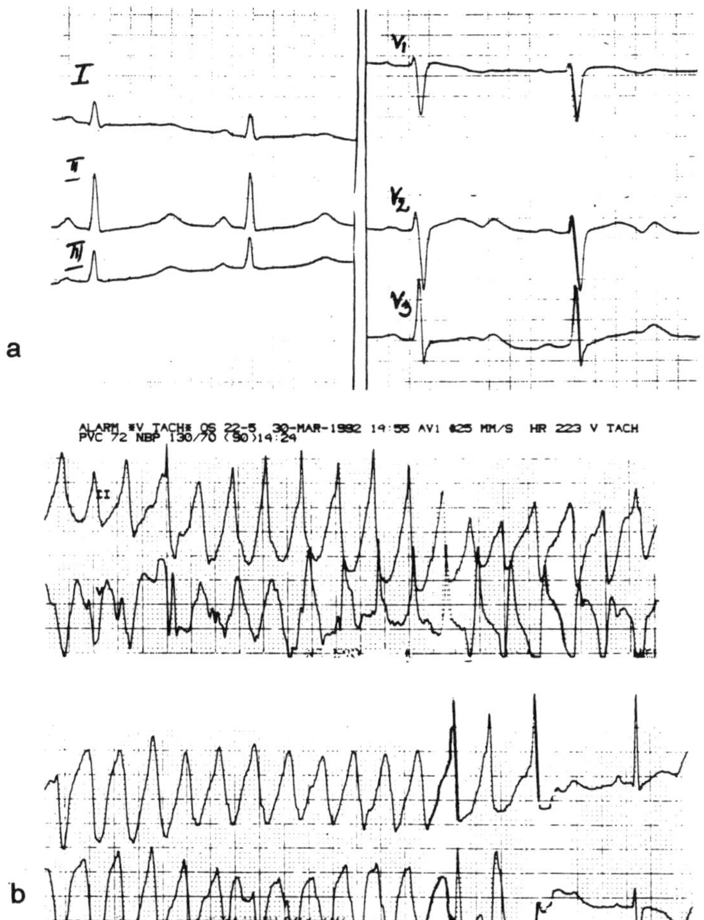

Figure 1. (a) A Q–T interval of 580 ms (heart rate 67/min), and (b) *torsades de pointes* ventricular tachycardia in a woman taking terfenadine and itraconazole. Reproduced from Pohjola-Sintonen *et al.* [11] by permission of Springer-Verlag

of unmetabolised terfenadine when it was used without ketoconazole. In contrast, all six had significant concentrations of parent terfenadine when it was co-administered with ketoconazole. In five subjects terfenadine was detectable in serum for 24 h after the last 60 mg dose and in some subjects even for two to three days (Figure 2) during the ketoconazole administration. The usual limit of quantification is 5 ng/ml. The estimated change in clearance of parent terfenadine ranged from 16- to 73-fold. There was a strong correlation between serum terfenadine concentration and the change in the Q–T$_c$ interval. Only two of the six subjects completed the

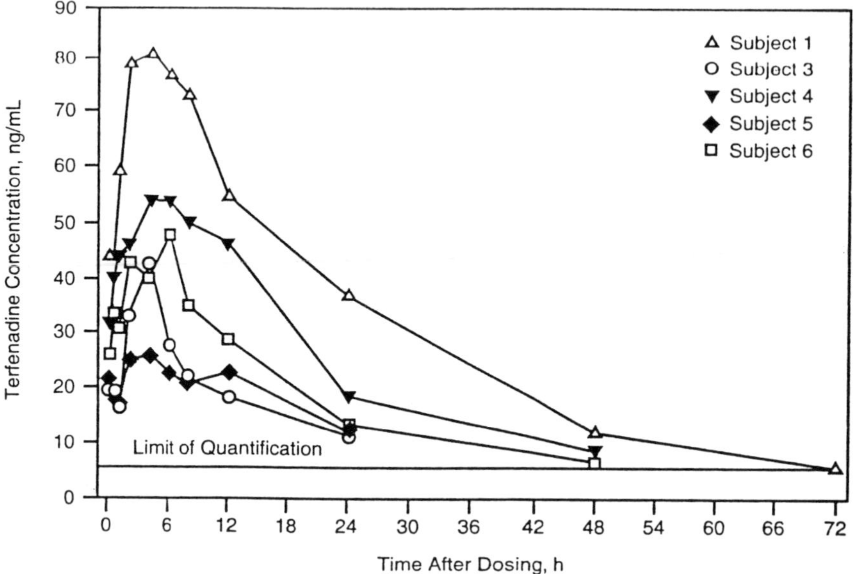

Figure 2. Serum concentrations of unchanged terfenadine in five subjects after the combined use of terfenadine and ketoconazole. Reproduced from Honig *et al.* [9] by permission of the American Medical Association. Copyright 1993, American Medical Association

planned seven-day course of ketoconazole. In the other four cases, administration of ketoconazole was terminated early because of significant electrocardiographic abnormalities.

Woosley *et al.* [12] have investigated the mechanism of the cardiotoxic effect of terfenadine. Their *in vitro* studies demonstrated that terfenadine is equipotent to quinidine as a blocker of the delayed potassium current in isolated feline myocytes. In contrast, the metabolite terfenadine carboxylate did not inhibit the potassium current even at concentrations 30 times higher than that of terfenadine producing a half-maximal effect. The antihistamine effect of terfenadine seems to be mediated by its carboxylate metabolite and not by the parent drug itself, whereas the cardiotoxic effects of terfenadine are caused by parent terfenadine which accumulates as a result of interactions.

The distribution of activity of the CYP3A4 enzyme is highly skewed, with a 30-fold difference between individuals at the end of the distribution range [13]. It is possible that those subjects with the lowest enzyme activity are at even higher risk of developing high concentrations of terfenadine as a result of an interaction. Ketoconazole, itraconazole, erythromycin, troleandomycin, verapamil, diltiazem and other potent inhibitors of CYP3A are obvious risk factors for terfenadine toxicity [10,14]. Furthermore, other drugs which themselves can prolong the Q–T interval, as well as hypokalaemia and liver disease, increase the toxicity. Thus, the clinical consequences of terfenadine–drug interactions depend on several factors.

Midazolam and triazolam

Midazolam and triazolam are widely used as short-acting sedatives and hypnotic agents and also for the induction of anaesthesia. They undergo extensive first-pass metabolism largely by CYP3A leading to an oral bioavailability of 50% or less. The *in vitro* activity of midazolam 1′-hydroxylase is inhibited by many commonly used drugs [15].

We have studied the effect of *erythromycin* on the pharmacokinetics and pharmacodynamics of midazolam in healthy volunteers using a randomised cross-over design [16]. During the erythromycin phase (500 mg t.i.d.) the plasma concentrations and area under the curve (AUC) of orally administered midazolam (15 mg) were more than four times higher than during the placebo phase (Figure 3). This was associated with profound decrements in psychomotor tests (critical flicker fusion, digit–symbol substitution, peak saccadic velocity and saccadic reaction time). There was a significant difference between the placebo and erythromycin phases as early as 15 min after ingestion of midazolam, and the difference lasted up to 6 h. In contrast, the effect of oral erythromycin on plasma concentrations of midazolam after intravenous administration was minimal.

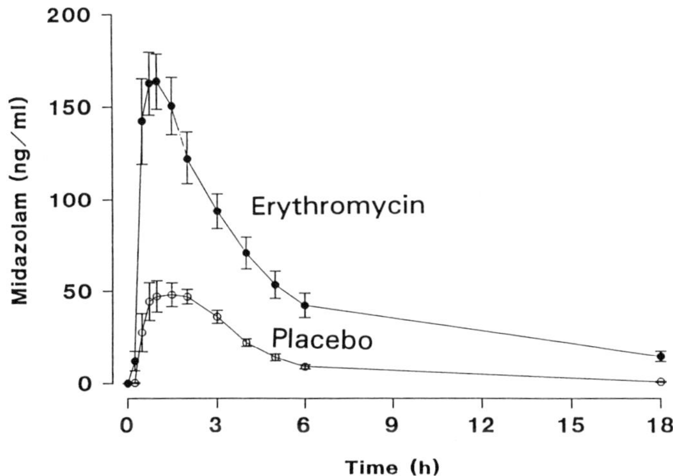

Figure 3. Mean (SEM) plasma concentrations of midazolam in 12 subjects after an oral dose of 15 mg, following pre-treatment with erythromycin 500 mg t.i.d. (solid circles) or placebo (open circles) for one week. Reproduced from Olkkola *et al.* [16] by permission of Mosby–Year Book, Inc.

The interaction between erythromycin and oral midazolam is of clinical significance. Erythromycin increases and prolongs the effects of oral midazolam to the extent that its hypnotic effect can no longer be regarded as of short duration. In one case report, deep unconsciousness and high plasma midazolam concentrations have been reported in a child receiving midazolam by mouth as pre-medication after intravenous erythromycin [17].

Some *calcium-channel blocking agents* are inhibitors of CYP3A. We have studied the effects of *diltiazem* (60 mg t.i.d.) and *verapamil* (80 mg t.i.d.) on the pharmacokinetics and pharmacodynamics of orally administered midazolam in healthy volunteers [18]. The peak plasma concentration of midazolam was doubled by co-administration of diltiazem and verapamil. The area under the plasma midazolam concentration–time curve was increased three-fold by verapamil and four-fold by diltiazem. The elimination half-life of midazolam was prolonged only slightly by these calcium channel blocking agents. The pharmacokinetic interaction between midazolam and the calcium channel blocking agents was associated with profound and prolonged effects on the pharmacodynamics of midazolam.

The antifungal agents *ketoconazole* and *itraconazole* are potent inhibitors of midazolam metabolism. Their effects on the pharmacokinetics and pharmacodynamics of orally administered midazolam (7.5 mg) have been studied in healthy volunteers using a randomised cross-over design [19]. During the ketoconazole phase (400 mg daily for four days) the peak plasma concentration of midazolam was more than four times higher, and the area under the concentration–time curve was more than 15 times higher than during the placebo phase. Itraconazole (200 mg daily) increased the peak concentration three-fold and the midazolam AUC by 10-fold. Up to 17 h the plasma concentration of midazolam during the ketoconazole phase was higher than the peak concentration during the placebo phase. All psychomotor tests indicated an increased and prolonged effect of midazolam when used with the antimycotics. It is clear that the metabolism of midazolam is inhibited both during its first-pass metabolism and during subsequent elimination. Therefore, ketoconazole and itraconazole may dangerously increase the depth and duration of sleep after oral midazolam.

Phillips *et al.* [20] have studied the pharmacokinetics of oral triazolam (0.5 mg) administered alone and after three days of erythromycin (333 mg t.i.d.). The peak plasma concentration of triazolam and its AUC were increased significantly by erythromycin.

It can be expected that the effects of oral triazolam and midazolam will be increased similarly in patients taking ketoconazole, itraconazole and other potent inhibitors of CYP3A. Such patients should be notified of this possibility, especially if they have to drive a car the next morning. If the patient has a sleep apnoea, an increased hypnotic effect may be dangerous.

Cyclosporin

Cyclosporin is a potent immunosuppressant used, for example, to prevent rejection of transplanted organs. After oral administration cyclosporin is rapidly and extensively metabolised during its first pass. It was thought previously that cyclosporin is metabolised exclusively in the liver. Recently, Kolars *et al.* [7] introduced cyclosporin into the small bowel of two patients during the anhepatic phase of liver transplantation. The pattern of cyclosporin metabolites in the portal blood indicated an extensive pre-systemic metabolism in the gut mucosa. In general, the contribution of the gut to cyclosporin metabolism may exceed that of the liver.

Concomitant oral use of ketoconazole, itraconazole, erythromycin, verapamil, diltiazem, danazol or other inhibitors of CYP3A can lead to a striking increase in the blood concentrations of cyclosporin [21–26]. The dose of cyclosporin may be reduced by one-third to one-half in patients receiving verapamil [27] or diltiazem but not in those receiving nifedipine. Thus, verapamil and diltiazem may provide a relative cost benefit to transplant patients also requiring calcium blocking agents for the treatment of hypertension. The concomitant use of ketoconazole or itraconazole allows reduction of the dose requirement of cyclosporin even further.

In contrast, phenytoin, phenobarbitone, carbamazepine, rifampicin and other enzyme-inducing drugs decrease blood concentrations of cyclosporin, by reducing its oral bioavailability and by increasing its rate of elimination [28–31]. Induction of intestinal cytochrome P450 isoforms appears to be more extensive than that of hepatic metabolism [28].

The therapeutic index of cyclosporin is narrow and its toxicity is concentration dependent. Therefore, interactions at the level of pre-systemic metabolism are clinically very important. They necessitate corresponding changes in the daily dose to avoid toxicity or organ rejection.

Calcium channel blockers

Felodipine, nisoldipine, verapamil and some other calcium blocking agents undergo extensive first-pass metabolism after oral administration. Their oral bioavailability is rather low even without enzyme induction, and the concomitant use of inducing drugs decreases it further.

The oral bioavailability of verapamil was lowered by more than 90% after 15 days of rifampicin therapy [32]. In epileptic patients using phenytoin, carbamazepine or phenobarbitone the relative bioavailability of felodipine was only 6.6% of that in normal subjects [33] (Figure 4). Less than 1% of the oral felodipine dose was bioavailable in these patients who were using enzyme inducers.

In contrast, ketoconazole, itraconazole and some other inhibitors of the CYP3A4 may increase the bioavailability of many calcium channel block-

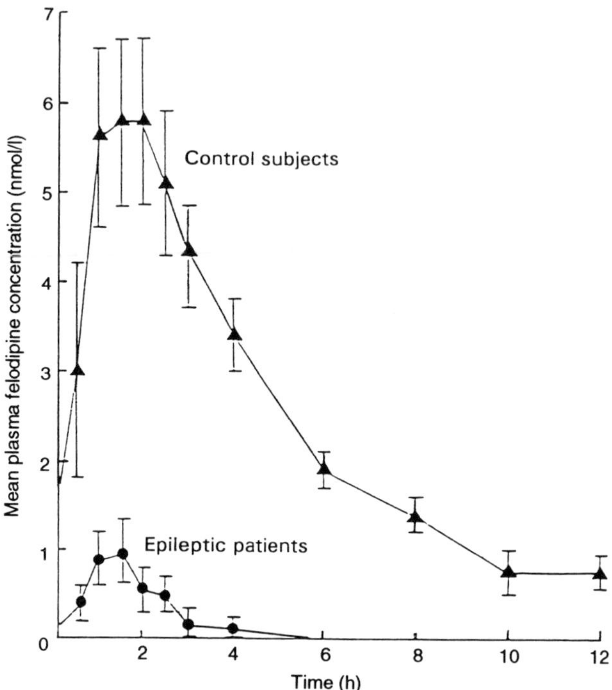

Figure 4. Mean (SEM) plasma concentrations of felodipine in 10 epileptic patients taking phenytoin, carbamazepine or phenobarbitone (circles) and in 12 healthy volunteers (triangles) after oral felodipine doses of 5 mg b.i.d. for four days. Reproduced from Capewell *et al.* [33] by permission of *The Lancet*

ing agents. Their effect on the bioavailability of felodipine and nisoldipine may be even more pronounced than their effect on verapamil, owing to their more extensive first-pass metabolism.

Beta blocking agents

Propranolol and other lipophilic beta blocking agents undergo extensive pre-systemic metabolism after oral dosage. Accordingly, some enzyme inducers and inhibitors can interact with them.

Herman *et al.* [34] found that steady-state plasma concentrations of propranolol were decreased by rifampicin (600 mg/day) given for three weeks. There was no significant change in the elimination half-life of propranolol, but its oral clearance was increased three-fold. The interaction between enzyme-inducing drugs and lipophilic beta blocking agents seems to be mediated mainly by increased pre-systemic metabolism.

According to a recent case report, addition of fluoxetine (20 mg/day) to a regimen of metoprolol (100 mg/day) caused a serious bradycardia [35]. It was suggested that fluoxetine may inhibit the metabolism of metoprolol.

Other drug–drug interactions during first-pass metabolism

Clinical reports suggest an interaction between fluoxetine—a selective inhibitor of serotonin reuptake—and the tricyclic antidepressants imipramine and desipramine [36,37]. Fluoxetine, after eight daily 60 mg doses, lowered the oral clearance of both imipramine and desipramine by tenfold and prolonged half-life by four-fold [38]. Fluoxetine causes an inhibition of tricyclic 2-hydroxylation and decreases both first-pass and systemic metabolism. Verapamil (120 mg t.i.d.), diltiazem (90 mg t.i.d.) and labetalol (200 mg b.i.d.) increased the relative bioavailability of orally administered imipramine (100 mg) as compared with placebo by 15%, 30% and 53%, respectively. Unlike verapamil and diltiazem, labetalol significantly decreased the formation of 2-hydroxyimipramine and 2-hydroxydesipramine [39]. Since these metabolic processes are dependent on CYP2D6, labetalol decreases the oral clearance of imipramine by inhibiting this system.

In addition to the above examples, there are many other studies and case reports in which enzyme induction or inhibition has caused clinically significant interactions in the pre-systemic metabolism of, for example, steroid hormones, digoxin [40], opioids, carbamazepine [41,42] and many other drugs. Further details are to be found in a number of reviews [4–6].

The concomitant ingestion of ethanol may also increase the bioavailability of some orally administered drugs, e.g. chlormethiazole [43] and propoxyphene [44]. On the other hand, the systemic availability of low-dose ethanol may be increased by enzyme inhibitors [45].

Grapefruit juice–felodipine interaction

A new type of food–drug interaction involving the calcium blocking agents felodipine, nifedipine and nitrendipine has been recently observed. In an initial report from Bailey *et al.* [46], the double-strength grapefruit juice tripled mean felodipine bioavailability in six patients with borderline hypertension. Also, the effect of felodipine on diastolic blood pressure and heart rate was increased by grapefruit juice. This interaction is probably caused by inhibition of pre-systemic metabolism and showed considerable inter-subject variability. Double-strength orange juice had no effect.

Normal grapefruit juice doubled the plasma concentrations of felodipine (Figure 5) and there was no change in the elimination half-life [47]. Felodipine has a single primary metabolite, dehydrofelodipine. Dehydrofelo-

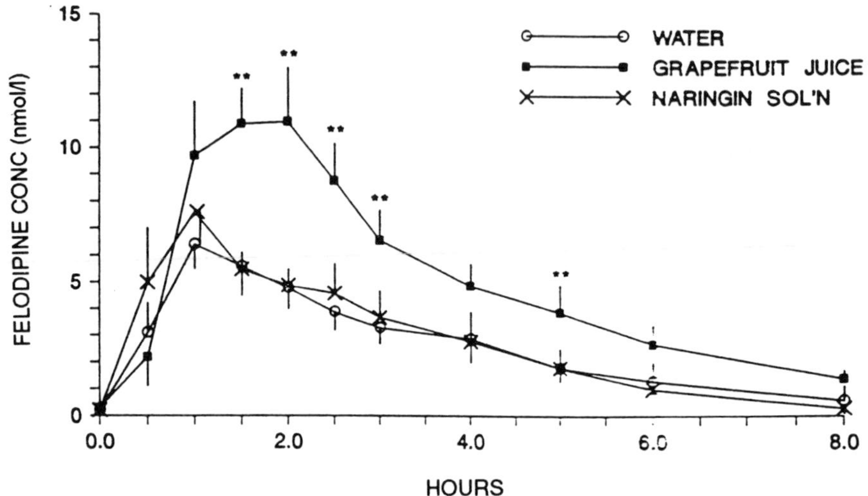

Figure 5. Mean (SEM) plasma concentrations of felodipine in nine subjects after an oral dose of 5 mg with 200 ml water, grapefruit juice, or naringin solution. Reproduced from Bailey *et al.* [47] by permission of Mosby–Year Book, Inc.

dipine/felodipine ratios in plasma were decreased by grapefruit juice, consistent with inhibition of pre-systemic felodipine metabolism. Grapefruit juice contains bioflavonoids which can inhibit P450-dependent activity. The most prevalent of these in grapefruit juice is naringin. Naringin is not found in orange juice. However, naringin in water produced much less interaction with felodipine despite the fact that it was given at the same concentration as that found in the grapefruit juice. Obviously, additional factors are important for this interaction.

Until now there have been only a few studies of the effect of grapefruit juice on other drugs undergoing extensive pre-systemic metabolism.

Summary and conclusions

- Interactions affecting first-pass metabolism may cause up to 20-fold changes in the bioavailability of certain drugs when these are used orally.
- If a drug undergoes extensive pre-systemic metabolism and has a narrow therapeutic index, interactions affecting first-pass metabolism can cause a clinically important variability in drug response.
- When a potentially interacting drug must be added to a patient's drug regimen, the doses should be modified according to the expected changes. The clinical response should be monitored carefully, and drug concentrations or biochemical effects should be measured if possible.

- If a new investigational drug undergoes extensive pre-systemic metabolism and if it is intended for oral use, its potential interactions with enzyme inducers and inhibitors should be studied during phase II or III trials, before its final approval for general use. This is a challenge to the pharmaceutical industry and to the drug regulatory authorities.

References

1. Pond SM, Tozer TN. First-pass elimination: basic concepts and clinical consequences. Clin Pharmacokinet 1984; 9: 1–25.
2. Greenblatt DJ. Presystemic extraction: mechanisms and consequences. J Clin Pharmacol 1993; 33: 650–656.
3. Lalka D, Griffith RK, Cronenberger CL. The hepatic first-pass metabolism of problematic drugs. J Clin Pharmacol 1993; 33: 657–669.
4. Somberg J, Shroff G, Khosla S, Ehrenpreis S. The clinical implications of first-pass metabolism: treatment strategies for the 1990s. J Clin Pharmacol 1993; 33: 670–673.
5. George CF. Drug metabolism by the gastrointestinal mucosa. Clin Pharmacokinet 1981; 6: 259–274.
6. Ilett KF, Tee LBG, Reeves PT, Minchin RF. Metabolism of drugs and other xenobiotics in the gut lumen and wall. Pharmacol Ther 1990; 46: 67–93.
7. Kolars JC, Awni WM, Merion RM, Watkins PB. First-pass metabolism of cyclosporin by the gut. Lancet 1991; 338: 1488–1490.
8. Monahan BP, Ferguson CL, Killeavy ES, Lloyd BK, Troy J, Cantilena LR. Torsades de pointes occurring in association with terfenadine use. JAMA 1990; 264: 2788–2790.
9. Honig PK, Wortham DC, Zamani K, Conner DP, Mullin JC, Cantilena LR. Terfenadine–ketoconazole interaction: pharmacokinetic and electrocardiographic consequences. JAMA 1993; 269: 1513–1518.
10. Peck CC, Temple R, Collins JM. Understanding consequences of concurrent therapies. JAMA 1993; 269: 1550–1552.
11. Pohjola-Sintonen S, Viitasalo M, Toivonen L, Neuvonen P. Itraconazole prevents terfenadine metabolism and increases risk of torsade de pointes ventricular tachycardia. Eur J Clin Pharmacol 1993; 45: 191–193.
12. Woosley RL, Chen Y, Freiman JP, Gillis RA. Mechanism of the cardiotoxic actions of terfenadine. JAMA 1993; 269: 1532–1536.
13. Yun C-H, Okerholm RA, Guengerich FP. Oxidation of the antihistaminic drug terfenadine in human liver microsomes: role of cytochrome P-450 3A(4) in N-dealkylation and C-hydroxylation. Drug Metab Dispos 1993; 21: 403–409.
14. Honig PK, Woosley RL, Zamani K, Conner DP, Cantilena LR. Changes in the pharmacokinetics and electrocardiographic pharmacodynamics of terfenadine with concomitant administration of erythromycin. Clin Pharmacol Ther 1992; 52: 231–238.
15. Gascon M-P, Dayer P. In vitro forecasting of drugs which may interfere with the biotransformation of midazolam. Eur J Clin Pharmacol 1991; 41: 573–578.
16. Olkkola KT, Aranko K, Luurila H et al. A potentially hazardous interaction between erythromycin and midazolam. Clin Pharmacol Ther 1993; 53: 298–305.
17. Hiller A, Olkkola KT, Isohanni P, Saarnivaara L. Unconsciousness associated with midazolam and erythromycin. Br J Anaesth 1990; 65: 826–828.
18. Backman JT, Olkkola KT, Aranko K, Himberg J-J, Neuvonen PJ. Dose of mid-

azolam should be reduced during diltiazem and verapamil treatments. Br J Clin Pharmacol 1994; 37: 221–225.

19. Olkkola KT, Backman JT, Neuvonen PJ. Midazolam should be avoided in patients receiving systemic antimycotics ketokonazole or itraconazole. Clin Pharmacol Ther 1994; 55: 481–485.

20. Phillips JP, Antal EJ, Smith RB. A pharmacokinetic drug interaction between erythromycin and triazolam. J Clin Psychopharmacol 1986; 6: 297–299.

21. Ferguson RM, Sutherland DER, Simmons RL, Najarian JS. Ketoconazole, cyclosporine, metabolism and renal transplantation. Lancet 1982; ii: 217.

22. Ptachcinski RJ, Carpenter BJ, Burckart GJ, Venkataramanan R, Rosenthal JT. Effect of erythromycin on cyclosporine levels. N Engl J Med 1985; 313: 1416–1417.

23. Pochet JM, Pirson Y. Cyclosporin–diltiazem interaction. Lancet 1986; i: 979.

24. Grino JM, Sebate I, Castelao AM, Alsina J. Influence of diltiazem on cyclosporine clearance. Lancet 1986; i: 387.

25. Ross WB, Roberts D, Griffin PJA, Salaman JR. Cyclosporin interaction with danazol and norethisterone. Lancet 1986; i: 330.

26. Lindholm A, Henricsson S. Verapamil inhibits cyclosporin metabolism. Lancet 1987; i: 1262–1263.

27. Tortorice KL, Heim-Duthoy KL, Awni WM, Venkateswara Rao K, Kasiske BL. The effects of calcium channel blockers on cyclosporine and its metabolites in renal transplant recipients. Ther Drug Monit 1990; 12: 321–328.

28. Hebert MF, Roberts JP, Prueksaritanont T, Benet LZ. Bioavailability of cyclosporine with concomitant rifampin administration is markedly less than predicted by hepatic enzyme induction. Clin Pharmacol Ther 1992; 52: 453–457.

29. Freeman DJ, Laupacis A, Keown PA, Stiller CR, Carruthers G. Evaluation of cyclosporin–phenytoin interaction with observations on cyclosporin metabolites. Br J Clin Pharmacol 1984; 18: 887–893.

30. Carstensen H, Jacobsen N, Dieperink H. Interaction between cyclosporin A and phenobarbitone. Br J Clin Pharmacol 1986; 21: 550–551.

31. Lele P, Peterson P, Yang S, Jarrell B, Burke JF. Cyclosporine and tegretol: another drug interaction. Kidney 1985; 27: 344.

32. Barbarash RA, Bauman JL, Rischer JH, Kondos GR, Batenhorst RL. The effect of enzyme induction on verapamil pharmacokinetics: verapamil–rifampicin interaction. Drug Intell Clin Pharm 1987; 21: IIA.

33. Capewell S, Critchley JAJH, Freestone S, Pottage A. Reduced felodipine bioavailability in patients taking anticonvulsants. Lancet 1988; ii: 480–482.

34. Herman RJ, Nakamura K, Wilkinson GR, Wood AJJ. Introduction of propranolol metabolism by rifampicin. Br J Clin Pharmacol 1983; 16: 565–569.

35. Walley T, Pirmohamed M, Proudlove C, Maxwell D. Interaction of metoprolol and fluoxetine. Lancet 1993; 341: 967–968.

36. Vaughan DA. Interaction of fluoxetine with tricyclic antidepressants. Am J Psychiatry 1988; 145: 1478.

37. Goodnick PJ. Influence of fluoxetine on plasma levels of desipramine. Am J Psychiatry 1989; 146: 552.

38. Bergstrom RF, Peyton AL, Lemberger L. Quantification and mechanism of the fluoxetine and tricyclic antidepressant interaction. Clin Pharmacol Ther 1992; 51: 239–248.

39. Hermann DJ, Krol TF, Dukes GE et al. Comparison of verapamil, diltiazem, and labetalol on the bioavailability and metabolism of imipramine. J Clin Pharmacol 1992; 32: 176–183.

40. Kauffman CA, Bagnasco FA. Digoxin toxicity associated with itraconazole therapy. Clin Infect Dis 1992; 15: 886–887.
41. Pearson HJ. Interaction of fluoxetine with carbamazepine. J Clin Psychiatry 1990; 51: 126.
42. Grimsley SR, Jann MW, Carter JG, D'Mello AP, D'Souza MJ. Increased carbamazepine plasma concentrations after fluoxetine coadministration. Clin Pharmacol Ther 1991; 50: 10–15.
43. Neuvonen PJ, Pentikäinen PJ, Jostell KG, Syvälahti E. Effect of ethanol on the pharmacokinetics of chlormethiazole in humans. Int J Clin Pharmacol Ther Toxicol 1981; 19: 552–560.
44. Girre C, Hirschhorn M, Bertaux L et al. Enhancement of propoxyphene bioavailability by ethanol. Eur J Clin Pharmacol 1991; 41: 147–152.
45. Guram M, Howden CW, Holt S. Increased blood alcohol levels with some H_2-receptor antagonists. J Pharm Med 1991; 1: 275–279.
46. Bailey DG, Spence JD, Munoz C, Malcolm J, Arnold O. Interaction of citrus juices with felodipine and nifedipine. Lancet 1991; 337: 268–269.
47. Bailey DG, Malcolm J, Arnold O, Munoz C, Spence JD. Grapefruit juice–felodipine interaction: mechanism, predictability, and effect of naringin. Clin Pharmacol Ther 1993; 53: 637–642.

INDEX

note: page numbers in *italics* refer to figures and tables

Index compiled by J. Halliday.

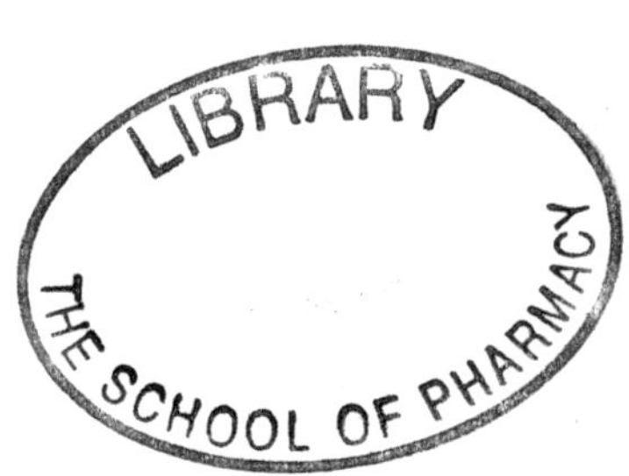